I.

THE MECHANISM OF DISLOCATIONS AND FRACTURE OF THE HIP

II.

LITHOLAPAXY; OR, RAPID LITHOTRITY WITH EVACUATION

BY

HENRY JACOB BIGELOW

A.M., M.D., LL.D.

MEMBER OF THE MASSACHUSETTS MEDICAL SOCIETY; EMERITUS PROFESSOR OF SURGERY IN HARVARD UNIVERSITY; SURGEON OF THE MASSACHUSETTS GENERAL HOSPITAL; MEMBER OF THE AMERICAN ACADEMY OF ARTS AND SCIENCES; MEMBER OF THE BOSTON SOCIETY FOR MEDICAL IMPROVEMENT; MEMBER OF THE BOSTON SOCIETY OF NATURAL HISTORY; FOREIGN HONORARY MEMBER OF THE CLINICAL SOCIETY OF LONDON; MEMBRE CORRESPONDANT ÉTRANGER DE LA SOCIÉTÉ DE CHIRURGIE DE PARIS; MEMBRE HONORAIRE DE LA SOCIÉTÉ ANATOMIQUE DE PARIS; MEMBRE CORRESPONDANT DE LA SOCIÉTÉ BIOLOGIQUE DE PARIS; SOCIUS EXTRANEUS SOCIETATIS MEDICÆ NORVEGICÆ; ETC., ETC.

LONGWOOD PRESS
BOSTON

Library of Congress Cataloging in Publication Data

Bigelow, Henry Jacob, 1818-1890.
I. The mechanism of dislocations and fracture of the hip ; II. Litholapaxy ; or, Rapid lithotrity with evacuation.

Reprint of the 1900 ed. published by Little, Brown, Boston.
Includes index.
1. Hip joint--Dislocation. 2. Hip joint--Fractur
3. Lithotrity. I. Title. II. Title: Litholapaxy.
[DNLM: WE B574me 1900a]
RD772.B53 1977 617'.15'8 77-81659
ISBN 0-89341-137-X

Published in 1977 by LONGWOOD PRESS INC.
P.O. Box 535, Boston, Massachusetts 02148
This Longwood Press book is an unabridged republication of the edition of 1900.
Library of Congress Catalogue Card Number: 77-81659
International Standard Book Number: 0-89341-137-X

Printed in the United States of America

THE First Part of this volume contains Dr. Bigelow's Treatise on the Mechanism of Dislocations and Fracture of the Hip, which has been long out of print. The Papers appended thereto comprise his other contributions to the literature of these subjects. They are reproduced with only such changes of the original text as their author had indicated a desire to have made.

The Second Part includes Dr. Bigelow's published articles on Rapid Lithotrity, arranged in chronological order, and unmodified except by his own annotations.

BOSTON, 1894.

CONTENTS.

Part I.

THE MECHANISM OF DISLOCATIONS OF THE HIP.

	Page
Introduction	3
Abstract	4
Dislocation of the Hip	9
The Y Ligament	16
Capsule of the Hip	20
Ligamentum Teres	20
Obturator Internus Muscle	21
Other Muscles	23
General Remarks upon Reduction	26
Position of the Patient and Surgeon	30
The Y Ligament, with Reference to Reduction and to Subsequent Treatment	30
How the Limb is to be Held	32
Capsular Orifice to be Enlarged	32
Fracture of the Neck	34
Flexion, Extension, Adduction, Abduction, and Rotation	34
Circumduction	35
Regular Dislocations	35
Dislocation upon the Dorsum Ilii	35
Signs	37
Dorsal Dislocation between the Rotator Muscles	42
Reduction of the Dislocation upon the Dorsum	44
Dorsal below the Tendon	56
Signs	59
The Mechanism of its Production, and Cause of its Irreducibility	61
Reduction	64

Regular Dislocations, — *continued.*

Page

Thyroid and Downward Dislocations 66
Thyroid 66
Signs 67
Vertical Downward Luxation 69
Dislocations near the Tuberosity or Perinæum 71
Reduction 75
Dislocation upon the Pubes 80
Dislocation below the Anterior Inferior Spine of the Ilium. — Sub-spinous 82
Reduction 84
Anterior Oblique Dislocation 87
Dislocations in which the Outer Branch of the Y Ligament is Broken. — Supra-spinous 90
Reduction 94
Everted Dorsal Dislocation 94
Reduction 96

Irregular Dislocations in which the Y Ligament is wholly Broken 97
Irregular Upward Luxation 99
Irregular Downward Luxation 100
Reduction 101

Special Conditions of Dislocation 101
Old Dislocations and their Reduction 101
Dislocation from Hip Disease 104
Dislocation of the Hip, with Fracture of the Shaft of the Femur 105
Spontaneous Dislocation 106

Fracture of the Pelvis 108
Fracture of the Rim of the Acetabulum 109
Fracture in which the Head of the Femur is driven through the Acetabulum 111
Asserted Fracture of the Acetabulum, without Crepitus, from a supposed Impossibility of keeping the Femur in Place . . 112
Fracture of other Parts of the Pelvis 113

Angular Extension 114

On Dislocation of the Hip 118

THE MECHANISM OF FRACTURES OF THE NECK OF THE FEMUR.

PAGE

FRACTURE OF THE NECK OF THE FEMUR 139
Impacted Fracture of the Base of the Neck, with Eversion . . 139
Anatomical Structure of the Neck of the Femur 141
Rotation 142
Shortening 142
True Neck 143
Remarks 145
Impacted Fracture of the Base of the Neck, with Inversion . 147
Impacted Fracture of the Neck of the Femur near the Head . 150
Comminuted Fracture of the Trochanters without Impaction . 154
Fracture of the Neck of the Femur resulting in False Joint . 155
Crack in the Neck of the Femur 156

THE TRUE NECK OF THE FEMUR: ITS STRUCTURE AND PATHOLOGY 158
Anatomical Structure of the Neck of the Femur 161
True Neck 162
Pathology: Impacted Fractures 167
Posterior Impacted Fracture of the Base of the Cervix . . . 167
Impacted Fracture of the Head of the Femur 170
Impacted Fracture of the whole Base of the Cervix, with Inversion 172
Unimpacted Fractures 172
Fracture of the Small Part of the Cervix of the Femur . . . 172
Comminuted Fracture of the Trochanters and Shaft 172
Treatment 173

FRACTURE OF THE NECK OF THE THIGH BONE 175

Part II.

RAPID LITHOTRITY, WITH EVACUATION.

	Page
Rapid Lithotrity	191
Rapid Lithotrity, with Evacuation	229
Litholapaxy	235
Litholapaxy	242
Litholapaxy	254
Litholapaxy	258
Litholapaxy	261
Litholapaxy; or Lithotrity with Immediate Evacuation	264
Litholapaxy. An Improved Evacuator	274
Litholapaxy	282
De la Litholapaxie: ou Lithotritie avec Évacuation immédiate en une seule Seance	285
Modern Lithotrity	296
Litholapaxy	320
Lithotrity, with Evacuaton	323
A Simplified Evacuator for Litholapaxy	332

Index 347

PART I.

DISLOCATION AND FRACTURE OF THE HIP.

INTRODUCTION.

SOME of the more important points in this paper are presented in the following abstract, which may serve either as a table of contents or as a list of propositions to be established by the evidence in the text. The comparatively few published autopsies of dislocation of the hip, and the still fewer conclusive ones, are perhaps insufficient for the complete analysis of its complicated mechanism; but the deficient evidence may in a great measure be supplied by experiments upon the dead subject, where the essential conditions are identical with those of the living and etherized patient, although the contrary has been alleged. The views here advanced may also be tested by the light they throw upon reported cases, of which I have carefully examined such as were accessible to me. If still deemed inconclusive, they must remain in doubt until established or confuted by further observation, but in the mean time it is certain that dislocated hips can be reduced upon the principles and by the rules laid down and explained in this paper. After reasonable attention to the subject, I confess that I can find no explanation so satisfactory as that here given.

ABSTRACT.

The points which were new to science in the first edition are here printed in italics.

1. The anterior part of the capsule of the hip joint is a triangular ligament of great strength, which, when well developed, exhibits an internal and external fasciculus, diverging like the branches of the inverted letter Y. It rises from the anterior inferior spinous process of the ilium, and is inserted into nearly the entire length of the anterior intertrochanteric line.

2. *The Y ligament, the internal obturator muscle, and the capsule subjacent to it, are alone required to explain the usual phenomena of the regular luxations.*

3. *The regular dislocations are those in which one or both branches of the Y ligament are unbroken; and their signs are constant.*

4. *The irregular dislocations are those in which the Y ligament is wholly ruptured; and they offer no constant signs.*

5. *In the regular dislocations of the hip, the muscles are not essential to give position to the limb, nor desirable as aids in its reduction.*

6. *The Y ligament will alone effect reduction and explain its phenomena, a part of those connected with the dorsal dislocations excepted. During the process of reduction, this ligament should be kept constantly in mind.*

7. *The rest of the capsule, except perhaps that portion beneath the internal obturator tendon, need not be considered in reduction, if the capsular orifice is large enough to admit the head of the femur easily.*

8. *If the capsular orifice is too small to allow easy reduction, it should be enlarged.*

9. *The capsular orifice may be enlarged at will, and with impunity, by circumduction of the flexed thigh.*

10. *Recent dislocations can be best reduced by manipulation.*

11. *The basis of this manipulation is flexion of the thigh.*

12. *This manipulation is efficient either by one method, because it relaxes the Y ligament, or by another method, because that ligament, remaining tense, is a fixed point, around which the head of the femur revolves near the socket.*

13. *The further manipulation of the flexed thigh may be either by traction or rotation.*

14. *The dorsal dislocation owes its inversion to the external branch of the Y ligament.*

15. *The so-called ischiatic dislocation owes nothing whatever of its character, or its difficulty of reduction by horizontal extension, to the ischiatic notch.*

16. *The ischiatic dislocation is better named* dorsal below the tendon, *and is easily reduced by manipulation. But the term "ischiatic" might better be suppressed. It is the dorsal dislocation with the least shortening.*

17. *The flexion of the thyroid and downward dislocations is due to the Y ligament, which, in the first, also everts the limb, until the trochanter rests upon the pelvis.*

18. *In the pubic dislocation, the range of the bone upon the pubes is limited by this ligament, which, in the sub-spinous dislocation also, binds the neck of the femur to the pelvis.*

19. *In the dorsal dislocation with eversion, the outer branch of the Y ligament is ruptured. In the absence of this fulcrum, this dislocation may need pulleys for its reduction.*

20. *In the anterior oblique luxation, the head of the bone is hooked over the entire Y ligament, the limb being then necessarily oblique, everted, and a little flexed.*

21. *In the supra-spinous luxation, the head of the femur is equally hooked over the Y ligament, the external branch of which is broken. The limb may then be fully extended.*

22. In old luxations, the period during which reduction is possible is determined by the extent of the obliteration of the socket, the strength of the neck of the femur, and the absence of osseous excrescence.

23. Old luxations may possibly require the aid of pulleys, in order by traction to avoid any danger which might result to the atrophied or degenerated neck of the bone from rotation.

24. *Right-angled extension, the femur being flexed at a right angle with the pelvis, is more advantageous than that which has usually been employed.*

25. To make such extension most effective, a special apparatus is required.

FRACTURES OF THE NECK OF THE THIGH-BONE.

1. *The terms "intra" and "extra" capsular, applied to these fractures, have little practical significance, because when a fracture near the head of the femur shows bony union, it is often impossible to say whether such a fracture was originally inside or outside the capsular ligament.*

2. *These fractures are therefore better divided, for practical purposes, into (1) the impacted fracture of the neck into the trochanter; and (2) other fractures of the neck.*

3. *In this impacted fracture, the limb is everted because the posterior cervical wall is almost always impacted, the anterior very rarely, and in a less degree.*

4. *These conditions mainly result from the relative thickness of the two walls.*

5. *While eversion is due to the rotation of the fractured bone on a hinge formed in the anterior cervical wall, shortening is generally due to the obliquity of this hinge.*

6. *In a well-formed bone, the posterior and thin surface of the neck of the femur is prolonged into the cancellous structure beneath the intertrochanteric ridge, and is the true neck.*

7. *The posterior intertrochanteric ridge is a buttress built upon the true neck, by which, when impacted, this ridge is sometimes split off.*

DISLOCATION OF THE HIP.

The original object of the following paper was to show that in dislocations of the hip the position of the limb depends chiefly upon a ligament which has been of late years imperfectly described, and that the reduction of these dislocations should be managed accordingly. In connection with this subject, I also attempted to show how the anatomical structure of the neck of the femur leads to a common variety of fracture of that bone.

These views have been, as I believe, so well established by repeated experiments upon the dead subject, and so corroborated by current pathological phenomena, and by the mass of reported cases and autopsies, that little doubt can exist of their correctness.

Since about the year 1854–55, the four dislocations of the hip, as usually described, together with the method of reducing them by manipulation alone, have been annually shown to the classes attending the lectures at the Medical School of Harvard University. These four luxations were made in each case upon a single dead subject, which, notwithstanding the great laceration to which the capsule of the hip had been subjected, in no instance failed to exhibit, and to demonstrate in a striking manner, the appropriate and well-known attitude of each dislocation. In fact, the firm and persistent position of a joint displaced under such circumstances is quite remarkable. In these experiments, the fixed attitude of the limb was at first attributed to the muscles, which when fully extended are capable of considerable resistance in the dead subject as well as in the living one; but it was supposed that the action of their complicated mechanism would hardly repay the labor of its study.

In the spring of 1861, having been led to expose a joint, the luxation of which had been the subject of a lecture, I was agreeably surprised to observe the simple action of the ligament, — a simplicity which subsequent experience has confirmed, and which strikingly explains the phenomena observed in the living subject.[1]

The dislocated joint alluded to presented on examination the following appearances: —

1. Great laceration of the muscles about the joint.
2. The ligamentum teres broken.
3. Laceration of the inner, outer, and lower parts of the capsule.
4. The anterior and upper parts of the capsule uninjured, and presenting a strong fibrous band, fan-shaped, and slightly forked.

The remaining tendinous and muscular fibres about the joint being now completely divided, with the exception of the strong fibrous band above alluded to, it was found that the four commonly described dislocations of the hip could still be exhibited without difficulty, and that in each of them the anterior portion of the capsular ligament, which alone

[1] Of the figures accompanying this paper, those of the Y ligament numbered 1, 6, 7, 8, 19, 24, 25, 27, 29, 31, and of the impacted fracture, 1, 2, 3, were reproduced, in the spring of 1861, from photographs made from this hip after dissection. In June, 1861, a paper upon the subject was read before the Boston Society for Medical Improvement; a second paper before the Massachusetts Medical Society, in May, 1864; another, in June, 1865, before the American Medical Association. In the present paper the rarer forms of dislocation have been added, with references to the more interesting reported cases.

remained, sufficed at once to direct the limb to its appropriate position and to fix it there.

Assuming that each of these dislocations does occur, and that, however much it may vary in degree, it uniformly exhibits its proper and familiar diagnostic signs; that the anterior portion of the ligament of the capsule far exceeds in strength any other part of it, and that on this account it not only is less likely to be torn, but generally remains intact; that when this alone remains, it is itself able to give position to the displaced limb: and that when it is divided, the other parts of the capsule, the muscles, and other tissues do this very imperfectly, as will be hereafter shown, — then the *a priori* evidence is strong that a luxated femur assumes its attitude chiefly in obedience to the traction of the tense fibres of this part of the ligament.

The resistance of a dislocated limb is unyielding, and unlike that of muscular action elsewhere, — in illustration of which a few cases may be cited, taken almost at random from Sir Astley Cooper.[1]

"CASE XXXVIII.— . . . He was bled thirty ounces in the recumbent posture, and small doses of tartarized antimony were administered, but without these means producing syncope. He was then placed upon a large table, and his pelvis fixed in the usual manner, by long jack-towels passed between the perinæum and the injured joint; the extending apparatus, composed also of a round towel, was then applied above the knee, and to it were attached weights to the amount of one hundred and twelve pounds, fastened to a rope, which was rove through a pulley. To the influence of this weight he was submitted for four hours, but without any effect being produced. He was therefore then sent to Guy's Hospital. At half past seven P. M. he was taken into the operating theatre. The pelvis was fixed by the common padded bandage, while to the knee was attached the circular bandage and pul-

[1] A Treatise on Dislocations and Fractures of the Joints. London, 1842.

leys, and gradual extension was made across the lower third of the opposite thigh for the space of twenty minutes, during which period he was given three grains of tartarized antimony in solution."

"CASE L. — John Cockburn, a strong, muscular man, aged thirty-three, was admitted into Guy's Hospital on the 31st of July, 1819. While carrying a bag of sand at Hastings on the 24th of July, he slipped, and dislocated the left hip-joint. The foot on the affected side was plunged suddenly into a hollow in the road, which turned his knee inward at the same time that his body fell with violence forward. On the day of the accident two attempts were made to reduce the dislocation by pulleys, but without success; and on the 27th of July a third, but equally unsuccessful, trial was made, although continued for nearly an hour.

"It was found, upon examination, that the thigh was dislocated backward into the ischiatic notch. The patient was carried into the operating theatre soon after his admission; and when two pounds of blood had been taken from him, and he had been nauseated by two grains of tartarized antimony, gradually administered, extension was made with the pulleys in a right line with the body, and the upper part of the thigh was raised, while the knee was depressed. The extension was continued at least for an hour and a half, during which time he took two grains more of tartarized antimony, by which he was thoroughly nauseated. The attempts at reduction, however, did not succeed." [1]

To a surgeon accustomed to the comparative ease with which the powerful muscles of a recently fractured thigh may be extended by a moderate effort continuously applied, these cases of enormous resistance in the reduction of a dislocated hip suggest a force more powerful and unyielding

[1] It is curious to remark that this case ultimately yielded, in the hands of Sir Astley, to the employment, unusual for him, of the flexion method, though combined with pulleys. In further illustration of the disadvantage of horizontal extension, let this case be compared with a similar one (dorsal below the tendon) where the reduction occupied three seconds (p. 69).

than that of muscular action. Indeed, the facility with which muscular contraction is overcome by ether, while the deformity and resistance of dislocation continue, should long ago have led to the conviction that muscular contraction is not a chief agent in this deformity.

But modern writers, with few exceptions, have adopted the theory of active or passive muscular resistance. Sir Astley Cooper says: —

"With respect to the fixed position of the head of the femur in the four dislocations which have been described, it is not to be considered as a mere matter of chance, but the natural result of the influence of the muscles, which draw the bone into these positions; and that therefore, under common circumstances, the condition is inevitable.[1] . . . The capsular ligaments, in truth, possess but little strength either to prevent dislocation or to resist the means of reduction. . . . The difficulty of reducing dislocations arises neither from the bones nor from the ligaments, but from the resistance which the muscles present by their contraction."[2]

Dr. Nathan R. Smith recognizes muscular contraction as the chief agent in effecting both dislocation of the hip and its reduction.[3]

That similar views are still entertained by distinguished surgical authorities is shown by the following reported remarks of M. Chassaignac at a meeting of the Société de Chirurgie in 1865: "The employment of chloroform in the reduction of dislocations had convinced him [M. Chassaignac] that obstacles to reduction said to be due to other causes than muscular contraction were chimerical,"[4] — an observation that seems to have passed unchallenged.

[1] A Treatise on Dislocations and Fractures of the Joints (p. 100). London, 1842.

[2] Ibid., pp. 20, 21.

[3] Medical and Surgical Memoirs (pp. 166, 167). By Nathan Smith, M. D. Edited by Nathan R. Smith, M. D. Baltimore, 1831.

[4] London Medical Times and Gazette, December, 1865 (p. 661).

Dr. Reid makes the following statement: —

"The chief impediment in the reduction of dislocation is the indirect action of muscles that are put upon the stretch by the malposition of the dislocated bone. . . . The limb or bone should be drawn in the direction which will relax the distended muscles." [1]

On the other hand, the theory of ligamentous resistance has been occasionally and distinctly recognized.

Boyer expresses his conviction of the importance of the ligament in this relation, but without proof.[2]

Professor Gunn maintains, in a paper [3] upon this subject, that different untorn or "undissected" portions of the capsular ligament are capable of producing the signs of hip and shoulder luxation; while, since the reading of the present paper, Professor W. Busch,[4] at the Bonn Clinic, has recognized the resistance to the reduction of dislocation as ligamentous and capsular, although he fails to identify the anterior ligament as its principal seat.

There is no doubt that in luxation as well as in fracture the muscles soon contract and adapt themselves to the new condition of things; so that the limb is steadied partly by the effort of the patient. In those luxations of the hip, for example, which exhibit great flexion, the muscles while active may contribute, when the patient is standing, to support the limb in a flexed position, while its own weight tends

[1] Dislocation of the Femur on the Dorsum Ilii reducible without Pulleys or any other Mechanical Power. (p. 41). By William W. Reid, M. D., of Rochester. Transactions of the N. Y. Medical Society. Albany, 1852.

[2] Traité des Maladies Chirurgicales, etc. (tom. iv. p. 282). Par M. le Baron Boyer. Paris, 1822.

[3] Luxations of the Hip and Shoulder, and the Agents which oppose their Reduction. By Moses Gunn, A. M., M. D., Professor of Surgery in the University of Michigan. Detroit, 1859.

[4] Year-Book of Medicine, Surgery, etc., for 1863 (p. 225.) Sydenham Society. London, 1864.

to straighten it; they may even help to convert a dislocation below the socket into one upon the dorsum, or into the foramen ovale,— or they may assist simply to reduce it. But there is no evidence that dislocations below the socket are capable of retaining their distinctive features in an erect posture of the body, when the muscles are relaxed, as in the dead or etherized subject.

Again, some of the muscles are stretched and elongated by the luxated bone; and their passive strength under these circumstances, which is greater than might be supposed, has been well illustrated by Dr. Reid. But it is unnecessary to dwell upon the tenacity of the muscular fibre passively stretched to its extreme limit, because this extreme tension does not occur in the usual dislocations, being prevented by the ligamentous action. It may be remarked, however, that muscle is far less strong than ligament; and that the muscles about the hip, which are inserted near the head of the femur, are acted upon at great advantage by this powerful lever, and might yield were they unsupported. Moreover, the dislocated hip can be shown equally well upon a subject in which the muscles have become soft by decomposition; and when the four classical dislocations have been produced upon a single subject, most of the muscular tissue immediately surrounding the joint will be found to have been torn away, while the rest may be divided without materially affecting the power of the limb to illustrate these four luxations. On the other hand,— a fact which is conclusive,— if the entire capsule of the hip joint be divided and the muscles left intact, these dislocations are but imperfectly represented.

Without denying, then, that muscular fibre exerts both an active and a passive force, it is here assumed that the muscles play but a subordinate and occasional part either in hindering reduction or in determining the character of the deformity, and that this is chiefly due to the resistance of a ligament the power of which will presently be illustrated, and whose simple mechanism will explain the phenomena both of luxation and its reduction. Out of twenty-two recorded autopsies, while in two only is there any allusion to the rupture of the anterior portion of the capsule, in fourteen it is distinctly mentioned that it remained wholly or in part unbroken,— a large proportion, considering that attention has hitherto not been directed to this point. It is not here maintained that this ligament will be found stripped clear of the remaining portion of the capsule,— the comparatively few autopsies on record showing that this is not the case; there is, however, reason to believe that the thinner portions owe their immunity from injury to the protection of the main ligament.

The theory here advanced recognizes the anterior portion of the capsular ligament as the exponent of the total agency of the capsule in giving position to the dislocated limb, and, what is more important, as so identified with the phenomena of luxation that reduction must be accomplished almost wholly with reference to it. It remains for future autopsies to show, by careful examination, how far the usual phenomena either of luxation or its reduction can occur after rupture of this ligament.

THE Y LIGAMENT.

The ilio-femoral ligament, known also as the ligament of Bertin, has been usually described as reinforcing the capsule by a single fibrous band extending from the inferior iliac spine to the inner extremity of the anterior intertrochanteric line, and playing no very important part in health or injury. This ligament is more or less adherent to the acetabular prominence and to the neck of the femur; but upon examination it will be found to take its origin from the anterior inferior spinous process of the ilium, passing downward to the front of the femur, to be inserted fan-shaped into nearly the whole of the oblique spiral line which connects the two trochanters in front, — being about half an inch wide at its upper or iliac origin, and but little less than two inches and a half wide at its fan-like femoral insertion. Here it is bifurcated, having two principal fasciculi, one being inserted into the upper extremity of the anterior intertrochanteric line, and the other into the lower part of the same line, about half an inch in front of the small trochanter. The ligament thus resembles an inverted Y, which suggests a short and convenient name for it.

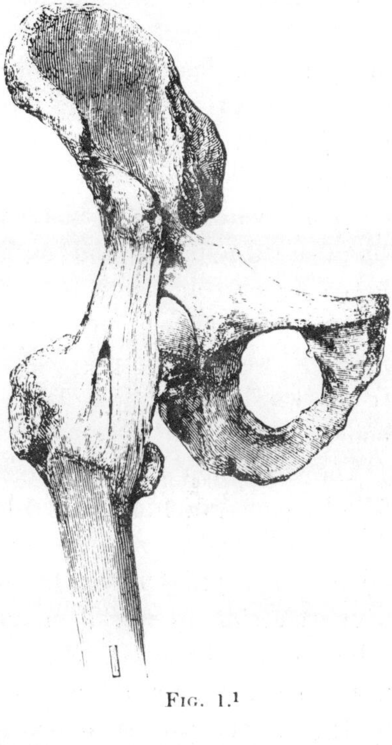

FIG. 1.[1]

The divergent branches of the Y ligament are sometimes well developed, with scarcely any intervening membrane. In other cases the intermediate tissue is thicker, and requires to be slit or removed before the bands are distinctly defined, and sometimes the whole triangle is of nearly uniform thickness. In the subject first dissected, and from which the accompanying woodcut was designed, the external fasciculus of fibres was nearly as well developed as the inner band, in two other subjects it was actually wider and thicker. But as

[1] The Y ligament, showing its inner and outer fasciculi. The former is known as the ilio-femoral ligament, the ligament of Bertin, etc. This specimen shows the interval between the two fasciculi.

the internal and external branches exercise somewhat distinct functions, — the one being chiefly concerned in limiting the extension, the other the eversion, of the femur, and also in producing inward rotation in dorsal dislocation, — it is fair to infer that in a normal condition they would exhibit greater development than the intermediate fibres.

The Y ligament is of remarkable tenacity and strength, being at some points, when well developed, nearly a quarter of an inch in thickness, and forming an unyielding suspensory band, by which the femur, when in a state of extension, as in walking, is forcibly retained in its socket.

In six by no means recent subjects, taken at random from the dissecting-tables and suspended by the shoulders, the lower limbs being united to the pelvis by the Y ligament alone, this ligament required for its rupture the attachment of weights to the foot, varying in the several cases from two hundred and fifty to seven hundred and fifty pounds.[1]

The dissection of the Y ligament here represented, taken from a photograph made in 1861, first directed my attention to the anatomical arrangement and strength of its fibres. Some seven years after this Y was photographed, I found upon referring to works in the library of my distinguished colleague, Professor O. W. Holmes, the following passages, which show that a bifurcation of this ligament was known to some of the earlier anatomists, although it has since been generally overlooked.

The first is from Winslow: —

[1] Although autopsies show that the whole of this ligament has sometimes been torn asunder, it may be assumed that such a lesion is likely to be of rare occurrence. Its strength probably insures its immunity in a large majority of luxations; while the constancy of their signs, which will be shown to be best explained by the action of this ligament, testifies to its integrity.

"It [the ligament] is very thick between the anterior inferior spine of the os ilium all the way to the small anterior tuberosity which unites, as it were, the basis of the great trochanter with the basis of the neck. It is likewise very thick between the same spine and the middle part of the oblique rough line observable between the tuberosity and the little trochanter; and here likewise it is strengthened by a bundle of fibres connected to the passage of the tendon of the iliac muscle and to the inferior portion of the oblique rough line. The disposition of the ligamentous fibres of which these two thick portions are composed forms a sort of triangle with the oblique rough line which terminates the basis of the neck."[1]

Weitbrecht, an excellent, perhaps the best, authority upon the ligaments, referring in this connection to Winslow, distinctly recognizes a forked arrangement, which he thus describes: —

"Partim anterius versus collum femoris et trochanterem minorem procedit, . . . partim vero lateraliter versus exteriora progreditur, et circa radicem trochanteris majoris in tuberculo laterali terminatur. Atque binae hae divaricationes, una cum linea obliqua, figuram . . . triangularem . . . constituunt."[2]

The Webers describe the ligament as triangular, laying stress upon its thickness, which, as they assert, is greater than that of the ligament of the patella or the tendo Achillis, and concluding thus: —

"With this great strength we should expect that every other part of the capsule would be ruptured before this ligament; and that even the bone itself would first yield."[3]

[1] An Anatomical Exposition of the Structure of the Human Body (sect. 2, pp. 138–139). By James Benignus Winslow. (Douglas's Translation.) London, 1776.

[2] Syndesmologia, sive Historia Ligamentorum, etc. (p. 141). Josias Weitbrecht, D. M. Petropoli, 1742.

[3] Traité d'Ostéologie, etc. (pp. 323, 324). S. P. Soemmerring, and G. and E. Weber. Paris, 1843.

CAPSULE OF THE HIP.

In a front view of the cleanly dissected capsule of the joint, the Y ligament is distinctly seen, the tissue occupying its fork being sometimes a mere membrane, and sometimes thicker. The external band hinders eversion, especially when the leg is extended. Both bands limit extension. In abducting the leg, a band is raised (pubo-femoral) between the bony ridge above the thyroid foramen and the prominence at the inner part of the intertrochanteric line, hindering abduction in every position of the limb. Between this band and the Y ligament the capsule is comparatively thin; and here the primitive pubic dislocation doubtless occurs. Behind and inside the pubo-femoral band, looking directly toward the thyroid foramen, is found the thinnest part of the capsule, which at this point resembles wet bladder, readily permitting the thyroid dislocation. Outside and behind the Y ligament, where the dorsal dislocations occur, the capsule is very strong, limiting adduction and rotation inward. There is also a fasciculus from the tuber ischii at its upper part to the upper part of the trochanter behind, arresting flexion and inversion. The principal ligamentous bands are the two first described, — no part of the capsule comparing in strength with the Y ligament and the tissue which lies immediately behind it, beneath the tendon of the obturator internus muscle.

LIGAMENTUM TERES.

Little can be added to the excellent paper of Mr. Struthers[1] upon the function of this ligament. When the limb is bent upon the body, it hinders eversion, — thus opposing the action of the sartorius muscle, and hindering, in this position, dislocation upon the thyroid foramen. It is not, however, possessed of much strength; is ruptured in all the complete and

[1] Edinburgh Medical Journal, November, 1858 (p. 434).

sudden dislocations, and, according to Cruveilhier, is often undeveloped and sometimes wanting.

OBTURATOR INTERNUS MUSCLE.

It will hereafter be seen that this muscle, with which the gemelli are practically identified, is materially concerned in one variety of hip dislocation, and is important in relation to its reduction. There is a peculiarity of the obturator internus, hitherto undescribed, which explains its strength. Its muscular belly is, in some subjects, mingled with tendinous fibres. This may be verified in dissection by reflecting the muscle from its pulley so as to expose its internal and fibrous surface. The four or five tendinous divisions which wind round the lesser sacro-sciatic notch, and which seem to disappear in the thickness of the muscular tissue, may then be traced in part to a bony origin, some of their minute and ultimate fibres arising from the margin of the obturator foramen. The muscle, when extended, thus practically becomes a ligament, and by the attachment of its combined tissues acquires great strength. Again, the friction of the tendon over the pulley lessens the draft upon the extended muscle, and so increases its power of resistance that it is the strongest, as in relation to luxation it is the most important, of the small outward rotators of the hip.[1] That portion of the capsule which lies directly beneath the tendon is also very strong; and while their fibres mutually reinforce one another, their mechanical action in the dorsal luxations is much the same.

[1] The average weight required to rupture this and the adjacent muscles in four subjects is as follows: —

Pyriformis	10 lbs.	Obturator externus	$36\frac{4}{5}$ lbs.
Obturator internus	$10\frac{4}{5}$ "	Gluteus medius	17 "

In the only recent subject among these, the obturator internus on one side parted at 64 lbs. and on the other at 60 lbs., the obturator externus at 52 and 44 lbs., and the pyriformis at 16 lbs.

Arising within the pelvis, the obturator internus emerges from the pelvic cavity at a point several inches behind the great trochanter, into the back and upper part of which it is inserted. By its contraction it draws the trochanter backward, everting the thigh when straight, and abducting it if flexed. Upon the dead or etherized subject it is rendered tense in the extended limb by rotation inward, adduction being then more limited; but in the flexed limb, and especially in extreme flexion, it is relaxed; so that in reducing a backward dislocation, when this muscle is still entire, it might be advantageous to flex the limb as much as possible.

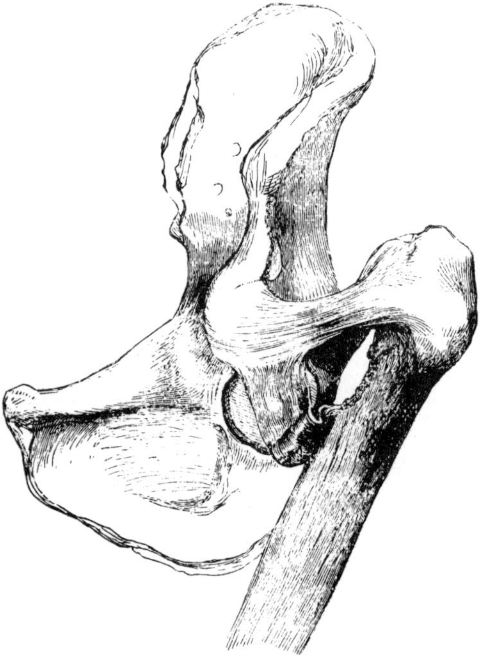

FIG. 2.[1]

A curious corroboration of the importance of this muscle, as well as of the external branch of the Y ligament, is seen in a preparation[2] of my own, the case having been one of old ununited fracture of the neck of the femur, in a subject the weight of whose body in walking had been suspended chiefly

[1] Ununited fracture of the neck of the thigh-bone, showing the hypertrophied outer fasciculus of the ligament supporting the weight of the pelvis in walking. The inner fasciculus is seen below.

[2] No. 2715, The Warren Anatomical Museum of Harvard University.

between the outer branch of the Y ligament in front and the obturator internus behind (Figs. 2 and 3). This is probably the usual condition of patients after this injury, where the shaft of the femur moves freely upon the detached head of the bone.

OTHER MUSCLES.

It has already been stated that the restricted movements of the thigh in the various luxations are in part due to the active and passive resistance of several muscles which (like the psoas and iliacus) connect the femur with the pelvis, and become more or less tense by its displacement; yet their action, in a practical point of view, is of secondary importance, whether considered in relation to its direction or its extent. Without the powerful ligament and the muscle already described, the regular femoral luxations would lose much of their present distinctive character; and regard being had to the action of these fibrous bands, the dislocations can be reduced with little reference to the muscles.

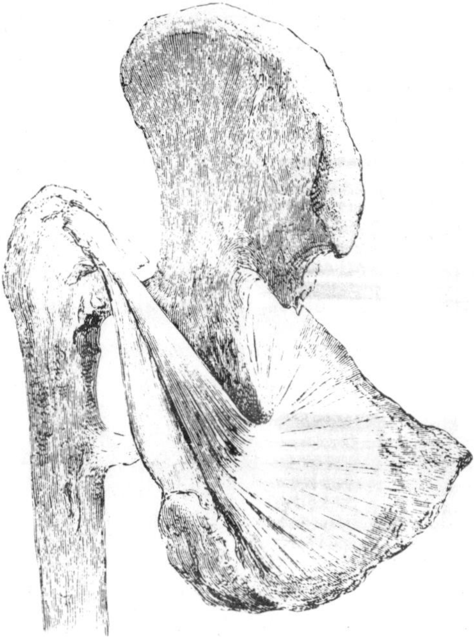

FIG. 3.[1]

[1] Fig. 2 seen from behind, to show the tense obturator tendon bearing its share of the weight of the body. The inferior gemellus, hypertrophied, is seen below it.

It may, however, be briefly stated that the gemelli are practically identified with the obturator internus, while the obturator externus below it and the pyriformis above it are also outward rotators, — the whole forming a deep muscular layer with interstices. The quadratus femoris muscle is below the usual range of dislocations, but is easily and frequently torn; and the three glutei have comparatively little efficacy in rendering the femur immovable, even when its head is engaged, for example, beneath the medius. The psoas and iliacus exert a force in the direction of the Y ligament, especially when that is ruptured; and if the limb is elongated, the adductors, the flexors of the leg, the tensor vaginæ femoris, and the muscular fibres arising from the anterior part of the crest of the ilium, may all become more or less tense.[1]

DISLOCATIONS.

MALGAIGNE is undoubtedly right in assuming that dislocation of the hip is sometimes only partial. These various degrees of dislocation give to the limb the slight differences of position observed in different cases of the same luxation. But the observation is not new. Hippocrates, in speaking of dislocation of this joint, remarks: "In a word, luxations and sub-luxations take place in different degrees, being sometimes greater and sometimes less."[2] Yet it cannot be denied that the general character of the deformity is the same for the same dislocation, and that the phenomena were on the whole well described by Cooper, and by preceding writers from the

[1] In a case of persistent flexion after reduction, I divided these fibres. (See p. 55 of this volume.)

[2] The Genuine Works of Hippocrates, etc. (vol. ii. p. 631). Printed for the Sydenham Society. London, 1849.

time of Hippocrates,[1] in three or four now familiar varieties, with three or four rarer forms of displacement considered to be anomalous.

Accumulated experience has justified the practical value of this general division, which should not be lost sight of either by exaggerating unimportant differences, or through needlessly obscuring what is plain by names of recondite derivation. Most surgeons have seen these dislocations in the living subject, and although the rotation, the shortening, or other displacement may have varied a little in each case, will concede that the general position of the limb is too constant and characteristic to be slighted either as a guide to the direction of the luxation, or to the force appropriate for its reduction. I have therefore adhered as far as possible to the familiar names of hip luxation, which as usually designated are those upon the dorsum, the ischiatic notch, the thyroid foramen, and the pubes. Great stress having been laid by most modern writers on a distinction between the first two, which if reduced by the flexion method are wholly unimportant variations of the same displacement, I shall endeavor to show how dorsal dislocations may be divided for practical purposes; also, that certain other less frequent luxations, hitherto classed as anomalous, are determined by the same mechanism as the rest, and with equal certainty.

Assuming that the Y ligament exerts a uniform influence upon the several dislocations, they will be here described with a view to their practical arrangement, according to the following classification: —

[1] Hippocrates describes the luxations on the dorsum, thyroid foramen, and pubes, justly including with the first variety that which has since been called "dislocation upon the ischiatic notch," most of the cases so described by modern writers being only dorsal. In a fourth variety, the dislocation "backward," — which has been, as I conceive, erroneously interpreted by his translators as "into the ischiatic notch," — Hippocrates describes at some length the dislocation directly downward.

I. THE REGULAR DISLOCATIONS, in which one or both branches of the Y ligament remain unbroken.

1. DORSAL.
2. DORSAL BELOW THE TENDON (ischiatic notch of Cooper).
3. THYROID AND DOWNWARD.
 Obliquely inward on the thyroid foramen, or as far as the perinæum.
 Vertically downward.
 Obliquely outward as far as the tuberosity.
4. PUBIC AND SUB-SPINOUS.
5. ANTERIOR OBLIQUE.

} Both branches entire.

6. SUPRA-SPINOUS.
7. EVERTED DORSAL.

} External branch broken.[1]

II. THE IRREGULAR DISLOCATIONS, in which the Y ligament is wholly ruptured, and whose characteristic signs are therefore uncertain.

GENERAL REMARKS UPON REDUCTION.

When the patient lies upon his back, especially if etherized, the dislocated limb gravitates, and the Y ligament becomes more and more tense as the limb approaches nearer and nearer

[1] Although the anterior-oblique, supra-spinous, and everted dorsal luxations resemble one another, it has been thought advisable to distinguish between them for the purpose of more accurately classifying recorded cases. In the anterior oblique luxation the outer branch of the Y ligament is still entire, as seen in the figure illustrating this luxation, where the ligament is of uniform thickness. This, indeed, is a form of supra-spinous luxation; but the limb cannot be brought down to a perpendicular, and corresponds in position with that in a case reported by Cooper. If the limb is forcibly brought to a perpendicular, the external branch is ruptured; and to such a case the term "supra-spinous" is here assigned. The term "everted dorsal" is intended to imply a power of eversion more or less complete. In such a case the limb may be everted at various angles, which can happen only after a rupture of the external branch of the ligament.

to a state of complete extension. If, now, as is here maintained, the chief obstacle to reduction of the luxated hip is found in this ligament, it follows that the method taught by Sir Astley Cooper, the weight of whose unquestioned authority has unfortunately availed to give it currency[1] during many years, is based upon an erroneous conception of the nature of the difficulty to be encountered. By that method the limb is placed as nearly as may be in the axis of the body, — thus rendering the Y ligament tense, and inviting its maximum of resistance before traction is made. Hence the necessity for pulleys, the tendency of which is undoubtedly to elongate or partly detach, at its femoral insertion, this powerful ligamentous band, at great sacrifice of mechanical force, with proportionate violence to the neighboring tissues and uncertainty as to the result. By the flexion method, which dates from a remote antiquity, the Y ligament is relaxed, its resistance annulled, and reduction often accomplished with surprising facility.

The following is the statement of Hippocrates on this subject: —

"In some the thigh is reduced without preparation, with slight extension, directed by the hand, and with slight movement; and in some the reduction is effected *by bending the limb at the joint, with gentle shaking*."[2]

[1] See Edinburgh Medical Journal, May, 1867, — "On the Reduction of Dislocations of the Hip-joint by Manipulation." By Thomas Annandale, Lecturer on Surgery, etc. "Its adoption in this country [reduction by manipulation] is as yet by no means general."

[2] Dr. Adams, in his Sydenham Translation of Hippocrates, renders this passage, "bending the limb at the joint, and *making rotation*" (vol. ii. p. 643). Mr. Sophocles, the distinguished Professor of Greek in Harvard University, has kindly furnished me the following conclusive note, defining precisely the character of this movement: —

"Your question has reference to the meaning of the word **κίγκλισις**, the formation of which is as follows: Κίγκλος, *wag-tail*, a well-known

In view of this observation of the Coan sage (450 B. C.), the indiscriminate use of pulleys hardly testifies to the progress of modern science.

Flexion lies at the foundation of success in the reduction of femoral dislocation; and compared with this the rest of the manipulation is of secondary importance. It may be taken as a safe and general rule that after the thigh has been flexed at a right angle the head of the bone is to be at once guided toward the socket, and that if the capsular orifice is large enough the operator will in general succeed; while it is equally certain that in the extended position of the limb the chances are all against him. When the femur is flexed, reduction may be effected in either of two ways. In the first (*traction*) the head is drawn or forced at once in the desired direction; in the second (*rotation*) the same result is accomplished by a rotation of the femur, which, in winding[1] the Y ligament about its neck, shortens it, and thus compels the head of the bone, as it sweeps round the socket, also to be guided toward the socket. In reducing a hip, the success of rotation, adduction, abduction, and extension depends upon this ligament, while the whole manipulation must be conducted with reference to it.

In modern times the flexion method has commended itself to the good judgment of various surgeons. Many cases of successful reduction by this method are to be found in the

bird in Greece, called also σεισοπυγίς, the Latin *motacilla*, κιγκλίζω, *to wag* (in the original sense of the term), as the bird aforesaid wags its tail.

"Κίγκλισις and κιγκλισμός, *a wag-tail movement*, *or shaking rapidly within narrow limits; gentle shaking*. The words *circumaction* and *rotation* are out of the question, — for the former is περιαγωγή, and the latter κυκλοφορία, — unless rotation be used in a peculiar sense.

"Erotian, in his Hippocratic Glossary, and Galen, define κιγκλισμός, the synonym of κίγκλισις, by βραχεῖα κίνησις, *short motion*, like that of the tail of the bird that furnishes the word."

[1] See Fig. 24.

journals, and many more have been unrecorded. Among the papers explicitly announcing it in this country is an original one, already mentioned, published by Dr. Nathan R. Smith in 1831, and advocating manipulation against pulleys in dislocation on the dorsum. His method, which has not been materially improved, consists of *free flexion, outward rotation, and abduction*, the employment of which he ascribes to his father, the late distinguished Prof. Nathan Smith, many years before.[1] In 1852, Dr. W. W. Reid, of Rochester, N. Y., published a paper also advocating manipulation to reduce the dorsal luxation (the only one described), by flexing the leg on the thigh, carrying the thigh across the sound limb upward over the pelvis as high as the umbilicus, and then abducting it and carrying the foot across the opposite sound limb,[2] — a method identical in its important features with that of Nathan Smith.[3] But these and other advocates of the flexion method in this country and abroad were anticipated by Hippocrates, so far as the essential principle of flexion is concerned.

It is desirable that before handling the limb the surgeon should accurately conceive not only the general object, but the details, of any movement he intends to employ, in order that the joint may not be injured by random, ill-devised, and fruitless manipulation. A slow, steady, well-directed movement will sometimes accomplish the desired result in a few seconds, while an ill-considered or uninstructed effort may be continued for a long time to no purpose.

In all the manœuvres the gentle shaking, oscillation, or rocking motion suggested by Hippocrates may be useful as the head approaches the socket.

The following points are worthy of note.

[1] Medical and Surgical Memoirs, p. 177.

[2] Ibid., p. 35.

[3] See also note, p. 65 of this volume.

POSITION OF THE PATIENT AND SURGEON.

The patient should be laid upon the floor, that the operator may command the limb to the best advantage, and should be etherized until the muscles of the hip are completely relaxed.[1]

THE Y LIGAMENT, WITH REFERENCE TO REDUCTION AND TO SUBSEQUENT TREATMENT.

Except in the supra-spinous dislocations, the two insertions of the Y ligament are most closely approximated when the

[1] Some writers have expressed a different opinion. As a result of the theory of muscular resistance, Dr. Reid concludes that etherization to a state of complete relaxation, instead of being an advantage, is a detriment, because it prevents the contraction of the muscles required to replace the bone. (See a paper entitled "Observations on Dr. Markoe's Report of Cases of Dislocation of the Femur treated by Manipulation. By W. W. Reid, M. D., of Rochester, N. Y." New York Journal of Medicine, etc., July, 1855, p. 72.) Dr. Reid seems here to add the theory of active muscular resistance to that of passive muscular resistance, already quoted from a previous paper written by him.

The British Medical Journal (Oct. 20, 1866) contains a paper read by Mr. Nunneley at a recent meeting of the British Medical Association at Chester, "On the Reduction of Dislocation (more especially of the Hip and Shoulder) by Manipulation," in which the following views are presented: "The most important condition to be insured is a relaxed but not perfectly helpless, flaccid, uncontractile condition of the muscles, as it is by the contraction of the muscles which are attached near to the head of the dislocated bone that reduction is mainly accomplished; . . . while, on the other hand, if they be incapable of any contraction whatever, it will frequently be found to be impossible for any manipulatory movements of the surgeon to replace the bone, or, being replaced, for its being retained in that position. I feel confident that I have seen both of these causes materially interfere with success, particularly the latter one, when the muscles have been entirely paralyzed owing to the anæsthesia having been too profound."

In 1844 a patient was made completely insensible by the administration of a bottle of port wine and half a bottle of rum in divided doses, and a hip reduction was accomplished during "a condition of muscular collapse." London Medical Gazette, 1844, p. 60; from Casper's Wochenschrift, No. 9, 1844.

thigh is flexed upon the trunk, carried toward the navel, and rotated inward.

But it has happened that after unsuccessful efforts a hip has been reduced when semi-flexed in the act of extension; which shows that in certain cases the ligament may be needlessly relaxed by extreme flexion, and may be advantageously drawn tighter by a little extension or outward rotation.[1]

I may here refer, in connection with the subsequent treatment of the patient, to the practical importance of preventing such a relaxation of the anterior ligament, whether by flexing the thigh or raising the body to a sitting posture, as may permit a recurrence of luxation. For this purpose, where the bone inclines to slip from the socket after reduction, certain cases may require not only that the limb should be kept straight, but also that the thigh should be confined for a time in the position which completed the reduction; namely, for the dorsal luxations, in abduction and eversion, or in vertical extension; for the pubic and thyroid, in a position of inward rotation and adduction, — thus taking advantage of the tense ligament to bind the bone to the socket.[2]

[1] Markoe, in an interesting paper upon this subject, states that he found it necessary to vary a little from the method by flexion, abduction, and rotation outwards, recommended by Reid in dorsal dislocation. He says: "It failed us so completely from the first that we were led to add the bringing down of the thigh to the straight position in a state of abduction, still keeping up the rocking motion; and it has been uniformly in the act of thus bringing down the limb that the reduction has been accomplished." (See "An Account of the Cases of Dislocation of the Femur at the Hip-Joint, treated by Manipulation alone, after the Plan proposed by W. W. Reid, M. D., of Rochester, which have occurred in the New York Hospital during the past Two Years. By Thomas M. Markoe, M. D., one of the Attending Surgeons." New York Journal of Medicine, etc., vol. xiv., January, 1855, p. 23.) See also note, p. 46 of this volume.

[2] See case, p. 53 of this volume.

HOW THE LIMB IS TO BE HELD.

The thigh should be bent upon the body, and the leg at a right angle with the thigh. With one hand the surgeon grasps the ankle from above, while with the other, placed beneath the head of the tibia, he lifts and guides the limb. In this way, by using the flexed leg as a lever, keeping it always flexed at a right angle for that purpose, great power is brought to bear upon the head of the femur, especially in rotating the thigh. It is therefore important to keep accurate account, during such manipulation, of the position of the head of this bone, which should not be moved at random, or indiscriminately urged when locked, lest it be broken from the shaft; and it may be convenient to remember that in every position the head of the femur faces nearly in the direction of the inner aspect of its internal condyle.

CAPSULAR ORIFICE TO BE ENLARGED.

Much stress has been laid by certain writers upon the difficulty of replacing the head of the bone, when it has escaped by a small aperture in the capsule. That this condition may occasionally occur seems probable; and it is suggested by Gellé,[1] in his elaborate paper upon the subject, that when the slit occurs close to the femoral insertion of the capsular ligament, it may be impossible to replace the head of the bone. This writer, with Malgaigne, Gunn, and others, urges the importance of placing the bone in the position it occupied when luxated, with a view to its re-entering the socket by exactly retracing its path. But while this path cannot always be known, any difficulty is easily obviated by carrying the head of the bone toward the opposite side of the socket, and thus enlarging the

[1] Étude du Rôle de la Déchirure Capsulaire, etc. Par M. Gellé. Paris, 1861.

slit, — a simple manœuvre, easily accomplished by circumducting the flexed thigh across the abdomen in a direction opposite to that in which it is desired to lead the head of the bone, which should be made in this way to pass across below the socket, and never, it is needless to say, above it, across the Y ligament. This expedient, of which I have had occasion to avail myself, will, as I believe, be in future generally adopted when any such difficulty is encountered in reducing the hip. The subcutaneous injury is trifling in comparison with that resulting from a protracted and ill-planned manipulation, or from the brute force of pulleys. It depends for its success upon the strength of the Y ligament, which, in firmly attaching the base of the neck of the femur to the inferior spinous process of the ilium, forms a fulcrum or pivot round which the shaft and the neck of the femur can be made to revolve, like opposite spokes in a wheel, — the Y ligament being strong enough to rupture, in this way, the whole of the rest of the capsule and the obturator muscle without itself yielding.[1]

When a slit has thus been made by circumducting the neck of the bone across the posterior aspect of the capsule, the head of the bone has traversed an interval reaching in some cases from the dorsum to the thyroid foramen, and slips readily from side to side. This laceration already exists in most cases of dorsal dislocation below the tendon, where the head of the bone has reached a secondary position after a previous luxation downward, and is also known to surgeons who have reduced dislocations by the old and awkward method of extension, where the bone sometimes slipped many times backward and forward from the dorsum to the foramen ovale; and yet I can find recorded only one instance of this familiar

[1] Reid, in the paper already quoted (New York Journal of Medicine, July, 1855, p. 69), proposes, in a similar case, "to make an incision down to the head of the bone, and open the capsular ligament sufficient to admit the return of the head into its place."

occurrence as being followed by any permanent injury, and even in that case there may have been a predisposition to the hip disease which ensued. It will hereafter be seen that when the head of the bone has thus been made to slip from side to side, rotation becomes a less efficient manœuvre for reduction, — the bone tending at the critical moment to slip laterally away from the socket instead of into it, especially where the rim of the acetabulum is prominent, or the Y ligament is relaxed. It is here that vertical traction, sudden or continued, is especially to be relied on. This will be further explained.

FRACTURE OF THE NECK.

Except in a very old subject, no apprehension need be felt of fracture from tolerably skilful manipulation, or from circumduction with a view to tearing the capsule. The femur has, indeed, in rare instances been fractured by manipulation as well as by pulleys ;[1] and if the head of the bone be forced into a position where it is confined by the Y ligament, and from which it cannot escape, it will be acted upon with great power by the shaft serving as the long arm of a lever, if force be still indiscreetly applied.

FLEXION, EXTENSION, ADDUCTION, ABDUCTION, AND ROTATION.

Of these terms the last two alone require notice. If a thigh abducted at a right angle be rotated outward, with the knee bent, this position of the limb has been sometimes

[1] Verneuil relates a case of fracture resulting from an attempt to reduce a dislocation on the pubes in a man eighty-one years of age, but only after the bone had resisted many attempts at reduction. (Medical Times and Gazette, December, 1865, p. 661.) Similar cases have been reported of fracture from the use both of manipulation and of pulleys. (See Cooper's "Treatise on Dislocations and Fractures of the Joints," Case XXXVII.)

erroneously described as one of flexion. It becomes so only as the knee is brought forward.

Rotation is here always intended to apply to the thigh, the inward or outward rotation of which, in a limb bent for reduction, carries the foot in an opposite direction, and may thus lead to doubt.[1]

CIRCUMDUCTION.

When the patient lies on the floor, circumduction carries the knee of the dislocated limb through arcs of a horizontal circle of which the Y ligament is the centre. In attempting reduction, the direction of this motion is of primary importance, as well as the point at which it begins. The following varieties of circumduction should be distinguished from one another : —

Circumduction of the	extended	thigh,	outward (continued by)
"	"	flexed	"	inward.
Circumduction of the	extended	"	inward (continued by)
"	"	flexed	"	outward.

The patella here always faces to the front. If it inclines outward or inward, rotation has been added to circumduction.

REGULAR DISLOCATIONS.

DISLOCATION UPON THE DORSUM ILII.

THE dorsal dislocations having a mutual resemblance, resulting from the regular outline of the bone upon which they rest, may be more readily grouped than the others.

[1] The *thigh*, abducted and a little flexed, was rotated ***inward***; the *leg* and the *foot*, on the contrary, were in forced rotation ***outward***. — OLLIVIER: *Archives de Médecine*, *1823*, *tom. iii. p. 545.*

They are found at various points of the continuously curved surface of the os innominatum, from the tuberosity of the ischium to the hollow of the ilium, — with the articular head well down beneath the external obturator muscle, or farther back in the same muscular interstice, behind the tendon of the internal obturator, or emerging above this tendon between it and the pyriformis muscle, or, lastly, above the pyriformis.

When the femur is flexed at right angles, and thrust directly backward, it tends to pass between the obturator internus and the pyriformis. At an angle of forty-five degrees it may be thrust upward above the pyriformis, while in extreme flexion it is directed downward and outward toward the tuberosity and between the obturators. Inward rotation luxates the bone at lower points, even though the limb be flexed at the same angles.

The dislocation below the internal obturator tendon and the subjacent capsule is probably common, because the neck of the femur is here first arrested in its ascent from the frequent downward displacement which occurs while the limb is flexed, as it is in the great majority of such accidents. The dislocation between this muscle and the pyriformis and the one above the pyriformis may be assumed to be more rare, these muscular fibres being probably more often torn; but future autopsies can alone show how often the other small outward rotators are lacerated[1] in the dorsal dislocation, when the internal obturator with its capsule has yielded, — or, indeed, how often the head of the bone escapes above the internal

[1] In an autopsy of dorsal dislocation by Mr. Todd (see Cooper's "Treatise," Case XL.; also Dublin Hospital Reports, 1822, vol. iii. p. 396), the dislocated extremity of the femur had occupied a large cavity between the gluteus maximus and medius; the pyriformis, gemelli, obturatores, and quadratus were completely torn across; the iliacus, psoas, and adductors were uninjured; the orbicular ligament was entire at the anterior superior parts only.

obturator tendon, and how often it ruptures it in reaching the same point.

With reference to reduction, however, these are not questions of essential importance.

The comparative infrequency of autopsies of hip dislocation, while it leaves us in the dark upon certain points which it would be desirable to have elucidated, bears evidence to the fact that this lesion is not a severe one. There can be little doubt that the small rotators near the joint are lacerated with comparative impunity, both by luxations and by their reduction. They may exert some influence upon the relative difficulty of reduction in different cases, and (as will hereafter be shown) the mutual conversion of the different varieties of dorsal luxation one into another probably depends upon the laceration of these different muscles, as well as upon that of the capsule.

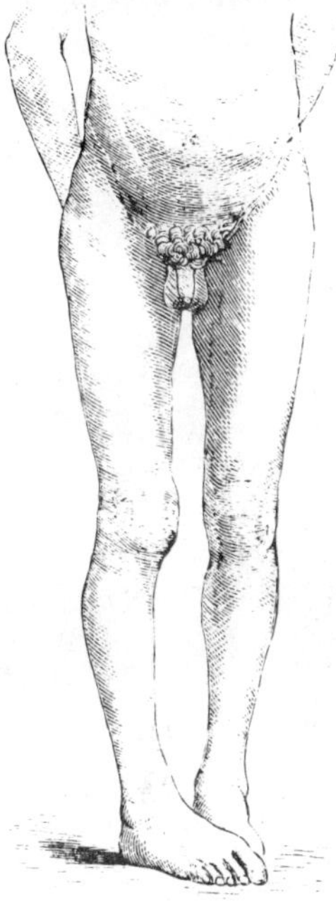

FIG. 4.[1]

SIGNS.

In this dislocation the limb is moderately inverted, a little shortened, and advanced. The toes cross the toes or the instep of the other foot, according to the degree of flexion and inversion, and the head of the bone may generally be felt upon the dorsum.

[1] Dorsal dislocation, showing the limb inverted, the toes crossing those of the other foot. The leg has been well brought down, and exhibits but little flexion. (See p. 41 of this volume.) It is often more flexed. (See Figs. 11, 13, and p. 102 of this volume.)

The inversion is chiefly due to the outer branch of the Y ligament, as is shown by the fact that the characteristic sign disappears when this branch is divided.[1] But other parts of the capsule, varying with its laceration, may assist the inversion of the limb; and when the latter is exaggerated, as when one thigh crosses the other at its middle or upper third, they may seem to be largely concerned in it. Thus, if the dorsal luxation is secondary to one below the socket, only the anterior and superior fibres will remain untorn; while if the femur has been thrust obliquely upward and backward, attachments may be found at both the anterior and inferior margins of the acetabulum. But it is unnecessary to consider these lesser and comparatively slender fibres. In such cases the knee can be depressed, as indeed it often is, by the forces to which it is subjected at the time of the accident, until the exaggerated flexion and inversion have disappeared; and if even a large part of the capsule, as shown in Fig. 5, is stretched tense across the socket, it may then be ruptured without diminishing the in-

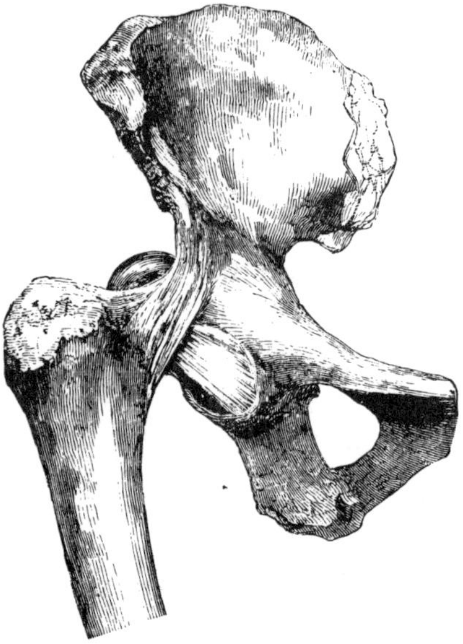

FIG. 5.[2]

[1] For an illustration of the condition of the anterior part of the capsule in a congenital dorsal luxation of this character, see Malgaigne's "Traité des Fractures et des Luxations" (Paris, 1847. Pl. XXVIII. Fig. 1).

[2] Dorsal dislocation, showing a comparatively sound capsular ligament. For the dissected Y ligament, see Figs. 6, 7.

version, which for all practical purposes is due to the outer branch of the Y ligament. Upon this, in fact, inversion ultimately depends; without its rupture there can be no eversion, and after its laceration the other fibres of the capsule have comparatively little strength. The rupture of the inner branch of the Y ligament does not materially change the attitude of the limb. The shortening varies with the position of the head of the bone. Sometimes there is little; sometimes it amounts apparently to two inches or more; but, as Malgaigne remarks, it is then complicated by flexion, and is more apparent than real.[1]

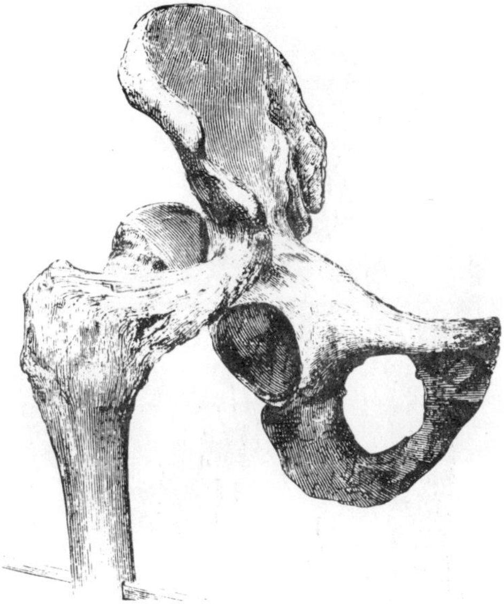

FIG. 6.[2]

The accompanying figures (6 and 7) are intended to illustrate the operation of the Y ligament in limiting the range of the femur, and the consequent amount of shortening. At its lowest point, the head of the bone corresponds to the lower part of

[1] The elongation or shortening of a dislocated thigh may, like that of the arm, be real or only apparent. If the head of the bone is luxated downward, the limb should be longer; but flexion or abduction of the shaft approximates the usual points of measurement. To this source of error should be added the tilting of the pelvis in the femoral luxations.

[2] Figs. 6 and 7, — dorsal dislocation. These two figures are intended to show the possible range of the dissected femur when limited by the Y ligament alone. (From photographs taken in 1861.)

the ischiatic notch, while it may rise upon the dorsum about an inch and a quarter above it. The former position is that most frequently occupied in dorsal luxations, the head of the bone being usually confined to the neighborhood of the socket by the unruptured muscles and by the capsular and Y ligaments (see Fig. 5). Should the femur have been thrust upward to a higher point, it might again gravitate to the level of the ischiatic notch unless engaged in the interstices of the small rotators. From examination of eleven specimens of dorsal dislocation, Malgaigne[1] infers that the head of the femur generally corresponds to the ischiatic notch, and that the iliac luxation of Cooper is a pure hypothesis, while his plate illustrating it is imaginary. It will be observed that the dorsal dislocations here given in woodcuts from photographs exhibit an inconsiderable shortening.

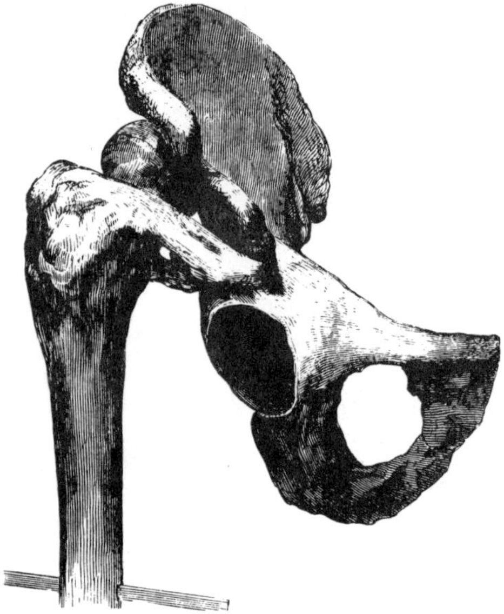

FIG. 7.

If, then, there be a fixed inversion of the limb with shortening, and the head of the femur is felt upon the dorsum, little desirable information is to be gained by measurement unless in exceptional or doubtful cases, inasmuch as a primary dislocation upon the dorsum practically signifies one and the same thing, whether directly backward behind the acetabulum, or

[1] Traité, etc., p. 820.

obliquely upward and backward to the full extent of the Y ligament, if this remain unbroken. A more useful indication is the degree of its mobility.

The thigh can always be flexed, and then its mobility varies with the extent of the laceration of the capsule and the adjacent tissues which bind the neck of the femur to the pelvis, — an important point, best determined by the extent to which the flexed limb can be abducted. If the bone has escaped by a large aperture in the capsule, perhaps with rupture of the obturator tendon, there will be a comparative freedom of motion and less inversion; while if the laceration is small, the movement will be restricted and the limb comparatively rigid.

By flexing and rotating the thigh, the head of the bone may be felt upon the ilium, unless the patient is very fleshy or the parts are greatly swollen; but when this sign is wanting, a differential diagnosis can be based on other indications. Thus, although it is practically needless to distinguish the dorsal dislocation from the one below the tendon, the latter is generally characterized by a more advanced position of the knee, the limb being more inverted, and crossing the sound thigh at a higher point. On the other hand, the other regular dislocations and the fractures exhibit eversion, if we except the fracture of the neck accompanied by inversion,[1] — an accident so rare that it need hardly be taken into account, — and some of the fractures of the pelvis.

In the dorsal dislocation, however much the knee may be advanced and the leg inverted, even when the head of the femur is below the tendon, the thigh may be depressed by manipulation until the knees lie almost upon the same plane; and in some cases, — where, as in a female, the legs are knock-kneed, or where the knee-joint is loosely articulated, or in an

[1] See p. 147 of this volume; and also a Practical Treatise on Fractures and Dislocations (p. 351). By Frank Hastings Hamilton, M. D., etc.

old dislocation, — the foot may seem not to be inverted. But the inversion of the patella, and especially the degree of resistance in everting the foot, betray the still unreduced luxation, even when the position of the limb has been much improved by efforts at reduction, which, though unsuccessful, have lacerated the capsule and loosened the muscles. This is especially true in the case of a fleshy subject, where the marks are obscure.

DORSAL DISLOCATIONS BETWEEN THE ROTATOR MUSCLES.

It has been said that the dorsal dislocation is often secondary, the head of the femur having first escaped below the socket. But the head of the bone may also reach the dorsum at once by a backward thrust in the direction of its axis, which is also likely to engage the head in the muscular interstices of the rotators. Autopsies have hitherto failed to show whether in such a high dorsal dislocation the internal obturator, with other inward rotators, is usually ruptured, or whether the head of the bone usually emerges above the internal obturator; but I have expressed the belief that the outward rotators are often ruptured, both by the original injury and by the protracted manipulation accompanying the use of pulleys, and that this lesion is by no means serious. It may, indeed, be difficult to distinguish between the flexion and inversion of a femur engaged above the obturator muscle and those of one in the act of ascending from the position of a luxation near the tuberosity to that below the tendon. But this distinction is practically unimportant, since, by circumduction of the limb, a way can be cleared for the head of the bone from any point of the dorsum within the range of the Y ligament round to the thyroid foramen.

The head of the femur has been found between the obturator internus and the pyriformis, which lies above it, and has even passed still higher beneath the pyriformis, emerging between it and the gluteus minimus.[1] The bone is then drawn so far backward by the obturator tendon that the outer branch of

[1] See an interesting case mentioned by M. Parmentier (Bulletin de la Société Anatomique, 1850, p. 177). The limb was "adducted and shortened three quarters of an inch. The femur was luxated between the pyriformis muscle and the obturator internus, the head reaching to the ischiatic spine. The button-hole thus formed opposed the reduction of the luxation in the dissected specimen." Another interesting and exceptional case has been reported by Dr. Servier. (See Bulletin de la Société de Chirurgie, 1863, p. 485. Report of M. Legouest.) The head of the femur, instead of escaping between the obturator internus and pyriformis muscles, as in the case described by M. Parmentier, was here found above the pyriformis, between this muscle and the gluteus minimus. The signs, so far as can be judged from the account given, were those of the dorsal luxation. The capsule was ruptured posteriorly. It has been remarked that there is great difficulty in producing these luxations in the dissected specimen without rupturing the slender outward rotators; but if the head is made to emerge between them, either by rotation or by a direct backward thrust of the shaft, it is so embraced by the muscles, and also by the capsular orifice, which is then likely to be small, that the movements of the limb are comparatively restricted, and the muscular obstacle to their reduction may be considerable. I do not know how such cases can be identified with certainty during life. If the head of the bone has escaped by rotation of the shaft inwards, it may perhaps be reduced by outward rotation, with previous or subsequent flexion of the thigh, and thus brought to a point below the socket; although the surer way is to take the risk of rupturing all these smaller muscles by outward circumduction of the flexed limb, accompanied with outward rotation, and then to reduce the bone as usual.

M. Guersant (Notices sur la Chirurgie des Enfants, Paris, 1864–77), reporting two cases which occurred under his own observation, and referring to a paper of M. Chapplain, proposes a distinction between superficial and deep iliac luxations. Such a difference would be difficult to discover in practice, either in a fleshy or a thin subject, but may have some foundation in the muscular complications just alluded to. Mr. Wormald reports a case of dislocation, *originally on the ilium*, in which, by the use of pulleys, the bone was "thrown" *upon the sciatic notch*, whence it "*could not be reduced*." (Medical Times and Gazette, Aug. 16, 1856, p. 170.) I am at a loss to explain this case, if the facts are accurately given, except upon the hypothesis that muscular button-holes, together with horizontal extension, determined the result.

In a case of "Dislocation of the Thigh-Bone upward and backward, the Y becomes very tense, producing great inversion in the extended limb, and adduction when it is flexed, the obturator limiting inversion. The occurrence, during life, of these varieties of dorsal luxation having been well attested, it is possible that they are comparatively common, and that many dorsal luxations occur above the internal obturator tendon,—a condition which would explain the reported "change" by pulleys of the "dorsal" dislocation into that "upon the sciatic notch," when the limb was drawn down. The subjoined methods will accomplish their reduction before, or at any rate after, the rupture of the internal obturator; and this muscle may be ruptured at will.

The strong outer or posterior part of the capsule, which offers a resistance nearly in the direction of the obturator tendon, may also be torn by circumduction,—the capsule requiring less effort for its rupture than the muscles, being inserted at the base of the neck, nearer to the centre of rotation.

REDUCTION OF THE DISLOCATION UPON THE DORSUM.

This dislocation may be equally well reduced by traction or rotation.[1]

primarily on the Dorsum Ilii, secondarily on the Sciatic Notch" (James Syme, F. R. S. E., etc., Contributions to Pathology and the Practice of Surgery, p. 277), the following passage occurs: "That excellent authority, Sir Astley Cooper, though he has warned against the risk of this occurrence in reducing dislocation into the foramen ovale, has not noticed it with regard to the more common case of dislocation on the ilium." Something must be allowed for a conventional surgical prejudice against the "sciatic notch," which labors under a bad name.

[1] In experiments upon the dead subject, I have twice found that the femur, after reduction by rotation, had accidentally engaged the sciatic nerve upon the front of its neck. The limb was flexed, inverted, and a little abducted, and the nerve tense and projecting in the popliteal space, as in a case of old contraction of the knee-joint. This would not have occurred if the weight of the limb had been properly sustained.

By Traction.—1. Lay the patient, when etherized, on his back upon the floor, bend the limb at the knee, flex the thigh upon the abdomen, adduct and rotate it a little inward, to disengage the head of the bone from behind the socket. The Y ligament is then relaxed. (Fig. 8.)

If the bone can now be abducted beyond the perpendicular, the capsule and other tissues are probably so torn or relaxed that reduction may be accomplished without much difficulty; the thigh need only be forcibly lifted or jerked toward the ceiling, with a little simultaneous circumduction and rotation outward, to direct the head of the bone toward the socket.

2. The surgeon's foot[1] may be placed on the anterior superior spinous process of the ilium, or on the pubes, to keep the pelvis down, while he pulls the flexed knee up. Or in the same way, while assistants suspend the pelvis a few inches from the floor by a strip of board passed transversely under the calf near the ham, the surgeon may with his foot thrust the pelvis down into its place.

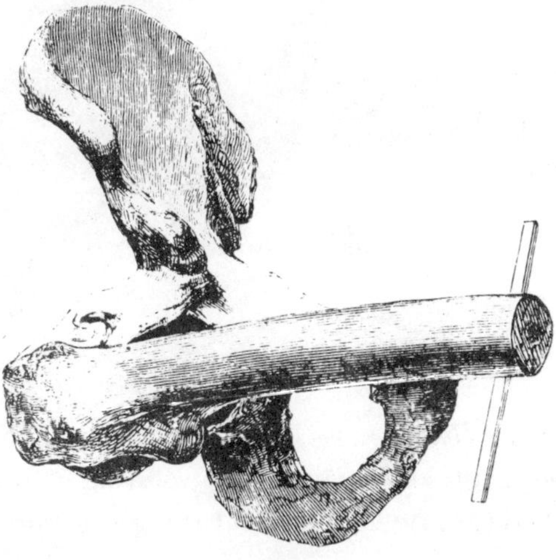

Fig. 8.[2]

3. Flex the thigh and circumduct it outward, across the abdomen. When it forms a large angle laterally with the trunk, the head of the bone, if it has not snapped into its

[1] Divested, it need hardly be said, of boot or shoe.

[2] Dorsal dislocation. The result of flexion in relaxing the Y ligament. (From a photograph taken in 1861.)

place, is in or near the thyroid foramen. The rent in the capsule being thus enlarged, restore the thigh to a perpendicular, and proceed as in the last method.

4. Place the patient face downward on a table, the thigh, flexed at right angles, hanging over its edge, and bear the limb downward, with or without rotation.[1]

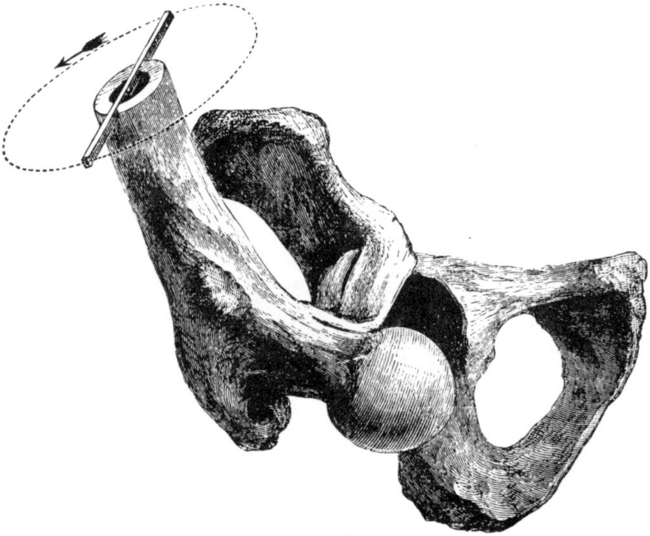

FIG. 9.[2]

By Rotation. — Flex the thigh and abduct or circumduct it outward, at the same time rotating it outward. The head of the bone, revolving about the great trochanter, which is fixed

[1] A little girl of twelve years, upon whom six or seven attempts of an hour each had been made to reduce this luxation by straight extension, was thus placed on a board, when the head of the femur immediately slipped in. (Collin, Thèse Inaugurale. Montpellier, 1833.)

In 1830 Colombot had employed this method with rotation. (Documents sur la Méthode Ostéotropique. Paris, 1840.)

[2] Dorsal dislocation. Reduction by rotation. The limb has been flexed and abducted, and it remains only to evert it, and render the outer branch of the Y ligament tense by rotation.

by the outer branch of the Y ligament, rises over the edge of the socket into its place unless the capsule is interposed, in which case enlarge the opening, as in the third method. This is a very effective manœuvre for the reduction of the dorsal luxations, and has been described in the words, "Lift up, bend out, roll out." An imperfect comprehension of this empirical rule has led to confusion in its application.[1] It should be remembered that if the thigh is everted before it is abducted, it may be locked below the socket. For this reason it is well, especially in an old dislocation where the parts are unyielding, to invert the limb until the final abduction, when it may be everted.

When the thigh is forcibly flexed upon the abdomen, the head of the bone is lifted out from beneath the socket.[2] A little inward rotation favors the same result. If the thigh be now slowly abducted or depressed outward, it is plain that

[1] An English journal terms this method "a knack." Mr. Cock, in a case of dorsal dislocation, gives the rule, "Lift up, bend out, roll *in*" (Medical Times and Gazette, June 30, 1855, p. 611), — a manœuvre which may succeed, although the method, also mentioned by Mr. Cock, of flexion, abduction, and rotation outward, is perhaps the more correct one. (Lancet, July 7, 1855, p. 6.)

The thigh being flexed, outward rotation and outward circumduction both carry the head of the bone toward the socket.

In a case of dorsal dislocation reported by Mr. W. J. Square, pulleys were applied for twenty-five minutes unsuccessfully; and again twenty-five minutes longer, with no better result, when they were abandoned. The thigh was now flexed at right angles, and easily reduced by circumduction outward. (Medical Times and Gazette, Nov. 13, 1858, and American Journal of the Medical Sciences, January, 1859, p. 258.)

[2] Dr. George Sutton of Aurora, Ind., relates a case of dorsal dislocation in which, after a failure from some cause to reduce the hip by the ordinary flexion method, a roll of cloth was placed in the groin, as a fulcrum, by which the head of the flexed femur was pried out from beneath the socket, and afterward reduced by abduction while the limb was lifted. (Western Journal of Medicine and Surgery, September, 1868. American Journal of the Medical Sciences, October, 1868, p. 588.)

the head of the bone, suspended by the Y ligament, must rise toward the socket; and that when the shaft is thus abducted, outward rotation assists the entrance of the head. If the head of the bone is above the tendon of the internal obturator, this outward circumduction also ruptures the small rotator muscles. It may be needless to say that were the head of the bone suspended by the dissected Y ligament alone, as shown in some of the annexed woodcuts, a lateral movement of the knee would perhaps cause the head of the bone to swing from side to side, instead of giving to it the desired upward tilt. This movement is hindered by the unruptured fibres of the capsule on each side of the Y ligament, which continue to a greater or less extent in the different dislocations, and contribute to the varying facility with which different cases are reduced. This is especially true of the dislocation behind the tendon of the obturator internus, where the posterior part of the capsule not unfrequently remains uninjured.

I have thus reduced the dislocated femur in living subjects by a single slow circumduction occupying from a quarter to half a minute, and also by a first rapid sweep of two seconds. The manœuvre may be perfectly accomplished without lifting the limb toward the ceiling, but is more effectual when terminated with an upward jerk.[1] If it fails, repeat the process once or twice, and then, if necessary, enlarge the opening. Or if the limb is too much flexed, and the Y ligament too much relaxed, then the limb may be slowly extended from the perpendicular position, when, as the Y ligament becomes

[1] This upward jerk is a very efficient manœuvre, both alone and when assisted by rotation. Annibal Parea is said to have availed himself of it. "He placed the patient on his back, the pelvis being confined by assistants; he flexed the knee, raised the thigh almost vertically, grasped its lower extremity with both hands, gave it a jerk as if to raise it perpendicularly, and the luxation was instantaneously reduced." (Malgaigne's "Traité," etc., p. 823.)

tightened, the head of the femur will rise into its place (see p. 31),[1] especially if the weight of the limb be sustained by the operator. The flexed femur is thus reduced by abduction and rotation with less flexion.[2]

If the laceration is large, and the head of the bone inclines to slip toward the thyroid foramen during abduction, this tendency is easily counteracted by the upward jerk or lift already described. But if upon examination the flexed thigh cannot be abducted beyond the perpendicular, the head of the bone has either escaped by a small orifice in the capsule (which is then comparatively sound), or has also passed above the obturator or pyriformis (which are then unbroken), and is suspended just behind the edge of the socket, midway between these muscles and the Y ligament. In the former case the luxation may perhaps be reduced by flexion with abduction and outward rotation; in the latter, it is possible, but not easy, to disengage it by traction across the symphysis, the bone being lifted by a towel round the thigh at its upper part.[3] If these attempts do not succeed, the obturator muscle and the capsule can be

[1] See a case of "ischiatic" dislocation treated in this way by George W. Callender, Esq., Assistant Surgeon and Lecturer on Anatomy at St. Bartholomew's Hospital. (Lancet, March 14, 1868, p. 343.) Mr. Callender believes, however, that the capsule "never can offer any obstacle to the reduction of dislocations of the hip."

[2] In the extreme flexed position of the limb, the Y ligament is so relaxed that it may not afford a firm centre of rotation. (See p. 31 of this volume.) A case reported by Mr. Jones (Medical Times and Gazette, April, 1856, p. 362) may serve to illustrate this point. In reducing a dorsal dislocation, the thigh was flexed as far as possible, abducted, and rotated outward. The attempt failed; but in gradually bringing the limb down while the same forces were applied, the head of the bone snapped into its socket when the thigh had reached a semi-flexed position. (See also Mackenzie, London Hospital Reports, 1866, vol. iii. p. 207.)

[3] To dislocate the bone above the obturator tendon in the dead subject, the posterior capsule should be divided high up toward the Y ligament, and the bone then strongly flexed, adducted, and rotated outward. By inward rotation it may be reduced.

ruptured by outward circumduction of the flexed limb, — an expedient also to be resorted to whenever the limb is especially fixed and unyielding, — after which the hip may be reduced as usual.

The following case will illustrate the method by traction. I was requested by Dr. E. A. W. Harlow, Oct. 5, 1861, to see, with him, a stout, middle-aged Irishman whose hip had been dislocated an hour or two before. In climbing the ladder of a freight car while the train was moving, his thigh was bent to a horizontal position just in time to be caught between this car and the next one. The flexed hip was thus dislocated backward primarily upon the dorsum, by a force very exactly applied to the knee in front and the pelvis behind, probably with slight laceration of the capsule. The limb was shortened, the toes were firmly inverted across the instep of the other foot, the head of the femur being felt upon the dorsum. On flexion the thigh could not be abducted as far as the perpendicular, and was unusually immovable, — the latter condition being perhaps due to the comparative integrity of the capsule. This would formerly have led to the belief that it was engaged in the ischiatic notch. It is also possible that the head of the femur may have escaped between the Y ligament and the obturator or pyriformis muscle. The patient being etherized, I flexed the limb, and made several efforts to reduce it by angular traction, but was unable to do so, the failure being doubtless due to the small size of the capsular and perhaps the muscular opening, which under the same circumstances I should now not hesitate to enlarge by circumduction. The attempt was abandoned till the next morning, when, the patient being again etherized and the limb flexed as usual, a rectangular metallic splint was applied beneath the knee, and so held by assistants as to suspend the pelvis a few inches from the floor. I then placed my foot upon the anterior superior spine of the pelvis, and at the first effort depressed the latter into its place.[1] During the patient's stay in the hospital this limb was a little longer than the other, — an appearance I have observed in several instances, and which is perhaps due to a portion of

[1] I venture to publish the following note from Dr. Mann, of Roxbury, in illustration of the above manœuvre: —

ROXBURY, Jan. 16, 1867.

PROF. H. J. BIGELOW:

DEAR SIR, — I take pleasure in sending you the following brief account of a case of dislocation of the right femur upon the dorsum ilii, in which I used the method for its reduction pointed out by you at the annual meeting of the Massachusetts Medical Society, in May, 1862. At that time you demonstrated a ligament described as the Y ligament, and the part performed by it in giving position to the limb and in preventing the return of the bone to its socket, together with the best means of overcoming that resistance. I was much surprised at the ease with which the reduction was accomplished, . . . for I am sure in no other way could it have been accomplished with so much ease to the patient and to myself.

I was called, July 10, 1862, to James Stump, a stout, muscular man, about fifty years of age, who while picking cherries lost his hold and fell from the tree, a distance of about twenty feet, to the ground. He complained of great pain in his hip, and was incapable of rising. He was picked up and conveyed to his home (a distance of three miles), where I saw him about an hour after the accident.

I found him lying on a mattress on the floor. The right leg was two inches shorter than the left, with the toes resting upon the opposite instep, the knee and foot turned inward, and a little advanced upon the other. The limb could be bent upon the other, but could not be moved outward. The trochanter major could be felt near the anterior superior spinous process of the ilium, and the head of the bone moving upon the dorsum ilii during rotation of the knee inward. He was just in the position I desired, and I determined to try your method of reduction.

Having etherized him, I placed my left foot (the boot having been removed for that purpose) upon the pelvis of the right side, and bending the leg of the patient upon the thigh, and the thigh upon the pelvis, thus relaxing the Y ligament, and placing my left arm under the knee, and grasping the ankle with the right hand, I had perfect command of the limb.

Keeping the pelvis firmly fixed with the foot, I made a firm and pretty forcible extension with the left arm, and with a slight rotatory movement with the right hand the bone instantly slipped into its socket with a smart snapping noise which could be distinctly heard by every one in the room.

In two days the patient was able to walk about his room and resume his work (which was that of fancy-basket maker). I met him upon the street three weeks after the accident, and he assured me he could walk as well as ever, saying that he had walked five miles that afternoon without fatigue.

Very truly yours,

BENJAMIN MANN.

the capsule being engaged between the head of the bone and the acetabulum, — but in 1869 it was shortened half an inch, everted, and the power of rotation impaired, apparently by dry chronic arthritis. In another case which I have lately examined, of dislocation reduced fifteen years ago by the late Dr. Hayward, this deformity of the hip from the same cause was much more strongly marked.

The subject of the following case of dislocation of four weeks' standing was sent to me by Dr. Thomas, of Scituate.

Four weeks ago a large door, weighing half a ton, fell upon the patient, — a man, aged fifty, — dislocating his left hip. An irregular practitioner etherized him, and with the assistance of two men drew the leg down, and told him that it was reduced. The left leg is now two inches shorter than the right, the foot inverted over the right instep, the trochanter higher and more prominent than it should be, and the head of the bone felt upon the dorsum ilii.

The reduction was effected as follows. The patient was etherized and laid upon the floor. The thigh was slowly flexed upon the abdomen, and then moved laterally, to loosen the tissues about the joint. It was then returned toward the perpendicular, and jerked upward, with a little simultaneous abduction and rotation outward, but without success. Recognizing the comparatively untorn or reuniting capsule as the cause of the failure of this effort, I slowly circumducted the flexed thigh outward until the head of the bone was carried from the dorsum nearly to the thyroid foramen. After the capsular orifice was thus enlarged, and the head of the bone replaced below the socket, the first upward jerk reduced the dislocation, — the whole manipulation having occupied scarcely a minute and a half.

The following cases were reduced by rotation.

In the first case the reduction was easy, and occurred in the wards of Dr. Cabot, who kindly submitted the case to me.

A man, aged twenty-four, had his left hip dislocated by the caving in of a bank of earth. The usual signs of dislocation on the dorsum were presented. To reduce it, the thigh was flexed to a perpendicular, and in order to enlarge the capsular orifice it was then slowly abducted with a little rotation outward, during which it snapped into its place. The manœuvre occupied scarcely ten seconds.

It will be observed that this movement is equally suitable for extending the capsular laceration in the direction of the thyroid foramen, or, if the laceration be already sufficient, for prying the head of the bone into the socket, with the aid of the Y ligament as a fulcrum.

The following was a case of dorsal dislocation of eight months' standing, which had occurred in consequence of a fall on the floor. The patient, a woman twenty-seven years of age, had remained in bed for several months, and afterward walked with great difficulty. The limb then presented the usual signs of dorsal dislocation, and was reduced by flexion, abduction, and eversion. I first saw her sixteen days after this operation, when the bone had again become displaced. The limb was an inch or more shorter than its fellow; and though its patella looked directly forward, and the foot was not inverted, yet the latter could not be everted like that of the sound limb, and the head of the bone was felt near the sciatic notch. By forcible flexion, abduction, and eversion I brought the head of the bone into the socket with a snap; but when the limb was again extended, a very slight inversion sufficed to reproduce the dislocation, — in fact, the limb could not be trusted to itself. After the bone had thus repeatedly slipped out, the patient was placed in bed on her back, and the dislocation again reduced by flexion, abduction, and eversion, which brought the flexed thigh and knee down to the mattress on their outer side. The knee was then tied to the bedstead in this position with a towel, and the foot secured to the knee of the sound side until the socket should be excavated by absorption. In two weeks she was allowed to sit up, and in two weeks more was discharged, well.[1]

In the following case of dorsal dislocation of the hip of six weeks' standing, after reduction a muscle was subcutaneously divided.

The patient while driving a railroad hand-car was thrown upon the track in front of it, the car passing over his body. On examination under ether, the head of the femur was felt "near the sciatic notch." After the thigh was flexed and rotated to break up the old adhesions, the dislocation was reduced by flexion, abduction, and extension. Eight days after this operation the bone had again slipped out; and at that time I first saw the patient, and made the following record in the Hospital books (vol. cxxxii., August, 1867):

"In the recumbent position the limb is flexed at an angle of about 40°, shortened the length of the patella, but not inverted. The trochanter is very prominent, the head of the femur being movable upon the dorsum. The dislocation is dorsal, but without inversion. The knee cannot be depressed without raising the loins. The patient, when erect, can bear about ten pounds' weight on the limb, which can be brought down by the side of the other, if the pelvis be laterally tilted to make up for the shortening, and thrown out behind to compensate the flexion. The buttock is flattened and widened, as in hip disease. The feet can be everted equally, each to an angle of about 45°."

At the close of the above examination, the bone was brought into the socket by flexion, abduction, and vertical extension, though it easily slipped out of place. The next day, as the record states, "the limb is found to be less flexed, and the head of the bone is in the socket. There is still, however, a

[1] Massachusetts General Hospital, Surgical Records, May, 1868 (vol. cxxxiii).

widening and flattening of the nates on the affected side, showing that the thigh is displaced laterally, as if the socket were partially occluded, although engaging the head of the femur, while the knee is still raised about four inches above its fellow, the tensor vaginæ femoris being quite tense. The knee can be depressed, but is flexed by some elastic force, rising again." Under these circumstances, it was decided to divide the last-named muscle subcutaneously, near the anterior superior spinous process, which, when done, allowed a considerable though not complete extension of the thigh. The limb was now brought nearly straight, and placed in a Desault's splint until the socket should be excavated by absorption. This extension was continued until September 8, when the patient began to sit up; on the 13th he was moving about on crutches, and on the 23d he left the Hospital, there being no lengthening of the leg, and only some atrophy of the muscles of the thigh. That the luxation was unequivocal in this case is attested by the presence of the head of the bone upon the dorsum, — the femur being flexed, although the foot was straight. If the bones were sound, this absence of inversion would indicate rupture of the outer fasciculus of the Y ligament. But the marked lateral displacement, resulting from the inability of the bone fairly to enter its socket, even when placed and held there, implies some anomaly, — either the callus of fracture, the remains of capsule, or the presence of cicatricial tissue, partially occluding the socket.

A little girl three and a half years old entered the Massachusetts General Hospital with unequivocal signs of dorsal dislocation of twelve days' standing. I flexed and abducted the limb, rotating it outward, and after some little effort, by pressing the head of the bone toward the socket, between the fingers applied to the superior spinous process and the thumb upon the trochanter, succeeded in reducing it.

DORSAL BELOW THE TENDON.

It has been before remarked that when the flexion method is universally adopted it will be practically needless to classify separately the dorsal luxations. Their varying relation to the small rotator muscles has, however, been already shown, and the strength of one of these muscles may entitle it to separate consideration.

The dislocation hitherto distinguished as "upon the ischiatic notch," and unnecessarily associated with it, is characterized by Sir Astley Cooper as differing from the dorsal displacement chiefly in producing less shortening of the limb. I believe that no dislocation upon the ischiatic notch is worthy of the name; that no satisfactory or practical result can be based upon this distinction alone; and that it is also an error to suppose that during reduction the femur ever notably "slips into the sciatic notch,"[1] or that the sciatic notch ever offers any obstacle to its reduction. A little more or less shortening and a varying degree of inversion depend both on the position occupied by the head of the femur upon the dorsum and on the degree of laceration of the capsule. In cases of this variety which have been recorded the signs were intrinsically the same, and reduction, if by pulleys, was usually effected in one and the same way, — unless we seek an exception to this statement in a slight variation of the angle of traction, quite as likely to occur in one case as another, and even to vary much in different attempts upon the same patient.

But there is one remarkable feature in some of the recorded instances of "ischiatic" dislocation. They were erroneously supposed to have been "irreducible." Sir Astley Cooper says

[1] See, for a recent statement of this erroneous notion, Holmes's "Surgery" (vol. ii. p. 644): "That in our attempts to reduce a dislocation upward [*on the dorsum*] the head of the bone may slip into the sciatic notch, there is abundant evidence."

"the reduction of this dislocation is in general extremely difficult;"[1] and this has thrown a shadow of uncertainty over a large number of other cases, where the observer, being persuaded that the reduction was more difficult than usual, or the limb less shortened, has taken it for granted that the head of the bone was engaged in the sciatic notch and forcibly detained there, but which were in reality simple dorsal dislocations.

In view of these facts, I propose to separate the dorsal dislocations into two varieties, of some practical importance in relation to their reduction. The first has already been considered. The second includes only those cases in which the head of the femur is engaged behind the internal obturator tendon and the capsule lying beneath it, and which sometimes absolutely require the flexion method for their reduction. This is also a secondary dislocation, in which the bone, by a movement of more or less inversion, reaches its final position behind the tendon after occupying one below it, and is doubtless of frequent occurrence, as this is the point at which the luxations below the socket are first arrested in their ascent upon the dorsum. I have ventured to call it, for simplicity, *dorsal below the tendon*, because, although the head of the femur lies behind the tendon, as it does in dislocation between the rotators, it is below it also, and not above it, as then happens (see p. 42).

The following are classical examples of this accident.

The first is from Sir Astley Cooper.

"Case XLIII. A boy sixteen years old had a dislocation of the thigh into the foramen ovale; he was placed upon his sound side, and an extension of the superior part of his thigh was made perpendicularly; the surgeon then pressed down the knee, but the thigh being at that moment advanced, the head of the bone was thrown backward, and passed into the ischiatic notch, from which situation it could not be reduced."

[1] Treatise, etc., p. 73.

It was probably this case that led Sir Astley to enjoin "great care," in reducing the thyroid luxation, "not to advance the leg in any considerable degree, otherwise the head of the thigh-bone will be forced behind the acetabulum into the ischiatic notch, from whence it cannot afterward be reduced; this accident," he says, "I once saw happen."[1] In other words, by flexing the thigh the Y ligament was relaxed, and the head of the bone was allowed to descend below the socket,[2] where there was an equal chance whether, in again extending the limb, the head would return inward to the thyroid foramen, or slip outward upon the dorsum behind the obturator tendon, as actually happened.

A second is from Malgaigne.[3]

A laborer, thirty-eight years of age, had dislocated his hip backward. The next day Lisfranc, with eight assistants, endeavored to reduce it by straight extension. At the end of an hour their efforts were abandoned, the patient being in a state of collapse. He died on the eleventh day of suppurative inflammation of the hip, resulting doubtless from the operation. At the autopsy the bone was found to lie behind obturator tendon, and was easily reduced by flexion.[4]

1 Treatise, etc., p. 63.

2 This movement is identical with that elsewhere described in connection with the three downward luxations. A similar result of relaxing the Y ligament by flexing the thigh occurred in a case of Verneuil, whose patient dislocated his hip a second time, fifteen days after the original accident, by suddenly rising to a sitting posture. The same thing happened also to a patient of Malgaigne ("Traité," etc., p. 840), and is not uncommon.

3 Traité, etc., Pl. XXVI.

4 For two autopsies of this dislocation see the cases of M. Bidard (Malgaigne, "Traité," etc., p. 835). In both these cases, of which the second seems to have been a more complete luxation than the first, the obturator internus was intact. In Queen's case, the sciatic nerve was engaged upon the neck of the femur (Medico-Chirurgical Transactions, 1868, vol. xxxi. p. 338). For a case in which the head of the bone had escaped just below the socket, and was arrested there on its way toward

SIGNS.

The distinctive signs of this dislocation, dorsal below the tendon, may be thus stated.

the obturator tendon, see Ollivier's "Archives Générales de Médecine," 1823, tom. iii. p. 545; also Lenoir, quoted by Malgaigne ("Traité," etc., p. 873).

In an interesting case, reported with its autopsy by Thomas Wormald (London Medical Gazette, 1837, vol. xix. p. 657), the dislocated limb was shortened and inverted, forming about half a right angle with the body, while the shaft of the femur, crossing the symphysis pubis, was fixed immovably in this situation. The head of the femur had escaped above the quadratus, through a rent of the capsule opposite the upper part of the tuber ischii, compressing the sciatic nerve, and had plunged beneath the obturator externus muscle so as to engage this muscle upon its anterior face. The obturator internus was completely ruptured; the pyriformis and gemelli were partially so; also the gluteus medius and minimus at their posterior edge. In this case the head of the bone, escaping between the two muscles, had passed forward beneath the external obturator, instead of retreating backward behind the tendon of the internal obturator. The luxation probably occurred when the limb was flexed and extremely inverted, to which position may also be referred the rupture of the obturator internus muscle. By depressing the knee the head of the bone would have been carried upward and backward, and the laceration so extended that reduction would have been easy. If the flexed knee had been circumducted outward, the external obturator muscle would have been partially ruptured; and this lesion probably occurs when the head of the bone is carried from the dorsum to the thyroid foramen, or *vice versa*. The regular thyroid luxation, however, occurs above this muscle, the upper edge of which only need then be ruptured. The external obturator and much of the quadratus are torn in the common dorsal dislocation.

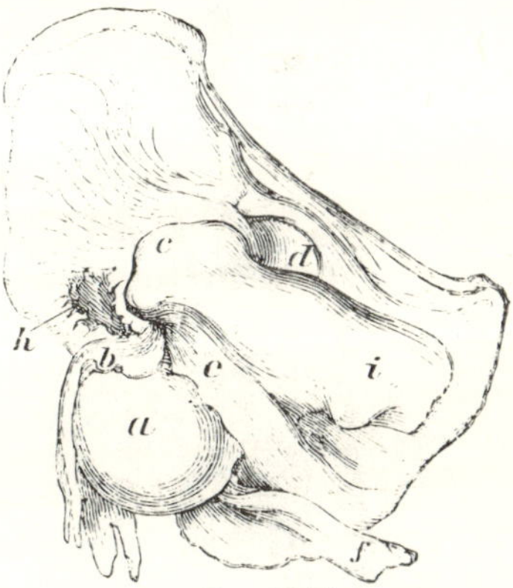

FIG. 10.[a]

[a] Wormald's case. Copied from the London Medical Gazette, 1837. The head of the bone, *a*, is seen engaged beneath *e*, the obturator externus muscle; *f*, sciatic nerve; *b*, obturator internus. *c*, *i*, trochanters; *d*, socket; *h*, gluteus.

The limb is extremely inverted. It crosses the opposite thigh, even as high as the middle of it, although in the

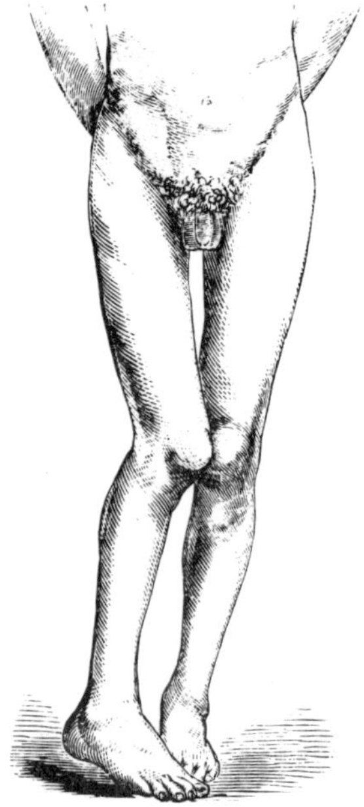

Fig. 11.[1]

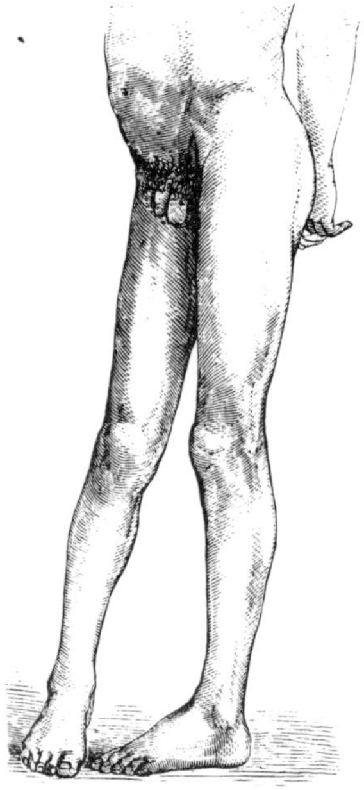

Fig. 12[2]

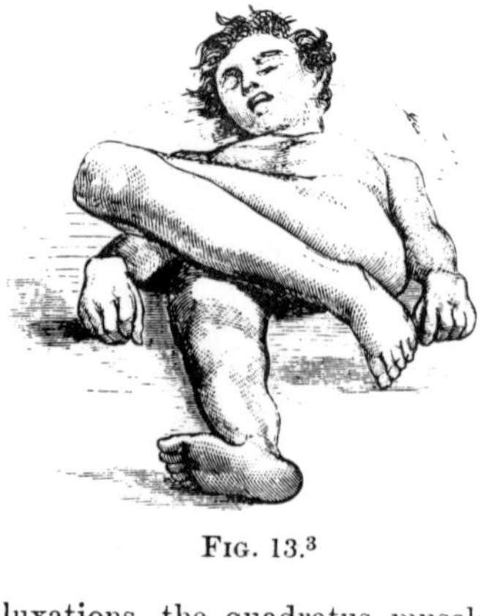

Fig. 13.[3]

[1] Dislocation below the tendon. The inversion is here seen to be greater than in the common dorsal luxation, and would be still further exaggerated in the recumbent position.

[2] Profile view of the same, showing the leg advanced.

[3] Dislocation downward and outward toward the tuberosity. This may be considered a first step to luxation behind the tendon, which it inclines to become when the patient is upright. The limb may occupy any interval between these two luxations, the quadratus muscle readily yielding. (See Fig. 10.)

upright position it may gravitate to a lower point. It is considerably in advance of the sound limb. By manipulation the capsular and muscular fibres may be so relaxed or torn that this dislocation may be made to resemble one higher up on the dorsum, or be actually converted into one by rupture of the obturator muscle.

THE MECHANISM OF ITS PRODUCTION, AND CAUSE OF ITS IRREDUCIBILITY.

In this luxation the bone first escapes below the socket, or on its thyroid aspect, when the thigh is flexed, as it generally is. The limb being extended by subsequent violence, while the neck of the bone is unyieldingly suspended beneath the socket by the Y ligament, the head slips upward, not only behind the acetabulum, but also behind the capsule and the internal obturator muscle. The fibres of the latter, instead of lying transversely behind the head, as when in place (Fig. 14), now lie obliquely in front of it, — a tendinous wall, interposed between it and the acetabulum (Fig. 15).[1]

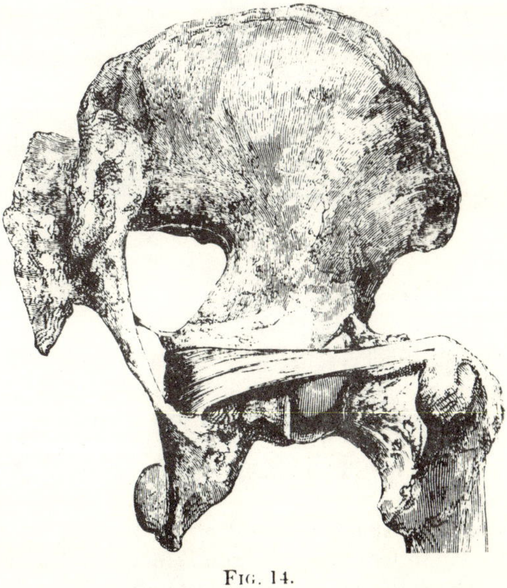

FIG. 14.

[1] A case of dislocation behind the tendon, with fracture of the socket, exhibited much the same signs: the right leg was two inches shorter than

The difficulty of reducing this luxation by extension in the axis of the body will be readily understood. In the absence of both posterior capsule and internal obturator muscle, the head of the bone might be slipped forward over the lower margin of the socket by rotation outward, after the pulleys had sufficiently elongated or detached the Y ligament, especially if the pulleys were then relaxed and the thigh flexed a little. But as the obturator tendon

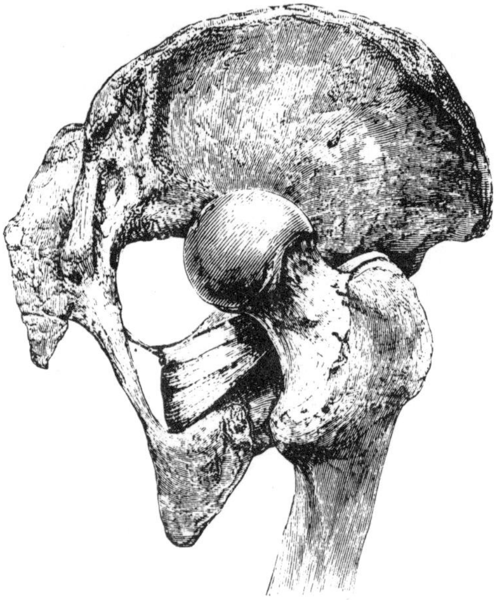

FIG. 15.[1]

the left, the knee and foot turned inward. An autopsy showed the posterior part of the acetabulum broken off, and the neck of the bone tightly embraced by the tendon of the obturator internus and the gemelli. (See Cooper's "Treatise," etc., Case LXXI. p. 113.)

[1] Figs. 14 and 15, — the mechanism of the dorsal dislocation below the tendon.

Fig. 14 shows the head of the bone in its socket, with the obturator tendon in its natural position behind it. The part of the capsule which lies beneath the tendon and behind the Y ligament has been slit, both to demonstrate its thickness and to allow the head of the bone to rise as high as the ischiatic notch.

Fig. 15 shows the head of the bone dislocated below the tendon into the neighborhood of the sciatic notch. If the tendon were not present, the capsule would produce much the same effect in binding the head of the bone close upon the ilium, without the interposition of the muscle.

and its subjacent capsule now lie between the head of the bone and the socket, they oppose the entrance of the head by a firm tendinous wall, which is drawn down as the head descends, and which no extension or rotation, short of its rupture, can displace or overcome.

The muscle is tense, and in its turn renders the ligament more tense, carrying the head of the bone backward and upward toward the ischiatic notch. The inversion, flexion, and adduction of the limb are thus augmented by the combined and reciprocal action of the ligament and the obturator muscle, — the latter being aided by the subjacent capsule, when that remains untorn.[1]

[1] It has been before said that if the neck of the femur be farther driven upward so as to rupture the obturator tendon and capsule, the luxation will become simply dorsal. Malgaigne correctly says that "the ischiatic luxation leads frequently to the iliac luxation;" but he fails to identify the mechanism of the change when he asks, "May not the former also be consecutive to the latter, in view of the fact that by flexion or strong traction the head of the bone may be drawn downward from the dorsum to the notch?" ("Traité," etc., p. 831.) In the high dorsal dislocation the small rotators would be so lacerated by the ascent of the bone or by drawing it down to reduce it, when engaged in their interstices, that the luxation "on the ischiatic notch" would lose its distinctive features. In an interesting discussion upon a pathological specimen of hip luxation of five months' standing, where an unsuccessful attempt had been made to reduce the bone by longitudinal traction, M. Tillaux maintained that "in backward luxation of the hip the capsule, and not the muscles [notably the obturator], limits the movement of the head of the femur." (Société Impériale de Chirurgie, 1er Juillet, 1868. L'Union Médicale, No. 79, p. 57.) It is true (see pp. 2, 63) that the obturator tendon and the posterior part of the capsule, which is next in strength to the Y ligament, mutually reinforce each other, so that when the head of the bone rises behind the socket it is generally engaged behind both these fibrous walls. But their mechanical action being identical, it is unnecessary to decide which under these circumstances would first be ruptured. The capsule yields fibre by fibre to the ascending bone, while the comparative elasticity of the tendinous muscle preserves it (Fig. 15), until at the moment of the final rupture of the tendon the dislocation has become practically iliac, and can now be reduced, though disadvantage-

REDUCTION.

The reduction is simple.[1] The head of the bone, having reached its present position by circumduction of the flexed limb inward, must be reduced by circumduction of the extended limb inward. When the thigh is raised perpendicularly to the floor, the head of the bone is unlocked and lies below the socket, and needs only to be jerked upward into its place; or the suspended pelvis may be depressed, or the thigh abducted and rotated outward, as in the common dorsal dislocation.[2] The laceration of the capsule is probably already sufficient, and will not need to be enlarged. It will be observed

ously, with pulleys, by straight traction through the slit thus made behind the capsule. It may be safely asserted, first, that the tendon is usually present in these cases of the iliac luxation by inversion, unless the bone has risen so high upon the dorsum that the posterior capsule also has been ruptured; and, secondly, that the tendon resists longest, and best characterizes the luxation.

[1] Mr. Nunneley, in the paper before quoted, expresses the contrary belief, that in this luxation reduction by manipulation will be more difficult, and will more frequently fail, than in any other form of dislocation to which the hip is liable.

[2] M. Lisfranc readily reduced a luxation "upon the sciatic notch" by the method of Després, twelve days after the accident. The pelvis being fixed, "he adducted the limb, at the same time flexing the thigh and leg; placing his fore-arm under the ham, and with his right hand grasping the ankle in order to use the leg as a lever, he instantaneously reduced the luxation by extension, outward rotation, and abduction."

For this case, which embraces the principles of flexion, abduction, outward rotation of the thigh, and the upward lift, see "Observations sur Luxations," etc., M. Malespine, Archives Générales de Médecine, Paris, 1839. See also Bulletin de la Société Anatomique, 1835, p. 4, and 1836, pp. 45, 169.

Mr. Travers (London Medical Gazette, Nov. 22, 1828) relates a case of dislocation "upon the ischiatic notch," of six months' standing, which was reduced by pulleys, but in which the bone slipped out again while the thigh was flexed in bed during the night, — the obvious result of relaxation of the Y ligament. In subsequent unsuccessful efforts at reduction, the neck of the bone was fractured.

that by the flexion method this luxation and that upon the dorsum are reduced in the same way, and with equal facility.

I have had but two opportunities of satisfactorily identifying this dislocation in the living subject. The usual extended position of the luxated limb so endangers the obturator that its condition must often be a matter of uncertainty, although this luxation cannot be uncommon compared with that higher up on the dorsum.

In the first case alluded to, which did not occur in my own practice, the patient (a middle-aged female) had fallen down stairs, and the limb had thus been subjected to a variety of forces. It was flexed, greatly inverted, and so advanced and adducted across the middle of the other thigh that I did not hesitate to recognize it at sight as a dislocation behind the obturator tendon; and yet it is possible that the bone may have been thrust between the rotators. With a view to its reduction, the limb was flexed, and a variety of movements were communicated to it, during which the bone slipped below the socket, — a change of position accompanied by a sharp report, probably due to the rupture of some fibrous band, or possibly the tendon of a rotator muscle.[1] It was afterward lifted into its socket.

The following case admits of no doubt. While correcting these sheets, I was called to the Hospital to see a middle-aged man who had three hours before been struck upon the hip by a bale of hay. Having fallen over on his left side, the bale dropped from the story above, striking upon his right femur below the trochanter a little in front, dislocating it outward and downward. He said that two physicians had unsuccessfully tried for an hour, with ether, to reduce it. He was in pain, sitting up in bed, the luxated thigh greatly inverted, and flexed so that it crossed the sound limb near the groin. (See Fig. 13.) After he was etherized and laid flat, the dislocated

[1] In the dead subject the muscular fibres yield noiselessly.

thigh, when drawn down, crossed the other at the junction of the middle and lower third, but still with great and firm inversion. This position of the bone, in connection with the facility of its reduction and the manner of the accident, indicated that the head, suspended at the trochanter by the Y ligament, was prevented from rising on the dorsum so as to permit the descent of the knee, by some obstacle, which could be no other than the obturator tendon and the subjacent capsule, stretched across its neck; also that the luxation was secondary, the bone having escaped below the socket before rising behind the tendon. After etherization, the knee came down somewhat, as the head rose behind the tendon. The hip was reduced by flexion, abduction, and eversion, with a slight upward jerk, at the first effort, and in three seconds from the moment the limb was grasped for flexion.

THYROID AND DOWNWARD DISLOCATIONS.

1. Obliquely inward and downward on the thyroid foramen.
2. Obliquely inward and downward as far as the perinæum.
3. Vertically downward below the acetabulum.
4. Obliquely outward and downward as far as the tuberosity.

These dislocations, if we except that upon the thyroid foramen, are comparatively rare. In view of the frequency of accidents dislocating the bone while flexed or abducted, this rarity may be explained by the readiness with which the extreme downward luxations are converted into those upon the thyroid foramen or the dorsum.

THYROID.

The bone escaping obliquely downward and inward beneath the socket by a laceration of the inner side of the capsule, where it is thin and membranous, tends to follow the inclined plane of the pelvis toward the thyroid foramen, where it finds a lodgement.[1]

SIGNS.

The limb is unequivocally flexed and abducted, the heel being raised from the floor, and the toe pointing outward and

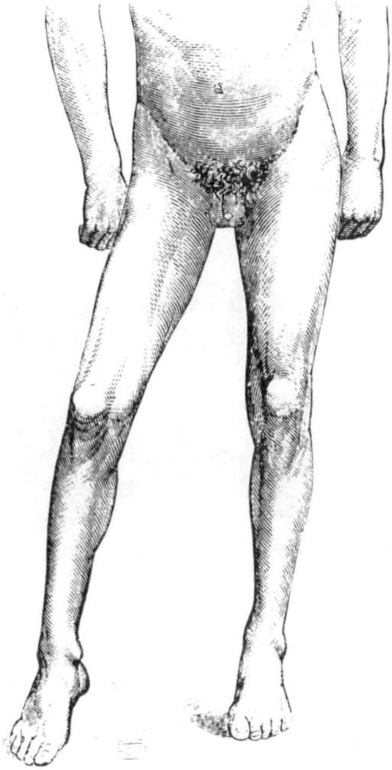

FIG. 16.[2]

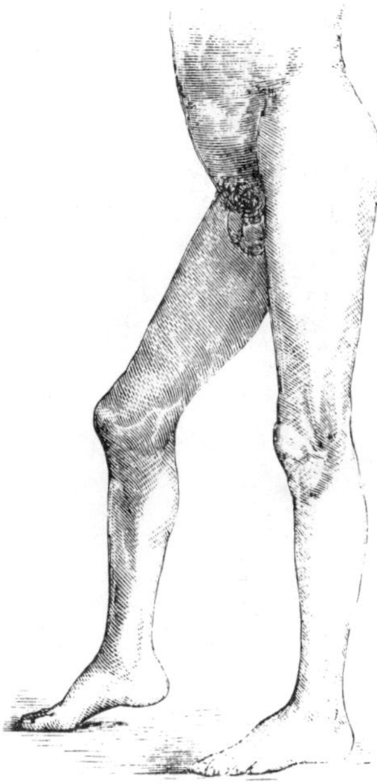

FIG. 17.

forward. The trochanters being arrested and suspended by the Y ligament, while the head of the bone descends from the socket, the thigh is flexed to an angle of about 35° and also abducted, until the great trochanter, by swinging outward,

[1] For a case of thyroid dislocation occurring in a child six months old, see Lancet, May 16, 1868.

[2] Thyroid dislocation. — Fig. 16 showing the front view, Fig. 17 the side view, and Fig. 18 the back view of the leg. The limb is seen advanced, abducted, and a little everted.

gets a bearing on the acetabulum, and the adductor muscles become tense. The head of the femur likewise rests upon the pelvis (enabling the patient sometimes to walk tolerably well), and is hindered from rising toward the pubes, and even from

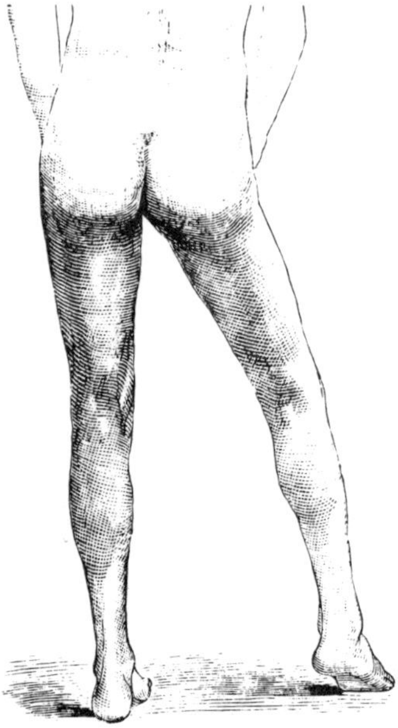

Fig. 18.

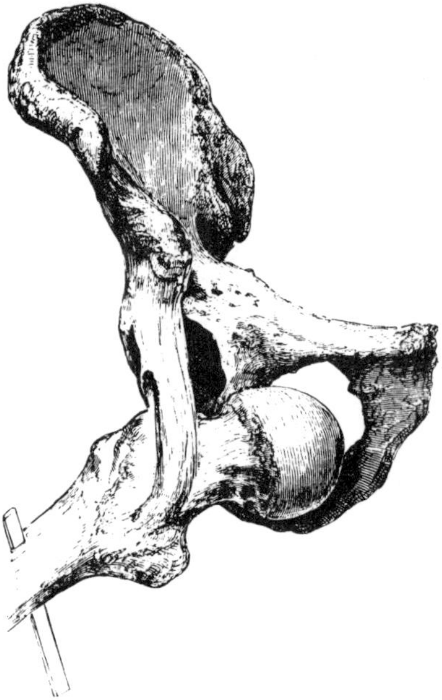

Fig. 19.[1]

re-entering the socket, by the inner margin of the acetabulum, the falciform edge of the lacerated capsule above, perhaps, contributing its resistance.[2]

[1] The mechanism of the thyroid dislocation, showing the Y ligament suspending the trochanters, while the head of the bone is lodged in the thyroid foramen, the trochanter resting on the acetabulum. (From a photograph taken in 1861.)

[2] In a case of M. J. Roux, the head of the bone had passed the thyroid foramen and reached the ischium; the leg was elongated, slightly flexed, and inclined outward. The thigh could be flexed, adducted, and abducted, but not extended. After unsuccessful traction, the luxation was reduced by flexion. (Revue Médico-Chirurgicale, tom. iv. p. 364.)

The internal obturator muscle is not necessarily broken even in the complete dislocation. That part of the capsule which is attached near the ilio-pectineal eminence may assist the Y ligament in suspending the limb, the thigh becoming in all cases more flexed when forcibly inverted. If the inner branch of the Y be ruptured, the bone is suspended by the great trochanter, and the eversion is diminished. Although it might be supposed that the extended psoas and iliacus muscles are concerned in the flexion, yet after the Y ligament is divided the tense fibres of these muscles produce a less degree either of flexion or eversion, and can be broken by depressing the knee. The long muscles of the anterior part of the thigh also become somewhat tense, and the head of the bone tends to escape toward the perinæum.

VERTICAL DOWNWARD LUXATION.

Escaping directly downward, the head of the bone may remain upon the lower margin of the socket, — the limb exhibiting less eversion than in the thyroid dislocation, but the luxation being practically of the same general character, provided the Y ligament be not ruptured. In Gurney's first case[1] the eversion was slight; the flexion moderate, but if carried beyond the sitting posture, painful; the knee lengthened by about an inch, standing and sitting; the foot capable of rotation inward and outward; and the limb able to support the weight of the body in walking, the patient having walked two hundred yards on the day of the accident and a mile six days after. In a second similar case the patient could walk; the foot could be rotated outward and inward freely, but the limb could not be flexed to the sitting posture; the head of the bone was felt behind and below the acetabu-

[1] See two interesting cases of dislocation of the thigh downward, by Edwin Gurney, Esq., Surgeon, Camborne, Cornwall. Lancet, 1845, vol. iii. p. 112.

lum. In these cases the bone obviously had a firm bearing below the acetabulum, which while it was capable of supporting the weight of the body in walking allowed rotation upon its convex surface. Flexion may have been hindered by the elongated extensors.

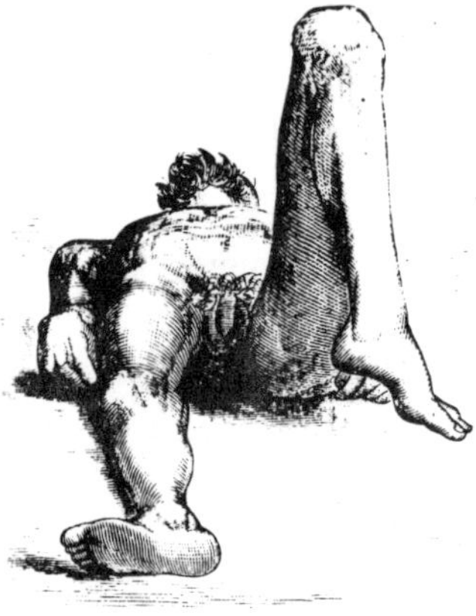

FIG. 20.[1]

Hippocrates probably refers to a case of this sort (and not, as has been supposed, to luxation on the ischiatic notch) when he speaks of "the leg and foot appearing pretty straight, and not much inclined toward either side; . . . the sole of the foot on its own line, and not inclined outward." Of the limb he says: "It becomes much shorter, and the patient can hardly reach the ground with the ball of his foot, — and not even thus, unless he bend himself at the groins, and also bend with the other leg at the ham; or, if resting upon the foot, the hips protrude backward far beyond the line of the foot." With a crutch the patient "will walk indeed more erect, but will not be able to reach the ground with the foot; or if he wish to rest upon the foot, he must take a shorter staff, and will require to bend the body at the groins."[2] This description indicates great flexion of the limb without inversion or eversion; and if it applies to a recent luxation, and not to an old one where the foot has been straightened by time, or unless we suppose the lesion here described to be the result of old hip disease, — an hypothesis which can hardly

[1] Dislocation downward. The bone has descended toward the tuberosity, the flexion of the thigh being proportionate to the descent of the bone.

[2] Hippocrates, "Genuine Works," etc., art. 71.

be considered possible in view of the practical experience of the writer, — these signs are compatible only with dislocation beneath the socket.

DISLOCATIONS NEAR THE TUBEROSITY OR PERINÆUM.[1]

When the thigh is thus strongly flexed, it is easy to imagine that the head of the femur, suspended by the Y ligament beneath the lower margin of the socket, pauses there, hesitating between the thyroid and the dorsal luxations. It has been found at various points in the interval

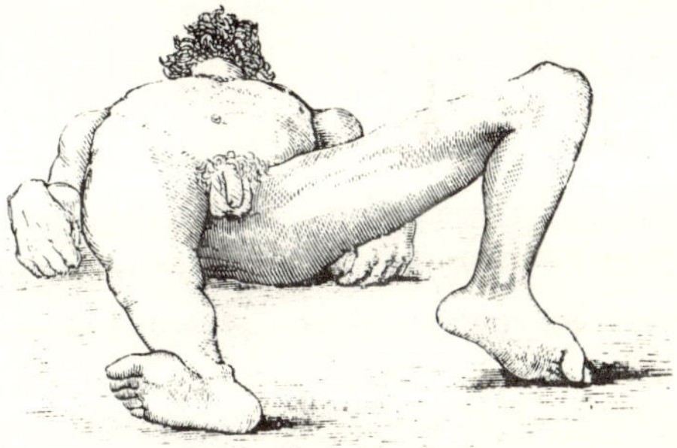

FIG. 21.[2]

[1] For a case of dislocation near the tuberosity, see Cooper's "Treatise," Case LXX. The limb was "considerably shortened and inverted," forming half a right angle with the body, — the shaft of the femur crossing the symphysis, and being fixed there. At the autopsy the head was found on the tuberosity; the obturator internus was ruptured, and the ischium and ilio-pubic symphysis were broken, — complications which would not, however, necessarily modify the character of this dislocation.

For a case of perineal luxation, with autopsy, see Transactions of the London Pathological Society, vol. x. p. 211. The thigh was much flexed and abducted, any attempt to adduct or depress it being met by resistance and pain. The head was felt in the perinæum. Reduction was effected by drawing the thigh vertically down from the pelvis, with lateral extension by a towel, aided by the knee of the operator in the groin. The capsular ligament was extensively detached, so that the head of the femur easily protruded. The "ilio-femoral ligament was detached at its outside, and partially separated from the neck of the femur; and a small rent extended from that point into the capsular ligament." Flexion here was doubtless due to the remaining inner band of the Y ligament.

[2] Dislocation downward and inward toward the perinæum. As in the other regular downward luxations, the flexion is proportionate to the descent of the head of the bone.

between these luxations, and directed into the one or the other in attempts to reduce it. In extreme flexion the head may reach as far as the tuberosity on one side and the ascending ramus of the ischium, and even the perinæum, on the other. In short, in the dead subject the ligament permits the head of the bone to descend until the edge of its articular surface sweeps the centre of the tuberosity and the ascending ramus of the ischium. When found in these positions in the living subject, — so far as may be inferred from the reported cases, — the ligament was not ruptured. Such being the position of the head of the femur in the dislocations with extreme flexion, the knee would occupy the extremity of the opposite spoke in an imaginary wheel of which the Y ligament should be the centre. The signs obviously vary with the position of the bone, the limb being always flexed[1] in proportion to the downward displacement of the head of the femur and the length of the ligament, — inverted when the femoral head is directed to the outside of the socket, and everted when it inclines to its inner aspect. If the head of the bone inclines a little to the inside, resting near the groove of the external obturator tendon, the limb is a little abducted, elongated, and rotated outward, this being a first advance toward the thyroid foramen. If the head of the bone rests a little

[1] In some of the reported cases of downward dislocation where the head was felt near the tuberosity, it is impossible not to recognize the fact that the flexion of the thigh was less than it should have been if the Y ligament was sound, — as it was in the case of Stanski, for example (see *note*, p. 73). Such a case is that of Bouisson, where the head was on a level with the tuberosity, and the thigh is said to have been but slightly flexed (Gazette Médicale, 1853, p. 664). The ligament may have been here ruptured in whole or in part, and if so the dislocation was irregular. On the contrary, in a fatal case reported by Mr. Luke (Medical Times and Gazette, vol. xvi. p. 12), the flexion of the leg is not alluded to, although the limb was lengthened one inch without inversion or eversion, and at the autopsy the head of the bone was found just below the acetabulum, and *the capsule was lacerated only below*. If so, the limb must have been flexed.

outside and behind the axis of the acetabulum, the rotation of the limb inclines proportionately inward, this being a step toward dislocation behind the tendon (Fig. 13), into which this luxation may be easily converted by depressing the knee. If the head of the bone is thrust down near the tuberosity, the limb is in extreme flexion, with perhaps adduction. If it is forced inward upon the perinæum, we naturally find also, with extreme abduction, the thigh standing out at right angles with the body;[1] and as there is no firm bearing for the trochanter in the perinæum, as in the thyroid foramen, the toes may be inverted or everted.[2]

[1] The following case of perineal luxation is reported by Willard Parker, in the New York Journal of Medicine, March, 1852, p. 188. A man was standing beneath a canal boat, his legs apart, and received the weight of the falling boat upon his back. The left leg and thigh were found extended at a right angle with the body, and a little inverted; while the head of the femur could be felt in the perinæum behind the scrotum. Extension outward and downward carried the head of the bone into the thyroid foramen, whence it was reduced by carrying the femur across its fellow.

A similar accident happened to Pope's patient (Ibid., p. 198), upon whom a bank of earth fell while he was standing under it with his legs widely spread. The thigh was found to be at right angles with the body, inclined a little forward, the head of the bone projecting beneath the skin in the perinæum. Reduction was effected by lateral extension applied with pulleys to the upper part of the thigh, the leg being used as a lever.

The case of Amblard (quoted by Malgaigne, "Traité," etc., p. 876) was attended with a good deal of local pain, and with retention of urine. The lesion was caused by a fall from a cart upon the leg, which is supposed to have been already luxated by some twist before the patient reached the ground. The thigh was spread at a right angle to the body, with a little outward rotation. To reduce it, the leg was drawn downward and outward, and the head of the bone lifted outward with a towel. The head entered its socket by the way of the foramen ovale.

The case of Amblard showed eversion, while that of Parker exhibited inversion.

[2] The annexed woodcut (Fig. 22) represents the specimen of Stanski (Bulletin de la Société Anatomique, 1837, p. 296), and is taken from Malgaigne ("Traité," etc., Pl. XXVII., Figs. 4 and 5), whose description is more complete than that of Stanski. It shows the anchylosed bones in a

The obvious affinity and resemblance between these downward luxations, of which the thyroid is frequent and the others

luxation of long standing, occasioned by the falling of a bank of earth upon a man while stooping. Although the dislocation is classed as thyroid by both these writers, the great flexion of the femur indicates that the head of the bone had passed downward and inward near the tuberosity, while the Y ligament remained entire, — "a mass of bony stalactites, which seem to prolong the inferior iliac spine downward to join the internal face of the femur, to which they adhere to the extent of four centimetres, bending round its anterior face, and even behind it, to join the great trochanter" (Malgaigne), being, if we may judge from the figure, the tense and anchylosed Y ligament, beautifully illustrating this form of luxation. (Compare with Figs. 19 and 20.) Or it may have been that in this case the external ligamentary band was broken, producing greater eversion and more flexion. I have examined only Malgaigne's lithograph of this specimen, in which the origin of the bony plate from the inferior spinous process is so clearly given that, if correctly represented, there can be little doubt of its real character. Yet it is proper to say that M. Houel alludes to it as a part of the tendon of the psoas muscle ("Manuel d'Anatomie Pathologique," etc., par Ch. Houel, Professeur Agrégé, etc., Paris, 1862, p. 231).

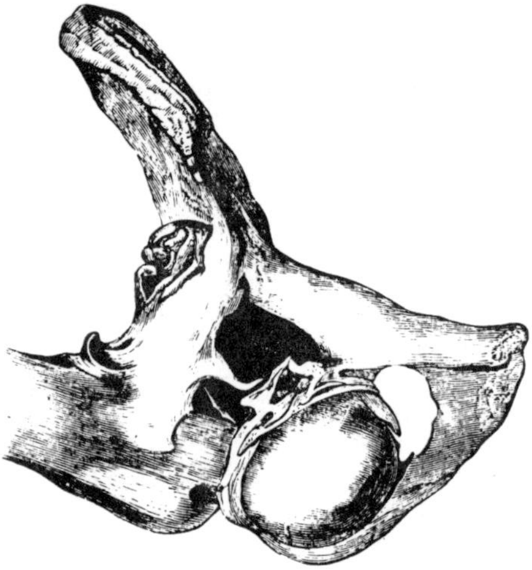

Fig. 22.

See also the case of Keate (London Medical Gazette, vol. x., p. 19). The accident happened to a gentleman, who while riding fell into a ditch, his horse falling upon him and widely separating his legs. The limb was three and a half inches longer than its fellow, "much flexed," with very great abduction and eversion. The head of the bone was close to the tuberosity, and freely movable. It was reduced by the way of the foramen ovale, — the route of the luxation, as stated by the patient. This case may have been "irregular," because the operator was able to elonrare, need not be urged. The bone is suspended by the Y ligament, and when the head is displaced to one side of the socket the limb passes to the other; or if the head is arrested directly beneath the cotyloid cavity, the limb is in simple flexion, — the position of the limb thus indicating that of the head of the bone, which can then generally be felt, sometimes very distinctly, as in the perinæum.

In the downward dislocations, if the inner fasciculus of the Y ligament is ruptured, the head of the bone is inclined downward by an inward rotation of the limb still suspended at the outer trochanter, — the head of the femur being then comparatively lower and the limb less flexed than if the inner fasciculus were unbroken. Such a state of the parts might exhibit the head of the bone in the neighborhood of the tuberosity without excessive flexion, but the limb would be greatly inverted.

REDUCTION.

The thyroid dislocation is usually not difficult of reduction; but the following methods will illustrate the variety of expedients to which the surgeon may have recourse, — it being remembered that the rent of the capsule, which is here thin, may be enlarged at discretion by circumduction of the flexed thigh inward.

1. *Rotation.* — Flex the limb toward a perpendicular, and abduct it a little to disengage the head of the bone; then rotate the thigh strongly inward, adducting it, and carrying the knee to the floor. The trochanter is then fixed by the Y ligament and the obturator muscle, which serve as a fulcrum. While these are wound up and shortened by rotation, the descending knee pries the head upward and outward to the socket. As in reducing the secondary pubic dislocation, the

gate or pull down the limb after reduction, — a circumstance which he attributed to a supposed fracture of the socket.

last half of this manœuvre is an inward circumduction of the flexed limb accompanied with rotation, and is practically the reverse of the flexion, abduction, and eversion by which a dorsal dislocation is reduced from the opposite side of the socket. In this manœuvre the action of the ligament may be aided, if necessary, by a towel passed round the upper part of the thigh, to draw the head of the femur upward and outward. Rotation outward may be substituted for inward rotation.[2]

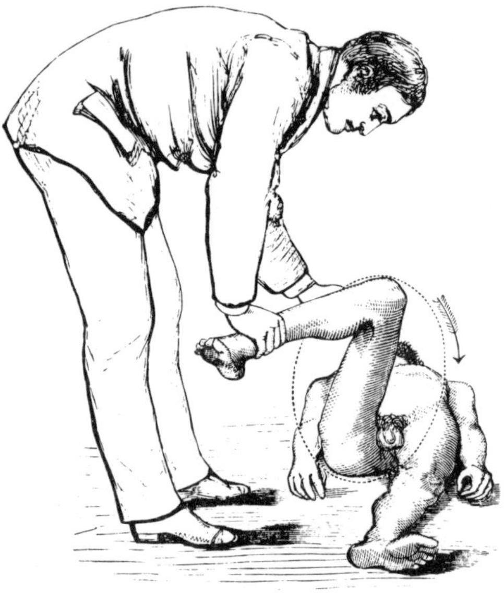

FIG. 23.[1]

[1] The surgeon is here represented in the act of rotating and circumducting the flexed thigh inward.

[2] In the paper already quoted, Dr. Markoe cites the two following cases of thyroid luxation reduced by rotation: —

(Case 8) Dr. Buck here reduced the bone by inward rotation, after two failures. In the third and successful attempt, the thigh was brought down from entire flexion to a little below a right angle, and again rotated inward, when the head of the bone slipped into its place.

(Case 9) Markoe, in imitating Buck's method by rotation inward, unintentionally carried the head of the bone round the socket to the sciatic notch, from which position it was returned to the foramen ovale, and reduced by rotation *outward*, the knee being at the same time strongly adducted toward and behind its fellow.

These cases are instructive, as showing that the head of the bone is directed toward the socket when the Y ligament is wound upon the shaft by rotation, *whether inward or outward;* and they correspond to the

2. *Traction.* — Flex the limb toward the abdomen, and draw the thigh outward by a towel passed round the upper part; or thrust it outward by applying the foot to the inside of the groin.[1]

3. Flex the thigh upward and outward, and drag or jerk it in that direction toward the socket. (Fig. 25.)

4. Lay the patient on his belly on the edge of a table, the injured thigh hanging, and the

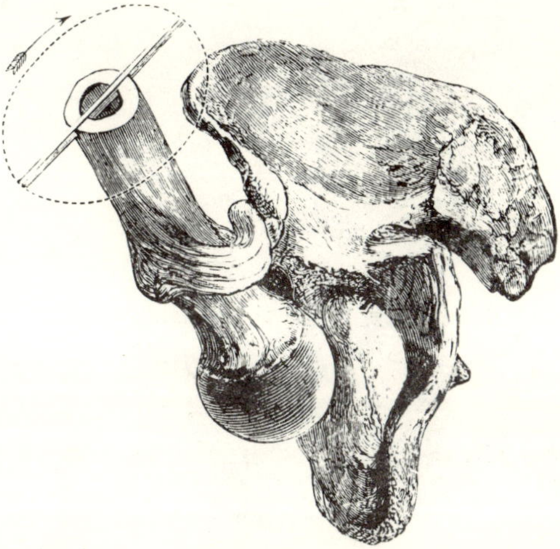

Fig. 24.[2]

results of my own experiments, made before I had read the report of these cases. In the first case, the operator in finally placing the thigh a little below a right angle tightened the ligament and directed the head upward, while at the same time a passage was left for the head of the bone between the trochanter and the socket. In the second, the surgeon, starting the limb at right angles, relaxed the ligament, engaged the head at its lowest point beneath the socket, and carried it by inward circumduction to the ischiatic notch. Had the thigh been now again placed in a vertical position it could have been jerked up into the socket. It was, however, returned to the thyroid foramen, and reduced by outward rotation. In these cases, the head entered the socket while the knee was being depressed obliquely inward. It may be superfluous to say that in Markoe's case inward rotation would probably have reduced the bone had the thigh been less flexed, or the manipulation been aided by oblique or vertical traction with a towel round the thigh at its upper part.

[1] In reducing a dislocation of this sort, flexion with lateral traction was successfully employed by M. Vertu. (P. A. Vertu, Thèse, No. 116, Archives Générales de Médecine, 1836, p. 379.)

[2] The mechanism of the manœuvre shown in Fig. 23 is here seen. The inner branch of the Y ligament being wound round the neck, the head must rise toward the socket as the femur is depressed inward.

leg bent to relax the flexors; then draw the head of the femur outward with the aid of a towel.

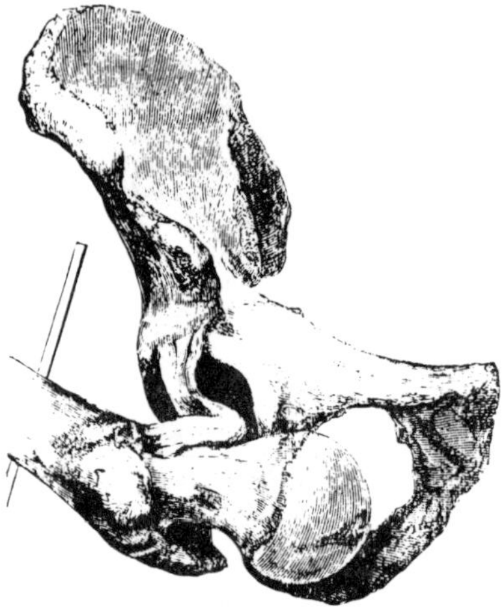

FIG. 25.[2]

5. Place him in a sitting posture, with a log or post or bedpost between his thighs, and pry the head outward over this fulcrum by means of the shaft of the femur as a lever.[1]

6. Let him lie on a table, the limb flexed as usual. Then let an assistant, turning his back to the patient, carry the flexed knee over his own shoulder, grasping the foot, and endeavoring thus to lift the pelvis, while the surgeon draws the thigh outward by a towel in the groin.

7. Let the surgeon, facing the patient, place the flexed limb upon his shoulder, and embracing the thigh near the pelvis, lift and direct the head of the bone toward the socket.[3]

[1] In illustration of the flexion method, see Cooper ("Treatise," etc., Case XLVI.) Eight hours after a thyroid dislocation, attempts were made to reduce it by traction in the usual way, and were continued unsuccessfully until late at night, when, the pulleys breaking, further proceedings were deferred until the next day. The patient, having then taken two doses of tartar emetic, was carried into the operating theatre at 2 P. M. Attempts at reduction were again made, and powerful extension employed for upward of an hour without success. The tartar emetic was repeated in large doses, and the man, becoming faint, was placed in a *sitting posture*. Extension was then made, and after a short time the head of the bone slipped into the acetabulum.

[2] Thyroid dislocation. Reduction by traction. The limb is flexed, abducted, and everted, relaxing completely the Y ligament. (From a photograph taken in 1861.)

[3] Method of Larrey. (See Malgaigne's "Traité," etc., pp. 853–855.)

8. Let the capsular orifice be enlarged by a little circumduction of the flexed thigh inward, as if to convert the thyroid into a dorsal luxation; and let the pelvis, suspended by the limb, be then depressed by the foot of the surgeon, while the thigh is drawn outward, if necessary, with a towel.

9. Convert the thyroid into a dorsal luxation, and proceed accordingly.

10. Most of these manœuvres may be executed while the patient lies on his sound side, if counter-extension be applied as a substitute for the weight of the body.

To reduce the other varieties of downward luxation, the femur should be flexed and its head drawn and guided toward the socket, — during which manœuvre these dislocations are sometimes converted into that upon the thyroid foramen, or upon the dorsum below the tendon.

For the dislocation downward we may employ vertical traction, rotating the femur a little inward to disengage the head; for the dislocation downward and outward, traction upward and inward, with abduction and rotation outward if required to tilt the head; for the dislocation downward and inward, traction upward and outward. In these three injuries the femur is of course to be kept flexed, its head drawn and guided toward the socket by local pressure, or lifted with a towel if necessary, with rotation outward, and abduction when the bone is directly below or outside the socket, and with circumduction at discretion when required to enlarge the capsular opening.

See also the methods, 6, 7, and 8.

DISLOCATION UPON THE PUBES, AND BELOW THE ANTERIOR INFERIOR SPINE OF THE ILIUM. (SUB-SPINOUS.)

DISLOCATION UPON THE PUBES.

In this dislocation the head of the bone is felt upon the pubes; the limb is a little shortened and everted, abducted

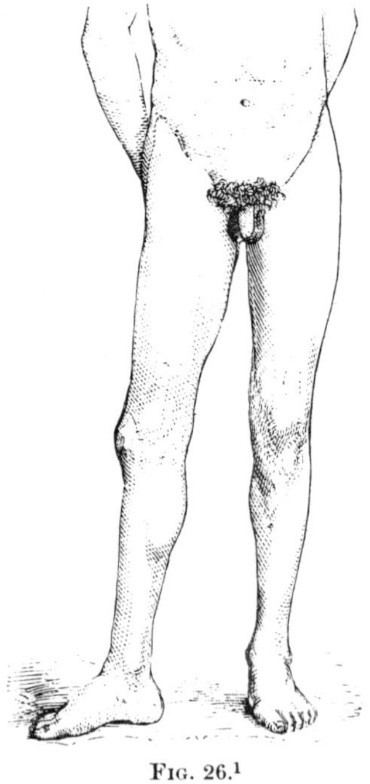

FIG. 26.[1]

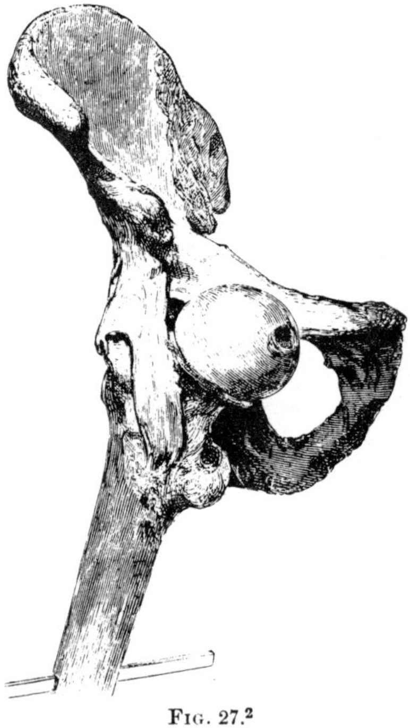

FIG. 27.[2]

and advanced. A laceration of the inner aspect of the capsule allows the bone to escape obliquely upward, to a point

[1] Pubic dislocation. The foot is everted, the thigh advanced and abducted.

[2] Pubic dislocation. The head of the bone is seen in the groin, suspended by the Y ligament. (From a photograph taken in 1861.)

upon the pubes distant in proportion to the violence of the force displacing it.[1]

Complete pubic dislocation is impossible unless the capsule beneath the obturator internus is ruptured,[2] after which this muscle everts the limb until the trochanter bears upon the pelvis. If this muscle is ruptured, the psoas and iliacus, binding the neck of the bone to the pubes, may produce a degree of eversion; but the principal agent of eversion even then is the Y ligament, which also embraces the neck. The untorn capsular fibres and the obturator muscle are agents in preventing flexion, their insertions being lower than the head of the displaced bone, which then becomes a fulcrum, the lever in flexion being the shaft; but in pubic dislocation nearer to the iliac spine, the obturator is not tense, and flexion is then probably hindered by the outer and inferior parts of the capsule, when they still exist. Both the muscle and the capsule act in preventing inversion. Dislocation to the neighborhood of the symphysis implies a rupture of the inner branch of the Y ligament.[3]

1 Larrey is said to have seen a case of pubic dislocation in which the femur was flexed at nearly a right angle with the body. (Hamilton, "Practical Treatise," etc., p. 655.) It is fair to suppose that it could have been brought down to the usual position.

2 In an autopsy of a case of pubic dislocation, recorded in a paper by Mr. Bransby Cooper (Guy's Hospital Reports, 1836, vol. i., p. 82), the gemini and quadratus femoris had suffered from laceration and subsequent ulceration, implicating all the outward rotators of the thigh.

3 A careful autopsy of pubic luxation is recorded in a communication of M. Aubry, read by M. Maisonneuve, to the Société de Chirurgie (Archives Générales de Médecine, Paris, 1853, p. 355). The head of the bone projected in the groin; the limb was rotated outward with flexion, a little abduction, and shortening to the extent of one quarter of an inch. The autopsy showed the psoas and the crural nerve upon the anterior surface of the neck. Half the anterior circumference of the capsule was torn at a quarter of an inch from its cotyloid insertion, the neck of the femur being held in a sort of button-hole between its fibrous edge and the cotyloid rim. Flexion of the thigh obviously relaxed this fibrous band, liberating the neck; extension produced the contrary effect, strangulat-

DISLOCATION BELOW THE ANTERIOR INFERIOR SPINE OF THE ILIUM, OR SUB-SPINOUS.

The head of the bone ranges along the pubes, displaced according to the violence and direction of the injury. If thrust

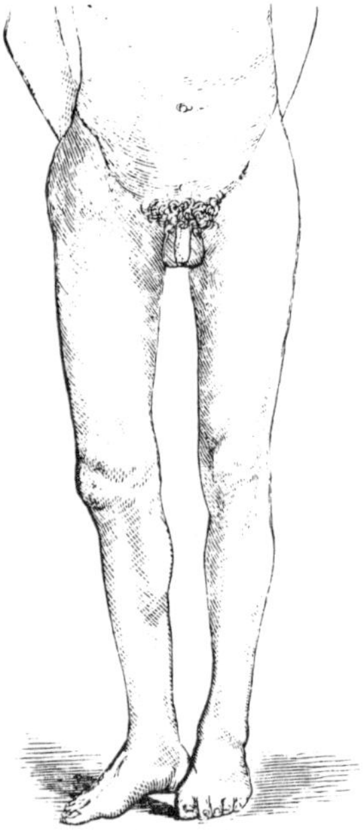

FIG. 28.[1]

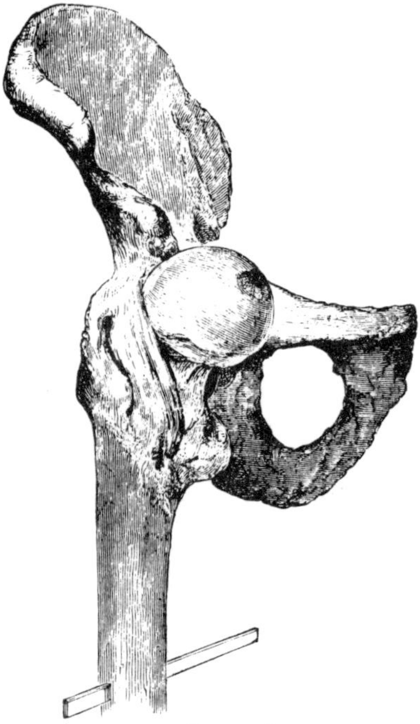

FIG. 29.[2]

directly upward, the bone may lie beneath the Y ligament and the inferior iliac spine; but this displacement requires that

ing the neck. Of the muscles, the external obturator was relaxed; the pyriformis, internal obturator, and gemelli appeared elongated.

1 Pubic dislocation nearer the spine. The limb is here seen everted, but is usually a little more advanced and abducted. Nélaton, however, describes a similar absence of flexion ("Clinical Lectures on Surgery by M. Nélaton," from Notes taken by W. F. Atlee, M.D., Phila., 1855, p. 213).

2 Sub-spinous dislocation. The neck of the bone is seen lying beneath the Y ligament, which is tightly stretched across it. (From a photograph taken in 1861.)

the upper part of the capsule should be completely detached from the edge of the socket. The firm bearing of the neck against the Y ligament may then explain how the patient has in some recorded cases been able to walk immediately after this accident.[1] The limb is still everted, but less abducted or advanced, and the head of the bone is plainly felt in its new position, — in the absence of which evidence the shortening and eversion might possibly be mistaken for fracture of the neck.[2]

When the bone has been thus displaced, the psoas and iliacus tendon is sometimes thrown off the neck of the femur toward the pubes where it then lies slack. But even when in place, the action of this tendon is wholly secondary to that of the Y ligament in producing either flexion or eversion, as may be shown by its division, after which the position of the dislocated bone

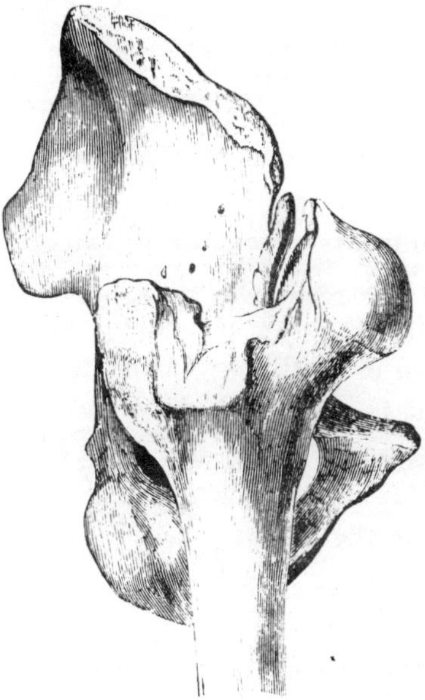

FIG. 30.[3]

[1] See Malgaigne's "Traité," etc., pp. 844, 845.

[2] The above figure (Fig. 30) from Malgaigne ("Traité," etc., Pl. XXVII. Fig. 1) represents a specimen elaborately described by M. Gely (Bulletin de la Société Anatomique, 1840, p. 303). The accident occurred to an insane person, a long time before death. The neck of the bone rides upon the inferior spine, and the leg is much everted. This eversion may perhaps be referred to pathological changes, but may have occurred at the time of the accident. Gely rightly supposes the weight of the body to have been supported by the upper part of the capsule, reinforced by the tendon of the rectus muscle (Bulletin, pp. 320, 327).

[3] Sub-spinous dislocation.

remains unchanged; while if the Y ligament be divided without the tendon, the bone drops to a position near the thyroid foramen, with little flexion, — an attitude of the limb resembling the irregular dislocation toward the perinæum or on the tuberosity.[1]

REDUCTION.

I have never met with pubic dislocation in the living subject, and am therefore unable to speak of the extent of a difficulty in flexion alluded to by some writers as characteristic of this luxation. But there is ample evidence that this difficulty is neither insuperable nor constant. The pubic dislocation has often been reduced by flexing the limb; and if the obturator tendon and its subjacent capsule resist flexion in the living as in the dead subject, the limb needs only to be drawn down toward the socket while in the act of being flexed.

If the bone has been thrust upward between the Y ligament and the pubo-femoral band, and the capsular orifice be small, this band may be ruptured by circumduction or even rotation of the flexed thigh inward. But well-marked pubic dislocation usually implies a rupture of the capsule which extends to its inner and lower aspects. (See p. 81.)

It is difficult to reduce the pubic dislocation by straight extension, and various accidents have happened in attempting it.

[1] If the head of the bone be still further displaced outward, it lies beneath the inferior spinous process, as in the case of Wormald (London Medical Gazette, January, 1837, p. 164), where the limb being somewhat everted, abducted a little, and shortened half an inch, the new cavity was formed in part by the upper portion of the cotyloid ligament. The patient, who died twenty-six years after the accident, was said to be able to walk well, being "engaged in carrying out beer for a publican in Portugal Street," — a statement which Malgaigne oddly translates, "*pour porter un mort au cimetière*" ("Traité," etc., p. 871).

The reduction may be accomplished in a variety of ways, among which are the following, combining angular traction and rotation.

1. *By Traction and Rotation.* — Flex the limb to a right angle, while drawing it down; rotate either inward or outward, and directing the head of the bone by its shaft, rock it downward into its place.[1]

[1] Two cases of pubic dislocation skilfully reduced by manipulation are reported by Dr. E. J. Fountain, of Davenport, Iowa, in the New York Journal of Medicine, etc., January, 1856, p. 69. In the first case, the patient was laid upon the floor on a quilt, made insensible with chloroform, and the limb was rotated outward. The leg was then flexed and carried across the opposite knee and thigh, the heel kept well up and the knee pressed down. This motion was continued by carrying the thigh over the sound one as high as the upper part of the middle third, the foot being kept firmly elevated; then the limb was carried directly upward by raising the knee, which was gently oscillated, when the head of the bone dropped into its socket. The time of this operation was from twenty to thirty seconds, and the force slight. In a second case, rotation and flexion produced greater pain, and the limb was less movable. Here also the knee and foot were rotated outward, the leg then flexed across the sound thigh, the heel kept up and the knee pressed down. The whole was carried in this position across the sound thigh directly upward to the flexed position, the operator holding the foot firmly up and making oscillations with the knee, when the head of the bone slipped into the socket. About twenty seconds sufficed for the operation, which was performed without the use of chloroform.

It will be observed in these cases that no real difficulty was encountered in flexion. The limb was flexed, and the vertical femur, rotated outward, was rocked down into its place. The outward rotation of the flexed femur made the outer branch of the Y ligament tense, with an interval through which the head of the bone, already rotated to a point just above the socket, descended into it. Perhaps, as Dr. Fountain recommends, the whole manœuvre should be commenced with an outward rotation, to be maintained till the reduction is accomplished; but it seems to me that this rotation is unnecessary until after the limb is flexed.

Devilliers and Aubry each reduced a pubic dislocation by flexion and rotation inward instead of outward, and Larrey by simple downward pressure at the groin, with the knee over his shoulder (Malgaigne, "Traité," etc., pp. 853, 854).

2. While extending the limb horizontally, with counter-extension by the foot in the perinæum, raise the patient to a sitting posture, counter-extend against the pubes, and rotate inward.

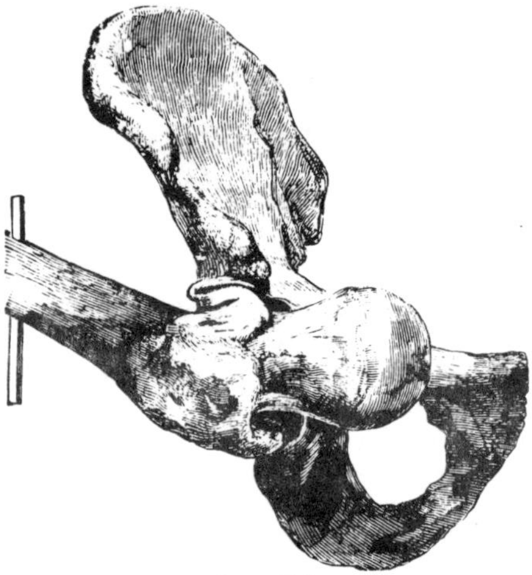

FIG. 31.[1]

3. The same method may be pursued, the patient lying on his belly on the edge of a table, or on his sound side.

4. See Reduction of the Thyroid Dislocation, Nos. 7 and 8.

5. Flex and abduct the limb and draw it outward, at the same time pressing the head downward and outward.

By Rotation. — Reduction by rotation is to be accomplished by much the same method as in the thyroid dislocation, except that in the pubic luxation the flexed limb should be carried across the sound thigh at a higher point. First, semi-flex the thigh to relax the Y ligament, at the same time drawing the head of the bone down from the pubes. Then semi-abduct and rotate inward, to disengage the bone completely. Lastly, while rotating inward and still drawing on the thigh, carry the knee inward and downward to its place by the side of its fellow. As in the thyroid luxation, this manœuvre guides the head of the bone to its socket by

[1] Pubic dislocation. Reduction by traction. The limb has been here flexed and abducted, for reduction by traction and local pressure. The abduction is represented as greater than necessary. (From a photograph taken in 1861.)

a rotation which winds up and shortens the ligament, enabling the operator, by depressing the knee, to pry the head of the bone into its place.

Briefly, while drawing upon the thigh, flex and abduct it to disengage the head; then rotate inward, and when the bone leaves the pubes, continue the rotation while straightening the limb; or circumduct the bent limb inward.[1]

Aid these manœuvres by drawing the flexed groin outward with a towel, or otherwise depressing it.[2]

If by these combined movements of traction, leverage, and rotation — of which the Y ligament and the obturator tendon, when it is unbroken, are the centre — the luxation is not reduced, it will perhaps be converted into one near the thyroid foramen, the rules for the reduction of which will then apply here.[3]

ANTERIOR OBLIQUE DISLOCATION.

The remaining luxations imply a free laceration of the tissues about the joint, and sometimes of a part of the Y ligament itself.

[1] See case of Dr. J. M. Irvine (British-American Journal, March, 1861, p. 282). A complete pubic dislocation of the right hip was reduced by flexing the thigh upon the pelvis, carrying the knee over the umbilicus to the left side of the body, and thence to a state of extension, when the head slipped in.

[2] Baron Larrey has reported a case of dislocation in front of the horizontal portion of the pubes, which he reduced by suddenly raising with his shoulder the lower extremity of the femur, while with both hands he pressed the head of the bone downward. (Hamilton, "Practical Treatise," etc., p. 657, and London Medico-Chirurgical Review, December, 1820, p. 500).

[3] Mr. Annandale, after some unsuccessful manipulation, succeeded by flexion in reducing a pubic dislocation of three days' standing, but used pulleys to withdraw the head of the bone from the pubes by outward extension. (Thomas Annandale, F. R. S. E., etc., Assistant Surgeon of the Royal Infirmary; Edinburgh Medical Journal, 1867, p. 997.)

In a common dorsal dislocation, let the leg be carried across the symphysis, so that the outer and convex surface of the

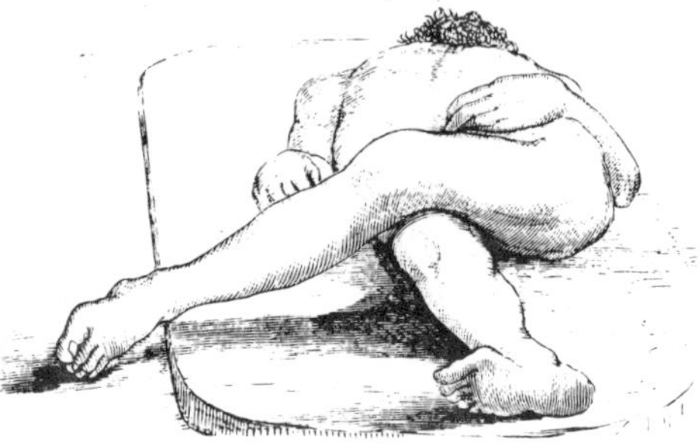

FIG. 32.[1]

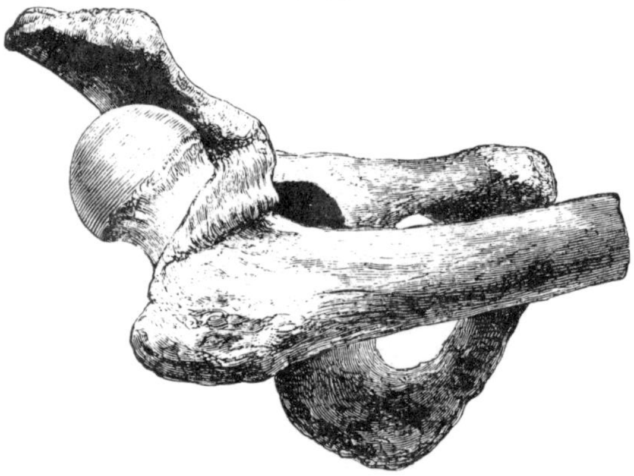

FIG. 33.[2]

[1] Figs. 32, 33, 34, — anterior oblique dislocation. The limb is here extremely everted, crossing the other above the knee. The general anatomical character of the luxation is seen in Fig. 33, where the Y ligament is still entire, the limb crossing the other high up. As the limb descends toward a perpendicular the outer fibres of the ligament yield, until, as it reaches the position seen in Fig. 37, only the inner fasciculus remains. The head of the bone is then hooked over this inner fasciculus, as seen in the dotted line (Fig. 37), and the supra-spinous luxation is complete. If now thrust back upon the dorsum, the dislocation is simply the everted dorsal, as shown in Fig. 40, where, however, the toes may be inverted at will.

[2] Anterior oblique luxation. By depressing the shaft of the femur the head rises over the inferior spinous process, as the external part of the ligament yields.

socket shall correspond to the hollow beneath the neck of the femur. With some force the thigh can now be everted, and afterward brought down across the upper part of its fellow. It is here firmly locked, with great shortening and some eversion, the limb facing forward and obliquely crossing the opposite thigh, while the toe points outward, — a position not wholly ungraceful, and suggesting some attitudes in dancing. (Figs. 32 and 33.)[1]

If in this position it is desired to bring the limb toward a perpendicular, the outer branch of the Y ligament must be ruptured. Thus liberated, it hangs suspended by the inner ligament, and becomes capable of lateral motion and of rotation; and this is probably the condition under which supraspinous luxation, although rare, usually occurs. (Fig. 35.)

The anterior oblique dislocation may be reduced by inward circumduction of the extended limb across the symphysis, with a little eversion, if necessary, to disengage the head of the

[1] For a description of the annexed woodcut, taken from Cooper, and which exhibits the position of the anterior oblique luxation, see case of Oldknow (Guy's Hospital Reports, No. 1, p. 97), also Cooper ("Treatise,' etc., Case LXVII.). The foot is said to have been very much everted, only the toes touching the ground. But the patient had lived twelve years after the accident, and something may be allowed for pathological changes. For a larger figure representing this dislocation, see a paper of Bransby Cooper, Guy's Hospital Reports, 1836, vol. i. p. 81.

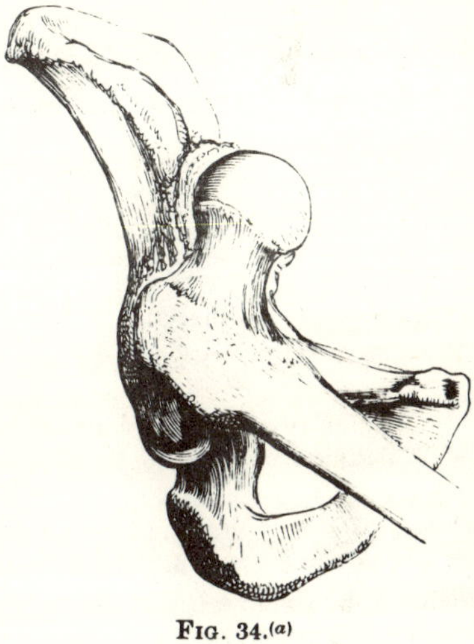

FIG. 34.[(a)]

[(a)] Anterior oblique luxation.

bone. Inward rotation then converts this into the common luxation upon the dorsum.

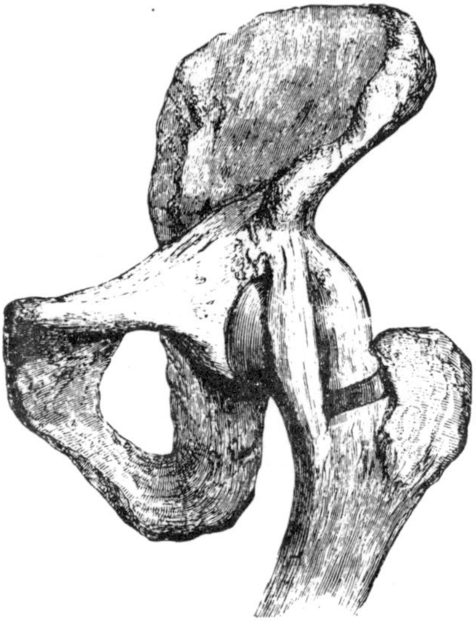

FIG. 35.[1]

DISLOCATIONS IN WHICH THE OUTER BRANCH OF THE Y LIGAMENT IS BROKEN.

SUPRA-SPINOUS DISLOCATION.[2]

THE head of the bone has been found above the inferior spinous process, the neck lying across the edge of the pelvis, the trochanter turned back, and — as is said — not readily discovered. The limb was shortened two or three inches, a

[1] This figure is intended to show in diagram the external portion of the Y ligament detached, as in the supra-spinous and everted dorsal luxations.

[2] See case of Cummins (Guy's Hospital Reports, vol. iii.). Cooper ("Treatise," etc., Case LXV.) cites this case as anomalous, illustrating it with a figure which represents the head of the bone as projecting farther upon the abdomen than the context indicates. The leg was shortened three inches, and could not be drawn down. The limb, which

little abducted, and everted, — this eversion being sometimes so great that the toes pointed backward, although in one of

was much everted, could not be rotated inward. Cooper considers this to be "a variety of dislocation hitherto unknown."

Travers (Medico-Chirurgical Transactions, vol. xx. p. 113) thus describes a case: "The trochanter is felt below and to the outer side of the anterior superior spinous process of the ilium. The neck of the bone lies apparently between the two anterior spinous processes, so that when the patient is erect the limb seems as it were slung or suspended from this point."

Sir Astley Cooper ("Treatise," etc., Case LXII.) cites a case of old dislocation "on the pubes." An accurate account of the autopsy, with the annexed figure, is given by N. Cadge, F. R. C. S., Norwich (Medico-Chirurgical Transactions, vol. xxxviii. p. 88). The left leg was full an inch and a half shorter than the right; the toes were turned outward; and while the body lay on its back the foot rested completely on the outer border. A large, globular, bony tumor was felt in the groin, close to the superior spine of the ilium. On dissection, the head of the femur was found in the interval between the anterior superior and anterior inferior spinous processes of the ilium. The head of the femur was covered with a complete bony cap, lined with a dense, pearly-white tissue, resembling fibro-cartilage (Fig. 36). The edge of the new cavity was connected with the neck of the thigh-bone by a thick capsular ligament. The rectus muscle, which had been torn from its origin, was inserted into the edge of the new cavity, — a condition that suggests the ascent of the bone above the inferior spinous process of the ilium at the time of the injury, with rupture of the Y ligament. This luxation may have been supra-spinous or irregular.

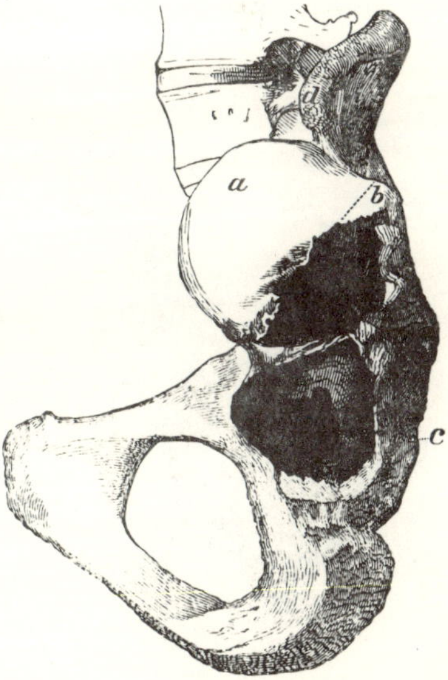

FIG. 36.[a]

[a] Supra-spinous dislocation. *a*, bony cap; *b*, fractured margin of ditto; *c*, socket; *d*, superior spinous process of ilium.

the cases related by Cooper they could be brought forward again to the side of the other foot. Another important feature was that the shortened limb could not be drawn down.

In this luxation the neck was doubtless hooked over the Y, and perhaps over the tendon of the rectus muscle also; so that direct extension, short of the rupture of this ligament, was worse than useless. The head of the bone had been thrust above and outside the Y ligament, upon which in its return the neck of the femur had engaged itself, the main

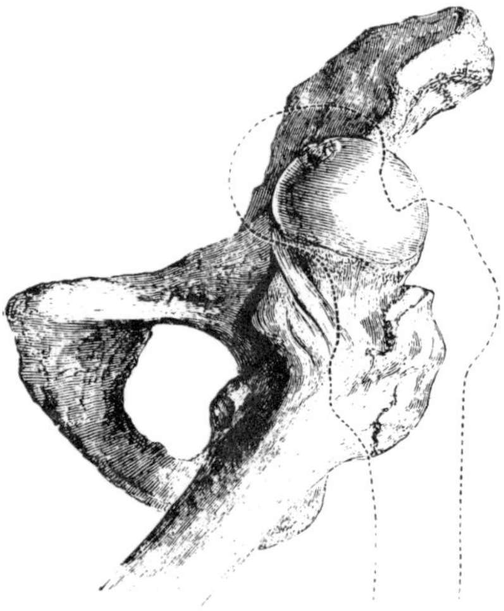

Fig. 37.[1]

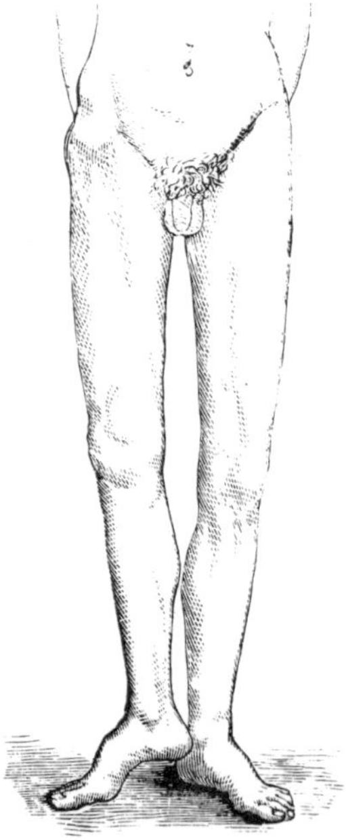

Fig. 38.

branch of the Y then lying behind the neck, and so wound around it as to produce great shortening.

In the supra-spinous luxations eversion is due to the internal obturator, when it remains entire, but also to the tense ligament.

[1] Figs. 37 and 38, — supra-spinous dislocation. (See *note*, p. 88.)

The muscles inserted into the back of the trochanter, especially the obturator internus, hinder the head of the bone from advancing upon the spinous process; but when they are divided, the head advances toward the abdomen. The first degree of supra-spinous luxation, which is represented in the woodcut (Fig. 37), requires the rupture of only the outer fibres of the Y ligament, and is but a slight exaggeration of the anterior oblique luxation (Fig. 33). But when the bone projects fairly upon the abdomen (as illustrated by the dotted line, Fig. 37), only the inner fasciculus remains.

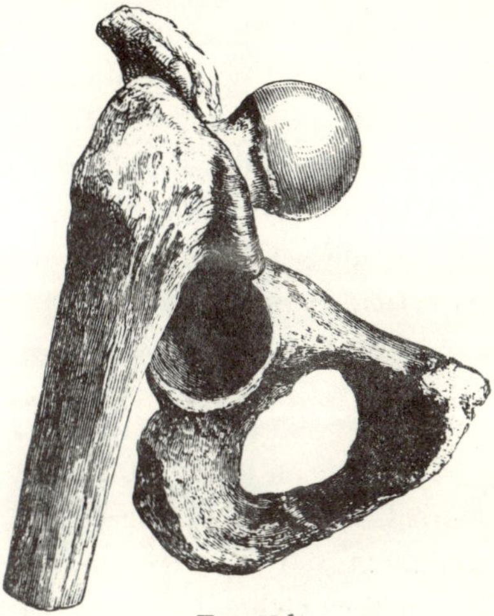

FIG. 39.[1]

It may be remarked that the anterior oblique dislocation, while it is also supra-spinous, differs from it in the comparative soundness of the ligament, which compels the limb to assume an oblique position. In the latter luxation the outer band is broken, and the limb is more movable; the term " supra-spinous " has been reserved for this, as probably the more common of these two rare varieties.

[1] This woodcut is intended to show the possibility of a posterior oblique luxation, the Y ligament being entire, the head of the bone thrust across it, and the shaft locked behind the tuberosity. In the dissected bones it will be found that the femur is firmly locked, the limb being directed backward, and the foot somewhat everted. But there is no authority, so far as I am aware, to show that such a position of the leg has been found in the living subject. By forcibly advancing the knee the outer branch of the ligament is ruptured, and the luxation then becomes supra-spinous.

REDUCTION.

After extension by pulleys in the axis of the body has failed, reduction of this luxation has been accomplished by extension downward and outward, with some manipulation of the head of the bone and probably with rupture of the ligament. It is obviously a better plan to unhook the neck by circumduction of the extended limb inward, with eversion enough to disengage it from the edge of the pelvis. The head then lies upon the dorsum, and if the outer branch of the Y is broken, is not inverted. The reduction may then be accomplished as usual in the dorsal dislocation, although rotation would be less effectual than if the ligament were entire.[1]

EVERTED DORSAL DISLOCATION.

It has been before stated that inversion of the limb in the dorsal luxations is due to the tense outer branch of the Y ligament. When the injury has been such as to rupture these fibres, the limb may still be inverted; but it can also be freely everted. Having escaped from the socket under

[1] The following case well illustrates the mechanism of the supra-spinous luxation, and is taken from Hamilton ("Practical Treatise," etc., p. 649): "Lente relates a case [of ischiatic luxation] under the care of Dr. Hoffman, in the New York City Hospital, in which, when the extension was suddenly relaxed by cutting the cord, and the thigh at the same instant was abducted and rotated outward, the head of the femur left the ischiatic notch and rose upon the dorsum ilii, assuming a position directly above the acetabulum and below the anterior superior spinous process, from which position it was with great difficulty subsequently returned to the socket."

If this luxation was really "ischiatic," as stated, and therefore "below the tendon," the forcible outward rotation of the thigh ruptured both the tendon and the outer part of the Y ligament, or in any case the latter; after which the head of the bone was free to turn forward and rise on the ilium toward the spine, the limb being of course everted, and the head of the bone perhaps engaged above the remaining ligament.

these circumstances, the bone may occupy any point upon the dorsum within the range of the inner fasciculus. The limb is then shortened in proportion to its upward displacement, the foot being sometimes everted a little, sometimes lying flat upon the bed, or even directed backward, the head of the femur facing accordingly, and — as has been elsewhere remarked — in the direction of its internal condyle. The femur is suspended midway between the inner branch of the Y and the obturator tendon. Theoretically it may be luxated either below or above this tendon; but in the former case the degree and nature of the force required to break the outer band would be likely to rupture the tendon also. If the head of the femur is driven upward and backward above the obturator tendon, the same forced eversion which would sever the inner branch of the Y ligament would relax this tendon, and so contribute to prevent its rupture. The tendon may then lend its aid in giving position to the limb.[2]

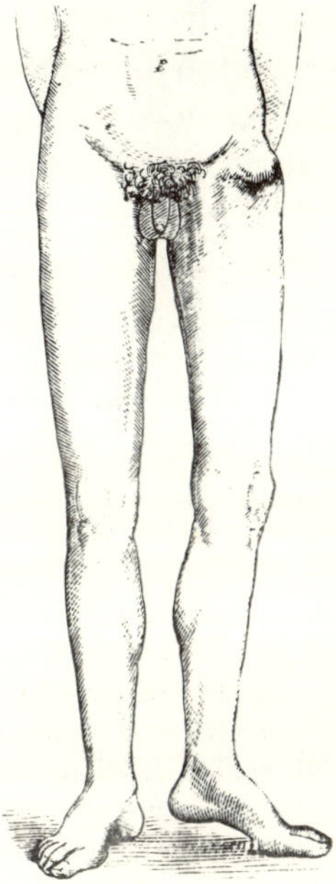

FIG. 40.[1]

[1] Everted dorsal dislocation. (See *note*, p. 88.)

[2] For an old case of this sort, with an analysis of the muscular action, see a paper by Dr. Gordon in the Dublin Hospital Gazette, Nov. 1, 1845, p. 87.

Mr G. R. Symes has described a case ("On an Unusual Form of Dislocation of the Hip Joint," by Glasscut R. Symes, one of the Surgeons of Stevens's Hospital, Dublin Quarterly Journal of Medical Science, 1864, vol. xxxviii.) in which the right leg was shortened two inches, the foot extremely everted, the buttock flattened, and the head of the femur two inches below the anterior superior spinous process of the ilium. The limb remained unreduced after protracted efforts by manipulation and

REDUCTION.

The limb should be flexed and inverted, with adduction if necessary, to make room for the head of the bone to slide upon the ilium; and the dislocation is then practically a simple dorsal dislocation, and easily reduced. Or if not, perhaps the whole upper part of the capsule is detached, making the luxation irregular.

The rupture of the outer fasciculus of the Y ligament deprives the operator of much of the advantage of rotation. The limb, after flexion and rotation inward, may be reduced by direct traction toward the socket, with local guidance.[1]

pulleys, during which it was repeatedly inverted and everted. The failure to reduce the limb was attributed by Mr. Symes to a "button-hole" laceration. In a similar case, or even if the head of the femur were engaged in the interstices of the rotators, I should attempt to liberate it by circumducting it to the thyroid foramen.

A case of everted dorsal dislocation has been reported by Dr. Van Buren ("Contributions to Practical Surgery," by W. H. Van Buren, M. D., etc., Philadelphia, 1865, p. 157). The limb was shortened an inch, and slightly everted, there being some obstacle to inversion. The trochanter was an inch and a half behind and above its usual position, and the head of the bone was obscurely felt in the back part of the sciatic notch. After repeated attempts at reduction by manipulation, the bone was reduced by pulleys applied to the thigh in a flexed position.

For a case probably everted dorsal, but classed by Cooper as anomalous, see Morgan (Guy's Hospital Reports, No. 1, p. 82). The left leg was shortened two inches, the foot excessively everted, so as almost to give the toes a direction backward, but when placed side by side with the other foot remained in that position. The leg was to some extent susceptible of all the natural motions, with the exception of rotation. The trochanter could not be felt; but the head of the bone was apparently lying between the anterior inferior spinous process of the ilium and the junction of that bone with the pubes. Traction was made from the knee against counter-extension with the foot in the perinæum. The patient was then directed to raise his shoulders from the bed, extension was suddenly increased with forcible inward rotation of the thigh, and the head snapped into the socket.

[1] The following interesting case (reported by Dr. Shrady in the New York Journal of Medicine, March, 1860, p. 255) occurred in the hospital

IRREGULAR DISLOCATIONS.

IN WHICH THE Y LIGAMENT IS WHOLLY BROKEN.

In rare instances the Y ligament may be completely ruptured by forced extension of the limb, or by an upward thrust, while the lower half of the capsule remains comparatively sound. But it has been shown that the position of the great majority of dislocations is determined by this ligament; and until it is likewise shown that when it is broken the luxated limb will be compelled, in obedience to other mechanical agents, muscular or capsular, to assume positions equally constant, it is fair to consider such luxations as irregular. When any mechanism shall be shown always to give to a luxated limb, after the Y ligament has been torn asunder, the same position under the same circumstances, the luxation may be withdrawn from the present category, and classed as "regular."

When the Y ligament is wholly broken, and the head of the femur is dislocated upward upon the edge of the socket, either

wards of Dr. Willard Parker. The patient was crushed to the ground by a gravel car falling upon the small of his back. The left limb was rotated outward and shortened three inches, the thigh slightly adducted and flexed, the knee slightly advanced and semi-flexed, and the toe so everted that the heel rested against the inner aspect of the opposite leg, just above the ankle. Passive rotation was very painful; the buttock of the affected side was much fuller than the other, and the post-trochanteric depression was obliterated. Only the tips of the toes touched the floor. The vertical distance from the trochanter to the crest of the ilium was shortened three quarters of an inch. (If this statement is correct, the apparent shortening of three inches was probably due to the flexed knee.) The head of the bone could be felt, but not very distinctly, in a direction forward and upward from the trochanter. Several efforts to reduce the limb by flexion and adduction were unsuccessful. The thigh was at last rotated inward, extension made in the direction of the socket, and the head of the bone guided by direct manipulation into its place.

inside or outside the iliacus tendon, there is little or no shortening, and no flexion; but the eversion of the foot is marked. The head is felt in the groin, and is reduced by flexion and inversion.

If the head of the bone under these circumstances be displaced toward the thyroid opening, there is abduction of the leg, produced chiefly by the fascia lata, with some flexion due to the adductors; but the flexion is less than in the regular thyroid dislocation, and the knee can be depressed, with a little effort, to the natural position. It is possible that such a dislocation might simulate the thyroid displacement; but it may be distinguished from this by the greater abduction and less considerable flexion of the limb.

If the head be now carried farther downward, the flexion becomes more considerable, though less than if the Y ligament were entire. Such may have been the condition of the parts in some of the cases of downward dislocation before referred to, where the head was said to have been felt near the tuberosity, and where the flexion was inconsiderable.

If the head of the bone be now carried behind the tendon of the obturator internus muscle, there is a flexion of the femur at an angle of 45°, but with such exaggerated inversion as to distinguish it from the regular dislocation below the tendon. The thigh then faces completely inward, and instead of crossing its fellow is even a little abducted. The leg, which is bent by the tense flexors of the thigh, stands at right angles with it.

If the head of the bone be carried upward upon the dorsum, the limb, while it faces directly inward toward its fellow, is no longer flexed, as in the regular dorsal dislocation, but lies flat upon the table. The head, being now detached from the socket, may be carried round upon the dorsum and hooked above the rectus muscle in front, — a position of the parts which, owing to the great strength of the Y ligament, is probably less frequent than the regular supra-spinous and everted dorsal luxations, where a portion of this same ligament still remains intact.

The Y ligament being destroyed, an upward and backward dislocation, if attended with accidental inversion, may be held in that position by the lower part of the capsule, which, however, is readily ruptured by outward rotation or circumduction.

IRREGULAR UPWARD LUXATION.

The bone may be thrust upward upon the inferior spine or above it, with rupture of the Y, but can then be drawn down as far as the remaining capsule will allow, unless detained by being hooked over the muscles arising from that point.[1]

[1] For several cases, of which the description is incomplete, but in which the limb was rotated outward, the head of the femur being outside the anterior inferior spinous process of the ilium, see Malgaigne's "Traité," etc., p. 869. In a patient at St. George's Hospital, the head of the bone was dislocated upward upon the inferior spine of the ilium, and a little to the outside, the upper half of the capsule being largely torn. (Lancet, 1840–41, vol. ii. p. 281.) In Gerdy's case, reported by Baron, the upper half of the capsule was torn, but the round ligament was only half broken. In this case the limb was reduced by flexion, the head of the bone being pressed toward the socket. ("Traité," etc., p. 870.)

See also the case of Adam Hunter (Edinburgh Medico-Chirurgical Transactions, 1824, p. 171.) The limb was shortened one inch, and the toes turned inward. The head of the bone was over the sciatic notch, the gluteus minimus, pyriformis, obturator internus, and other small muscles being ruptured. The capsule was entirely detached from the femur, so that when the ilio-femoral muscles were divided the limb was separated from the trunk. The head was said to have been bound down firmly on the sacro-sciatic notch by the gluteus medius, which passed over the neck of the bone. In the absence of the capsule, it is quite possible that the gluteus medius, beneath which the head of the bone was found, together with the anterior flexors of the thigh, exercised a certain controlling influence on the position of the limb; and yet after dividing the whole capsule in a recent subject, and engaging the head of the femur fairly under the gluteus medius muscle, I have found that rotation ruptured its fibres with little effort.

IRREGULAR DOWNWARD LUXATION.[1]

This variety should be distinguished from that in which the Y remains entire, — described in connection with the thyroid luxation. In the latter case the thigh will be forcibly flexed by the Y, and either adducted or abducted, while the head descends even to the tuberosity or perinæum, — afterward, perhaps, returning to be lodged near the thyroid foramen, or on the dorsum. But if the Y be wholly broken, the limb is suspended by the remaining and comparatively slender capsule, which in such a case would probably be ruptured, thus abandoning the limb to the muscles. Of these, the psoas and iliacus offer a resistance most resembling that of the capsule, and produce an imperfect flexion. The biceps and other extensors may in certain positions interfere with flexion, as they doubtless do in the regular dislocation downward, while the adductors and flexors are also put upon the stretch when the limb is extended or abducted. It has been elsewhere stated that the muscles inserted immediately about the hip are subjected to the very powerful leverage of the femur, and are readily ruptured when unsupported by the ligament of the capsule. The same is true in a less degree of the long muscles, which are liable to laceration from the great violence necessary to sever the entire capsule. When this happens, the bone may be considered as fairly torn from the socket, — a grave accident, which rarely occurs, and in which the limb assumes no uniform position. The head of the bone might possibly, in such a case, be found on the tuberosity or in the perinæum, even when the limb is extended.

[1] The case of Keate (see p. 74) may have been irregular, because the operator was able to "elongate or pull down the limb" after reduction, — a possibility supposed to depend on a fracture of the socket, but which may have resulted, if correctly reported, from a rupture of the Y ligament.

REDUCTION.

An irregular dislocation, with rupture of the Y ligament if not the whole of the capsule, cannot be reduced by any rotation which depends for its efficiency upon the integrity of these ligaments. On the other hand, their ligamentous fibres can no longer interfere with a direct traction of the femur toward the socket, aided by local guidance if required.

SPECIAL CONDITIONS OF DISLOCATION.

OLD DISLOCATIONS AND THEIR REDUCTION.

COOPER[1] cites a case of dorsal dislocation said to have been reduced after the lapse of five years by a fall from a berth on shipboard. Such an occurrence is by no means impossible, but would depend upon the condition of the acetabulum, and of the head of the bone, the changes in which would be influenced by the age and tendencies of the patient.[2] So long as the socket was still excavated, and the bones were not deformed by osseous growths, I should feel quite confident of breaking any adhesions, lacerating the newly formed capsule, and replacing the bone by the great power of the femoral shaft as a lever, and of the flexed leg in rotating the head of the bone around the main ligament.[3] I am unable to understand why Malgaigne,

[1] Treatise, etc., Case LXIV.

[2] For a case of dorsal dislocation reduced after eight months, see p. 53.

[3] The following passage corroborates the views here advanced, although its writer does not recognize the capsule as a source of resistance to reduction: —

"It is doubtful if the capsule is ever an obstacle to the return of the dislocated bone. Certainly the altered shape of the head of the bone never can prevent the return of the head to its articular cavity; and it is probable that where the articular cavity is partially obliterated, it is as quoted by my distinguished friend M. Broca,[1] in the discussion elsewhere alluded to, should assign an indefinite period of two years or more as the limit for reducing a dorsal dislocation, and only fifteen days for that upon the ischiatic notch. By the flexion method, the latter luxation should, theoretically, be reduced with even more facility than the former, and after as long an interval.

A difficulty that may be seriously considered is the risk of breaking the femoral neck, if it has undergone fatty degeneration or atrophy from long disuse; and it might be well in such a case to rely rather on traction, or other force exerted longitudinally upon the bone, than on rotation, where from the immense power thus laterally applied the neck is taken at great disadvantage. The angular traction, to be hereafter described, would be especially suitable, — although, from the greater facility of such an application of power, a better result might be anticipated in a dorsal or downward than in an old pubic or even thyroid luxation. Yet should fracture of the neck, or separation of a previous fracture, occur during such attempts at reduction, it may be fairly said that the patient will generally have a better limb after its inversion has been thus corrected than with an unreduced luxation.

An illustration of these points is afforded by a case in the Chelsea Marine Hospital, under the charge of Dr. Graves. The patient, a man twenty-three years of age, about six

the result of extraordinary violence and consequent inflammation. I have found the cotyloid cavity retaining its depth and covered with cartilage after the head of the femur had been dislocated for three years; and Fournier has placed a dissection on record where the head of the femur had been dislocated during thirteen years, and in which the acetabulum retained its form and depth and cartilage. (Bulletin de la Société Anatomique, 1855.)" — BERNARD E. BRODHURST: *On the Reduction of Old Dislocations* (St. George's Hospital Reports, vol. iii. 1868. London.

[1] Union Médicale, No. 79, p. 57.

months before entering the Hospital, had fallen from the mast-head, seventy-five feet, striking the thwart of a boat (which was broken by the fall) and dislocating his left hip. No attempt was made, at the time of the accident (Nov. 8, 1862) to reduce the displacement. At the time of entering the Hospital the patient was wholly unable to walk, being carried and placed in bed, where he remained. The limb was shortened about two inches, slightly flexed, and inverted to such a degree that the patella faced the inside of the opposite thigh, and the toes of the affected limb were more easily placed behind the heel of the other foot than upon the instep. The patient could partially flex the thigh, and also extend it nearly flat upon the bed, and could rotate the limb inward, but could not evert it. The head of the bone was readily felt upon the dorsum. Dr. Graves having kindly placed the man under my charge for the reduction of the dislocation, I flexed the limb once slowly upward upon the abdomen, — a movement which was attended with a continued fine crepitation about the hip. Upon examination, the head of the bone was now felt to be detached from the neck, and freely movable, like a grape-shot, among the muscles of the haunch. The patient was thereupon placed in bed, the position of the extended limb being much the same as before manipulation. In the course of a week the foot was gradually everted, after which extension was applied and maintained during three months, being increased by degrees from seven pounds to about twenty-one. In two weeks from this time the patient began to move about on crutches, which after six weeks more were abandoned, and at the end of two years he was able to walk without a cane. The limb is now, six years after the accident, an inch and a half shorter than its fellow, but otherwise in proper position, and moves freely in all directions, although it cannot be everted much beyond the perpendicular. The head is firmly attached to the femur behind the trochanter.

and seems with the latter to cover the acetabulum. The manipulation in this case was conducted in the presence of a considerable number of medical gentlemen; and the manner in which the head was detached from the shaft left no doubt upon their minds that the neck, as the result either of an original fracture or of subsequent inflammatory action, had not its normal strength. On the other hand, the present condition of the patient is much better than it would have been had not the dislocation been treated. He walks freely and firmly, with but little lameness, runs up and down stairs, and can swing the limb in all directions.

DISLOCATION FROM HIP DISEASE.

In the dorsal luxation which follows aggravated hip disease, the anterior part of the capsular ligament usually supports and inverts the shortened limb. On the other hand, the head of the femur, which rests upon the dorsum of the ilium, produces, when disintegrated by disease, less inversion than if it were of normal size. Again, the displacement is generally a sub-luxation; but it may sometimes be complete. In a case of hip disease, occurring in a boy about ten years of age, which terminated fatally, I excised the head of a femur (the first instance of this operation in the United States) that was completely dislocated upon the dorsum.

The following is an instructive case of dislocation, perhaps connected with hip disease, and reduced by manipulation.

The patient was a feeble and slender boy thirteen years of age, who was said to have dislocated his hip upon the dorsum by a fall upon a barn floor about three months before, and whom I was requested to see in consultation. The head of the bone could be plainly felt upon the dorsum, the limb being as usual inverted, shortened, and a little flexed. I found that in abducting the limb after it was flexed, a very considerable force was required to raise the head over the socket, and still more in outward rotation to make it enter, which it did only after the capsule and other attachments had been freely lacerated. After reduction, the head of the bone readily and repeatedly escaped, and could be kept in place only by the expedient, elsewhere alluded to, of confining the limb. The foot was secured to the inside of the sound knee, and the limb, thus flexed, was abducted down to the level of the bed, where it was bound to the side of the bedstead by a folded sheet under the knee. In this constrained position of flexion, abduction, and eversion, the patient remained for two and a half weeks, when I again saw him, and found the bone in place. But soon the hip-joint became stiff and painful, and sinuses slowly formed and opened in the groin, as if from hip disease. Upon inquiry, it was ascertained that the child had suffered from pain near the hip after a fall the preceding year, and had also lately recovered from protracted and grave disease of the bone near the ankle. The dislocation may or may not have been facilitated by this tendency to disease of the bone; but there can be little doubt that serious inflammatory action was awakened by the presence of the reduced femur in the socket.

DISLOCATION OF THE HIP, WITH FRACTURE OF THE SHAFT OF THE FEMUR.

Cases have been reported of fracture, even of the upper third of the shaft, in which an accompanying dislocation was reduced by manipulation. There seems to be no good reason why, after the firm application of lateral splints to the thigh, the attempt should not be made with entire success,[1] — reliance being especially placed upon flexion and the local management of the head of the bone, which may be guided into its socket by the hands of the operator applied directly to it, or by a towel in the groin. Angular extension of the lower

1 See Hamilton's "Practical Treatise," etc., p. 666.

fragment of the femur may draw upon its upper muscular insertions, and likewise make room for the upper fragment to follow it; but it is obvious that nothing can be effected by its rotation.

SPONTANEOUS DISLOCATION.

Cases have been cited of individuals who could partially luxate and reduce the head of the thigh-bone at will, by the action of the muscles of the hip. Hamilton has collected three such cases.[1] I have had an opportunity of examining two, and Dr. Lyman, of Boston, has communicated to me the details of a third, all of which were dorsal luxations.

In the first of these cases, — that of a soldier under the charge of Dr. Langmaid, to whom I am indebted for the opportunity of examining it, — the hip was dislocated while the legs were crossed, a wagon in which the man was riding having pitched into a hole. In a few hours the hip was reduced by flexion. Eight days after the accident, in attempting to walk upon the limb, it was again partially luxated, — when the patient himself replaced it by pushing against it with one hand and pressing with the other against his knee. Since that time both luxation and reduction have been comparatively easy, and the patient now displaces the head of the bone backward upon the edge of the socket by muscular action, and reduces it by "throwing the leg out sideways." The luxation is sometimes attended with pain, and the prominence caused by the head of the luxated bone is sensitive to the touch. In this and the following case, the displacement is rather a sub-luxation; and the limb exhibits slight flexion, shortening, and inversion.

In the second case, — that of a gentleman formerly of Boston, — the phenomena are much like those just described; the bone being slipped out and in upon the dorsal edge of the socket by muscular action at will.

[1] Practical Treatise, etc., p. 644.

A third case was under the care of Dr. E. M. Moore, of St. Mary's Hospital, Rochester, N. Y., who has published photographs of it, from which the annexed figures are taken. The following account of this case has been kindly furnished me by Dr. G. H. Lyman, of Boston, who obtained it from Dr. Moore: —

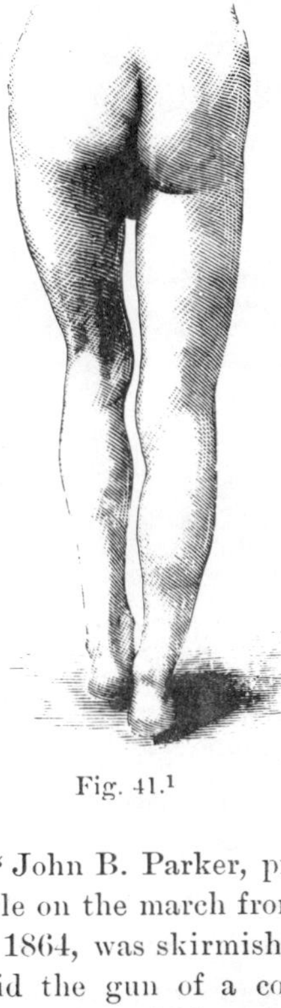

Fig. 41.[1]

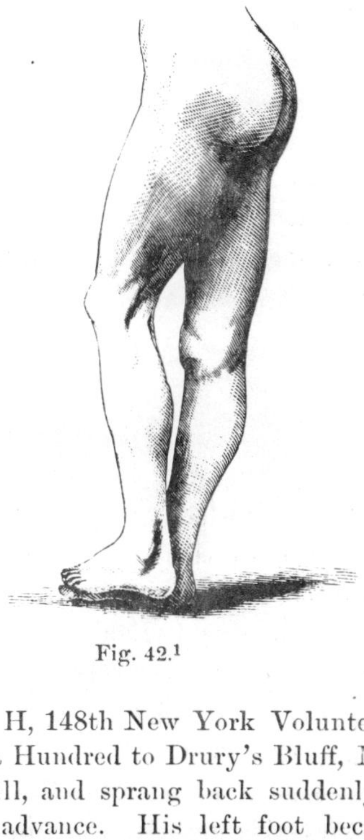

Fig. 42.[1]

"John B. Parker, private, Co. H, 148th New York Volunteers, while on the march from Bermuda Hundred to Drury's Bluff, May 13, 1864, was skirmishing up a hill, and sprang back suddenly to avoid the gun of a comrade in advance. His left foot became entangled, and his weight dislocated his hip. He felt the injury, and supposed it out of joint. Some comrades pulled it in. He immediately resumed his skirmishing, and marched seven miles, from 10 A. M. till 6 P. M. He lay down at night, and went on duty the next day, sharp-shooting, crawling all day. He con-

1 Spontaneous luxation of the thigh. Dr. Moore's case.

tinued this kind of duty five days, and returned to camp, when he was immediately put on intrenchments, and worked two days and nights. Afterward he went on picket, and entered the hospital May 28. At present he can luxate the hip-joint at any time, and does it by pressing the foot on the floor to fix it firmly, contracting the adductors, and throwing out the pelvis. The head suddenly leaves the acetabulum, and goes on the dorsum ilii."

Although the lateral displacement and slight inversion show that this is only a sub-luxation, with the head upon the edge of the socket, yet the flexion of the limb, due to the elasticity and comparative integrity of the living tissues, makes it perhaps a better representation of a common dorsal luxation than Fig. 4, which was photographed from the dead subject, and where the limb was purposely extended as far as the Y ligament would allow.

FRACTURE OF THE PELVIS.

THE following remarks on fracture of the pelvis are introduced here, chiefly with the view of showing how far this injury may be mistaken for regular dislocation of the hip. With this view the subject has been divided into four heads, comprising, respectively: (1) Fracture of the rim of the acetabulum; (2) Fracture in which the head of the bone is driven through the acetabulum into the pelvis; (3) Suspected fracture of the acetabulum; (4) Fracture of other parts of the pelvis. A few cases are given in illustration of each of these lesions. The more instructive of these are, of course, such as have been verified by autopsy. But there are some which are authenticated only by well-marked crepitus, and perhaps by mobility of the detached fragment; and it is then important that crepitus should not be confounded with the grating which results from the attrition of unbroken bone or cartilage.

Finally, there are still others, and by far the most numerous, in which a fracture of the socket has been inferred only from a supposed impossibility of reducing the luxated femur, or of retaining it in place after reduction. It need not be said that these last cases are more conclusive to the observer than to the reader.

FRACTURE OF THE RIM OF THE ACETABULUM.

To afford satisfactory evidence, cases of this sort should have been identified by autopsy, or at least by crepitus. Unfortunately, but a small part of the reported cases are thus elucidated, and fracture has been generally inferred because the head of the bone could not be restored to the socket, or could not be kept there. It is probable that when the rim of the socket is broken on the side either of the dorsum or of the foramen ovale, the signs of the displacement do not vary materially from those of the regular luxations. The regular backward displacement, for example, may be complicated with a detached rim, which, if enough be left to engage the head of the bone, in no way interferes with its conditions as a luxation, except that the bone tends to slip backward after being reduced. The same principle probably holds true in the case of fracture of the rim on the side of the foramen ovale, and also of the upper part of the socket, unless the fracture involves the upper insertion of the Y ligament, in which case the detached fragment might be so displaced as materially to modify the position of the limb, especially so far as its flexion or inversion was concerned. Such a luxation would be irregular.

These displacements, especially the displacement backward, demand the usual attempts at reduction by flexion. Although the bone inclines to slip from the socket, it can be retained there, in cases of a sort heretofore considered difficult of treatment, by angular extension, with an angular splint attached to the ceiling or some other point above the patient; or if any manœuvre has reduced the bone, the limb should be retained, if possible, in the attitude which completed the manœuvre.[1]

The following case occurred at the Massachusetts General Hospital, under the care of Dr. Gay. The patient, aged thirty-six, a robust and healthy man, fell from the roof of a building, striking upon the right hip. In the recumbent position the leg was shortened and inverted, the toes crossing the opposite instep. Being etherized, the thigh could be flexed at a right angle with the abdomen, there being crepitus in the region of the neck of the femur. The limb, when drawn down, was still shortened half an inch. The patient having died of other injuries, the autopsy showed the head of the bone partially dislocated backward, and resting upon the posterior fractured edge of the socket, the whole posterior wall of the socket having been broken away in a mass. The detached fragment measured one and a half inches square. The posterior surface of the head of the bone was deeply indented by the fractured edge of the acetabulum, against which it had impinged after displacing the portion broken off. A transverse crack extended through the acetabulum from the upper sciatic notch to the foramen ovale. The position of the limb in this case did not differ from that in the usual partial dislocation behind the tendon, and was determined by the same mechanism.[2]

[1] See p. 53.

[2] In a case of dorsal luxation with inversion, reported by Maisonneuve (Clinique Chirurgicale, 1863, p. 168), the autopsy showed fracture of the posterior part of the border of the socket.

Sir Astley Cooper's Case No. LXXI. is one of regular dislocation below the tendon of the obturator internus, which tightly embraced the neck of the bone, with shortening and inversion of the limb, although the posterior part of the acetabulum was broken off, and there was other extensive fracture of the pelvis.

Dr. M. Tyer's third case was shown by the autopsy to be a regular backward dislocation with inversion, — the posterior and inferior margin of the acetabulum being detached, and displaced toward the coccyx.

On the other hand, in Dr. Tyer's first case, the limb was *everted* while

FRACTURE IN WHICH THE HEAD OF THE FEMUR IS DRIVEN THROUGH THE ACETABULUM.

In regard to this accident Hamilton well remarks: —

"There seems to be no certain rule in relation to the position of the limb; but it is found to take the one direction or the other,

flexed and shortened, an inch and a half of the rim being completely detached at the upper and posterior margin of the acetabulum. The remaining portion of the rim may not have been sufficient to turn the head backward, and thus compel inversion of the limb. In a second case, the toes crossed the tarsus of the other foot, and the autopsy showed a fracture of the upper margin of the rim of the acetabulum. (Glasgow Medical Journal, February, 1830; American Journal of the Medical Sciences, 1831, vol. viii. p. 517.)

For a case of dorsal luxation with shortening, inversion, crepitus, and difficulty of retaining the reduced bone in the socket, see Cooper's "Treatise," etc., Case XXXIX.

In the following case of fractured acetabulum, the upper insertion of the Y ligament was detached. The patient, fifty-eight years of age, was caught by a revolving belt. The right limb was shortened a quarter of an inch, and so far everted and straight that the internal condyle of the left femur lay in the popliteal space of the injured one. The right groin was filled up. Toward its middle, and outside the femoral artery, was a hard, resisting, and obscurely spherical tumor, masked by the glands and swollen tissues. Flexion with outward rotation and local downward pressure failed to reduce the luxation; but on a third trial, flexion and downward pressure during slight abduction, instead of outward rotation, succeeded. Seven months afterward, the death of the patient from another cause showed a united fracture of the socket, comprising the external and anterior third of the rim with the two anterior spinous processes of the ilium. (M. Beraud, Bulletin de la Société de Chirurgie, 1862, tom. iii. p. 185.)

In the above case reported by M. Richet, the trochanter was rotated toward the median line, with the head of the femur facing directly forward, and probably with displacement of the detached bone. But the fact that the round ligament was unbroken would seem to indicate that the luxation was only partial, as might indeed have been inferred from the position of the limb, which, though everted, was not much displaced.

In this connection, M. Richet (Bulletin, p. 226) refers to a case of luxation of Maisonneuve (Revue Médico-Chirurgicale, tom. xvi. p. 48) in which a fragment of a broken acetabulum had in twenty-seven days united with the rest of the rim so firmly that the fracture could hardly be discovered.

probably according to the direction of the force which has inflicted the injury, and perhaps in obedience to circumstances not always to be explained."[1]

In two of the recorded cases the patients recovered, being able to walk; in one of these the head of the femur had become almost completely inclosed in a bony shell. In two other cases the patients died of the injury, which in all was the result of great local violence.[2]

It may be remarked that when the head of the femur is thus thrust completely within the pelvis, the capsule and surrounding muscles are relaxed, and would not determine the position of the bone.

ASSERTED FRACTURE OF THE ACETABULUM, WITHOUT CREPITUS, FROM A SUPPOSED IMPOSSIBILITY OF KEEPING THE FEMUR IN PLACE.

It has been already remarked that the evidence in this class of cases is unsatisfactory; and it is not unlikely that the bone could have been kept in place by angular extension when other means had failed, or by confining the leg in the position of the final manœuvre by which it was reduced, as before described.[3]

[1] Practical Treatise, p. 343.

[2] In the case of Lendrick, and that of Morel-Lavallée, the accident was supposed to be that of fracture of the neck, from which it may be inferred that the foot was everted. In Case LXXII. of Cooper, the appearance was that of dislocation backward, probably involving inversion. In that of Moore the limb was shortened two inches, slightly flexed and abducted, but without rotation in either direction. Cooper, "Treatise," etc., Cases LXXII. and LXXIII.; Lendrick, American Journal of the Medical Sciences, August, 1839, vol. xxiv. p. 481 (from London Medical Gazette, March, 1839); Morel-Lavallée, Malgaigne, "Traité," etc., tom. ii. p. 881; Moore, Medico-Chirurgical Transactions, 1851, vol. xxxiv. p. 107.

[3] See p. 53. In the case of Keate (Cooper, "Treatise," etc., Case LXIX.), the fact that the limb could be drawn down, together with doubtful crepitus, was regarded as evidence of fracture of the socket. For a

FRACTURE OF OTHER PARTS OF THE PELVIS.

A fracture of the pelvis not especially involving the acetabulum can hardly be mistaken for luxation of the hip; and yet the following case under my care may be cited as an instance of a limb the position of which, when first seen, was identical with that of a dislocation, and as in similar cases was probably due to an effort of the patient to relieve the pain of injured tissues.[1]

The patient, a young man of seventeen years of age, entered the Massachusetts General Hospital, having been caught beneath a heavy piece of machinery which fell from a wagon, striking upon the front of his left thigh just below the groin. Upon examination the thigh was found to be flexed upon the pelvis, and the foot everted. The knee was widely separated

case of Mr. Brodie, of twelve weeks' standing, where failure to reduce a dorsal dislocation was attributed to fracture of the socket, although none of its indications were present, see the Lancet, vol. xxiv. p. 671.

The following case of supposed fractured socket without crepitus is one of several reported by M. Richet. A young man fell in dancing, while endeavoring to fling up his leg to the level of his partner's face. The leg was much inverted, and three quarters of an inch shortened, the head of the femur being felt upon the dorsum. The bone was repeatedly reduced, and as often escaped. The patient was ultimately placed in a fracture apparatus with extension, and two years after walked lame, the head of the bone rising upon the ilium at each step. No crepitus was felt, the diagnosis being based upon the supposed impossibility of keeping the head in the socket. (Bulletin de la Société de Chirurgie, 1862, tom. iii. p. 251.)

[1] A case of fracture of the ilium yielded crepitus under pressure upon the anterior and upper part of the ilium, the leg being shortened three quarters of an inch, and the foot slightly everted. After extension by the double inclined plane for several weeks the deformity disappeared. (Lancet, vol. xliv. p. 877.)

In a case of fracture of the ilium, the right leg was half an inch shorter than the left, and slightly everted, with flattening of the region of the trochanter, the knee being also abducted. Pressure on the anterior superior spine produced crepitus attended with acute pain in the joint. (Lancet, vol. xv. p. 575.)

from the other, any attempt to approximate them causing pain. The pubes was tender when pressed. Under ether the leg resumed its normal position. No crepitus was discovered, although the patient had complained of a sense of grating in the perinæum. A broad strap was placed around the pelvis, and in six weeks the patient was well enough to be discharged, walking on crutches. It is difficult in this case to account for the position of the limb before etherization, except on the supposition that it may have afforded relief to pain. To the eye its position was that of a thyroid luxation.[1]

ANGULAR EXTENSION.

Pouteau[2] first remarked upon the disadvantage of traction with counter-extension in the perinæum, which brings the thigh into a straight line with the trunk. Most surgeons have observed the tendency of the pelvis, when pulleys are used, to escape from the counter-extending bands in the direction of the applied traction. It is believed that the apparatus here described will be found efficient, both in confining the pelvis and in enabling the operator to apply extension to a limb which has been flexed for the purpose of relaxing the Y ligament. Lateral extension, with or without pulleys, can then be made in any desired direction by a towel passed round the thigh at the groin.

The patient being laid upon his back, the pelvis is secured to the floor by a T band passing across it laterally in front, between the superior and inferior spinous processes of each side, and vertically over the pubes and perinæum. The three extremities, each terminating in a strap and buckle, are fastened to the floor beneath the margin of the pelvis by

[1] Massachusetts General Hospital Records, vol. cxxvii. p. 210.

[2] Malgaigne, "Traité," etc., p. 867.

common dislocation-hooks. The entire band, with the exception of its extremities, is cylindrical, about two inches in diameter, well padded and covered with buckskin. It firmly holds the pelvis by its pressure between the spinous processes on each side and upon the pubes. To apply it, the three pointed hooks are screwed into the floor, one near each tro-

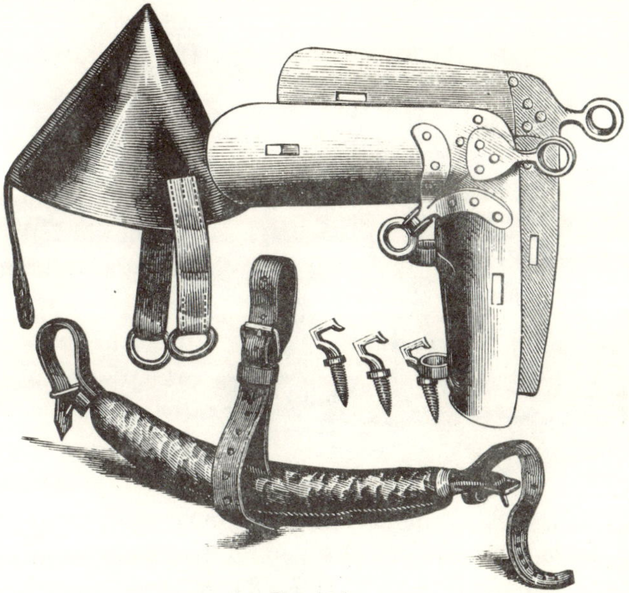

FIG. 43.[1]

chanter, and one near the perinæum; the band is then adjusted, and the pelvis buckled to the floor, after which it will be found that the thighs can be freely flexed. A tripod is now erected over the pelvis, consisting of three stiff poles about eight feet high, and held together at the top by a coni-

[1] Apparatus for angular extension. This woodcut represents the conical leather cap and rings, the angular splint, with rings above and below the knee for the passage of a transverse wooden lever, and of a longitudinal one beneath the calf, the padded T pelvis band, and the hooks to attach it to the floor.

cal leather cap, with three short, dependent straps and rings from which the pulleys are suspended. It remains only to attach the pulleys to the limb. This is effected by means of a strong right-angled splint of sheet-iron, extending nearly from the hip to the ankle, made concave so as to embrace the under surface of the thigh and leg, and padded, within which the limb, flexed at right angles, is confined by bandages or straps. Two iron rings riveted to the splint near the condyles of the femur receive a wooden rod about two feet in length and an inch in diameter, which crosses the ligament of the patella transversely above the head of the tibia; and to this rod, between the rings, the pulleys are attached by a strap or cord. Vertical traction is thus made exactly in the axis of the shaft of the femur.

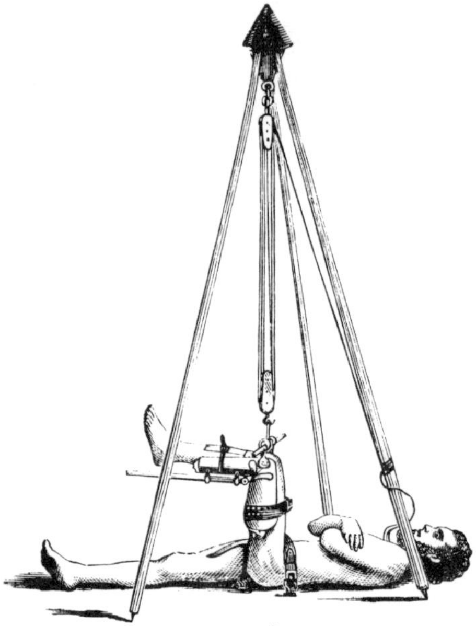

FIG. 44.[1]

Powerful rotation can be made by grasping the extremities of this transverse rod, while another useful movement, called by the French *bascule*, or tilt, may be effected by a similar

[1] Angular extension. The pelvis is buckled to the floor. The flexed leg is suspended from the cap at the summit of the tripod by pulleys which are attached to a transverse wooden rod across the patella. This rod passes through rings on the angular splint, and serves to rotate the limb. A similar rod is seen beneath the leg.

rod in the axis of the leg below the knee, passed through two rings beneath the splint, — one near the ham, the other near the heel, beyond which it projects a foot or more, — to afford a handle. By vertically raising this rod at its extremity we carry the head of the bone from the dorsum, or pubes, in the direction of the tuberosity.

Oblique extension may be made by changing the position of the tripod.

Although the need of this apparatus may be rare, it will prove occasionally efficient in reducing a luxation of long standing or complicated with fracture. At any rate, I cannot believe that the period is remote when longitudinal extension by pulleys to reduce a recent hip luxation will be unheard of.

ON DISLOCATION OF THE HIP.[1]

THE simplicity of the principle which controls hip reduction is as yet scarcely appreciated by the majority of practitioners into whose hands the scattered cases fall. Writers also, until very lately, have seemed disposed to consider "manipulation" as but one of several means of reduction of equal value, — occasionally available, indeed, but complicated with many methods, and by conflicting opinions regarding its essential features, — by perplexing talk of abduction and inversion, of flexion and partial flexion, of rotation and circumduction. I have, perhaps, myself unintentionally contributed to this erroneous belief. But my paper upon this subject[2] was based upon the analysis of a large number of dissections, experiments, and cases of reduction, which could neither be condensed advantageously nor yet omitted; while its object was to show the relation between hip dislocation and the ilio-femoral ligament, then generally unrecognized. The whole matter is really very simple. The word "manipulation" is an unfortunate one; "flexion" is better. The modern method of hip reduction, whether by lifting or by mere abduction, is the "flexion method;" and it supersedes all others.

A common way of describing dislocation is by the terms "backward," "forward," "in front," and "behind." It should be borne in mind that when the body is erect the pelvis is oblique, — the acetabulum standing in like manner obliquely, at an angle of about 45°, facing the front and outside of the thigh, at a point an inch or two below the trochanter; so that what

[1] The Lancet, June 15, 22, 29, 1878.

[2] The Mechanism of Dislocation and Fracture of the Hip. (Henry C. Lea, Philadelphia, 1869.)

is behind the socket may be either below or outside of it. In fact, it is not easy immediately to place an os innominatum, or even a pelvis, in the normal erect attitude to which alone these terms should refer.

As preliminary to reduction, the patient should be etherized to relaxation, and, in order to give the surgeon control of the limb, laid on the floor. It is well to remember that the head of the femur always faces the same way as the internal condyle.

If there is any single and best rule for reducing a recent dislocation of the hip, it is to get the head of the femur directly below the socket by flexing the thigh at about a right angle, and then to lift or jerk it forcibly up into its place. This rule applies to all dislocations except the pubic, and even to that when secondary from below the socket. I have taught it many years. A case reduced by this method under the care of the distinguished surgeon, Mr. Erichsen, will be found in "The Lancet" for 1872 (vol. i. p. 10). Of the various ways which incorporate the essential principle, this one was placed first in my paper in connection with the common dorsal dislocation; and I elsewhere showed how it was applicable to other dislocations. The reduction by the lifting method is usually instantaneous; and flexion is at the basis of its success.

But if after one or two trials it should appear that the hip cannot be jerked into place, let the rent in the capsule be enlarged a little by moving the flexed thigh, not up and down, but from one side to the other, so as to sweep the head of the femur across below the socket.[1] No danger need be appre-

[1] The following case is interesting in this connection: A short and very fat elderly woman was suspected of thyroid dislocation. Attempts already made to reduce the bone had so loosened the capsule that the limb was now lying parallel with the other. While the foot could be everted or inverted, the head of the bone could be nowhere felt. In

hended from this expedient of circumduction; the added injury is a very slight one. So long as air is not admitted to the wounded parts the lesion is no more serious than often occurs in a simple fracture of the thigh. The laceration which resulted from the old longitudinal traction with pulleys was often much greater, and that from ill-planned and protracted efforts by flexion is always so. Indeed, such additional laceration may sometimes advantageously occur without the knowledge of the surgeon during unsuccessful efforts to reduce the bone, especially in executing the manœuvre described in the rule "Flex, abduct, evert."[1]

consultation I was quite unable to satisfy myself about the lesion until it occurred to me to flex the limb and circumduct the head of the bone, as if it had been dislocated upon the thyroid foramen to the dorsum. Then the characteristic inversion at once demonstrated the dislocation. The thigh was again brought to a perpendicular, and readily lifted into place, — circumduction here affording a valuable means of diagnosis as well as of reduction.

[1] Flexion dates from Hippocrates. He combined with it a movement which, by a literal translation of the original, is the "wagtail shake" (κίγκλισις). (See "The Mechanism of Dislocation," etc., p. 27, footnote). But Hippocrates seems to have relied mainly on direct extension, aided by the rude application of levers and other mechanical expedients. The method concisely expressed in the words "flex, abduct, evert," a method the paternity of which has sometimes been in doubt, belongs to an investigator of fifty years ago, a man of highly original mind, — the late Nathan Smith, Professor of Medicine in Dartmouth College, New Hampshire, and afterward Surgical Professor in Yale College. He attended lectures in Edinburgh under the elder Monro and Dr. Black, and studied also in London. In a Biographical Memoir published in 1831, soon after his death, it is stated that "his mode of reducing dislocations of the hip is new, philosophical, and ingenious." In a posthumous volume of "Medical and Surgical Memoirs" (Baltimore, printed by William A. Francis, 1831), edited by his son, Nathan R. Smith, M.D., twenty pages are devoted to a detailed description of his method, from which the following is taken (pp. 180, 181): "The first effort which the operator makes is to flex the leg upon the thigh, in order to make the leg a lever with which he may operate on the thigh-bone. The next movement is a gentle rotation of the thigh outward, by inclining the foot toward the ground and rotating the knee outward. Next, the thigh is to be slightly ab-

This familiar rule, until I explained its mechanism, was an empirical one. Flexion is indeed the essence of it; but besides this, the femur is rotated around the ilio-femoral ligament as a centre. When the knee, abducted by this rotation, descends on the outside, the head of the femur rises on the inside, like an opposite spoke in the wheel, and is thus pried into place by the shaft of the bone as a lever, with the outer band of the ligament as a fulcrum. Eversion is of less importance, but helps the movement by inclining the head of the abducted femur toward the socket. It is best effected by keeping the foot of the flexed limb stationary while the knee is pressed outward. By the great power it gives the operator, this method, or rather the circumduction connected with it, is especially useful in breaking the adhesions of an old dislo-

ducted by pressing the knee directly outward. Lastly, the surgeon freely flexes the thigh upon the pelvis by thrusting the knee upward toward the face of the patient, and at the same moment the abduction is to be increased. Professor N. Smith regarded the free flexion of the thigh upon the pelvis as a very important part of the compound movement. He believed that it threw the head of the bone downward, behind the acetabulum, where the margin of the cup is less prominent, and over which, therefore, the adductor muscles would drag it with less difficulty into its place. The operator may slightly vary these movements as he increases them, so as to give some degree of rocking motion to the head of the os femoris, which will thereby be disengaged with the more facility from its confined situation among the muscles." This covers the ground of priority of invention. It belongs to Nathan Smith. But surgeons were not as yet prepared for so considerable an innovation. In the words of Professor N. R. Smith (p. 174), "the propriety of employing pulleys, for the purpose of multiplying power in the treatment of dislocations of the hip, appears to be so tacitly and universally admitted at the present time that one who contends against it can scarcely expect to obtain a favorable hearing." The method by flexion and abduction had been taught by Nathan Smith long before 1831. In 1835 Després, and in 1852 Dr. Reid, of Rochester, N. Y., enunciated the same views. The practice was good; but both Professor Smith and Dr. Reid based the method and sought its mechanism in the erroneous theory of muscular resistance. The rule, it should be added, applies only to dorsal dislocation.

cation. It might be called the abduction method, to distinguish it from the lifting method.

Abduction sometimes succeeds at once. It does not answer, however, when there is much laceration of the capsule. Then the head of the bone will not rise. Suspended by the ligament which is attached at the trochanters, it slips backward and forward below the socket, from the dorsum to the foramen ovale. The upward lift then becomes absolutely essential. In one of the figures of a standard and very excellent modern English surgical work, which has done me the honor to refer to my views, the engraver has placed the hand of the surgeon above the knee, adding to the weight of the limb, and bearing the head down below the socket, where it might even hook up the sciatic nerve. The weight of the limb should be sustained with the hand in the ham.

Such are the simple principles of hip reduction, which are still often buried beneath unimportant details, and sometimes under a flood of technical language.

By the lifting method I have reduced, without haste, a dorsal dislocation of both hips in the same man in less than two minutes. With an effort to do it quickly, I reduced in two seconds a dorsal dislocation that had just been vainly "manipulated" under ether by two medical practitioners for an hour. A few months ago I forcibly lifted into its place from the dorsum, in a few seconds, a dislocated hip, which required traction with the whole strength of the elbow engaged under the knee, against the foot upon the pelvis.

By the lifting method combined with abduction I have lately, in the case of a little girl of seven years, reduced a dorsal dislocation of five months' standing, said to have occurred during the delirium of typhoid fever. To keep the bone in place when reduced it was necessary to tie the knee to the side of the bedstead, in extreme abduction, after securing the foot to the knee of the sound side, in order to maintain the limb in the final position that reduced it.

Since this occurred I have reduced by simple abduction, and in a moment, a recent dorsal dislocation in a little boy of four years.

From these and other cases may be gathered the following rules for reduction. In the dorsal dislocation, —

1. Flex, and forcibly lift. If this fails, —

2. Flex, and lift while abducting. If this fails, it will be found that abduction has carried the head of the bone from the dorsum nearly or quite to the thyroid foramen, and that the capsular rent has been so enlarged that the first method may now prove successful. Lifting the femur abducts it if it raises the pelvis on the lifted side. In thyroid dislocation adduction of the flexed thigh reverses this movement and carries the head from the thyroid foramen to the dorsum, also enlarging the opening and making the first rule effective. The pubic dislocations may be generally brought down, after flexion, without difficulty from above the socket. If they are secondary, the head of the bone will fall, after flexion, to its previous position below the socket, and may be reduced from there like the thyroid.

My belief has long been expressed that the flexion method is the only rational one, and that pulleys are practically obsolete, unless perhaps to steady the limb in some rare case, by rectangular, not longitudinal, traction. Then alone is the tripod apparatus possibly useful. But why flex the thigh? Because it relaxes a part of the ilio-femoral ligament. When the limb is straight, this ligament is rigid and the bone fixed; when it is flexed, the inner band is slackened, — as also the whole ligament if the limb be lifted, — and the head is brought down below the socket, level with the capsular rent, becoming movable for reduction as it was previously for escape.

Now, flexion, with adduction or abduction, is the habitual attitude of the thigh, especially in action or for self-defence; and the ligament is thus habitually relaxed. On this account, and also because the capsule is weak and thin below "like wet bladder," and the socket margin notched on that side, the dislocation downward is the most common one. All this I have elsewhere shown, and also that the head of the bone, thus escaping primarily below the socket, generally at once slides up to a second position on one side of it or the other. In fact, downward dislocation is so frequent, and the route from below to the dorsum is rendered so easy both by muscular contraction and by the conformation of the bone,—by the latter especially,—that in a very large proportion of cases the displacement is found to be dorsal. The result has been to extend the application of any rule for reduction which applies to dorsal dislocation, and to make it comparatively familiar.

These secondary dislocations from below the socket are well known; and all the regular dislocations (if we except those between the small rotator muscles) may be secondary. On the other hand, there can be no question that the bone may be primarily dislocated in various directions. Flexion does not in all dislocations return the limb to a point below the socket without increased laceration of the capsule, as it would if they had all come from there. Just as the downward dislocation may take place during extreme flexion, especially with rotation inward, and through a comparatively small aperture, so the dislocation on the pubes may occur during extreme extension; and it is usually reduced from above the socket. A direct thrust backward may produce dislocation upon the dorsum when the ilio-femoral ligament is relaxed. Primary dislocations are not rare, in various attitudes of the limb.

But in order to compare the regular dislocations more readily, let us for the time consider them all as secondary from a common point below the socket, and follow the progress of the bone from the moment of its original escape downward to this point.

The femur is, then, sometimes held below the socket in extreme flexion, firmly, as if the neck were embraced in the capsular rent. Such dislocations have been considered anomalous, and described as "upon the perinæum," and "upon the tuberosity." I have shown them to be regular. But it oftener happens that from after-violence, or by its own weight, the knee falls, the thigh is straightened, and the head of the bone, suspended at the trochanters, is pried upward on one side or the other of the socket, lacerating the capsule. In this view the downward dislocation is a first stage of the others, the head pausing below the socket and hesitating which side to go, — whether to the thyroid foramen, or above it to the pubic region, or even to a higher point, where the dislocation is still a regular one (the sub-spinous), all these being internal to the socket; or, which is more common, external to and behind the socket on the dorsum, where, as I have shown, the limb is at once inverted by the outer band of the ilio-femoral ligament. The first serious obstacle the bone then encounters in its dorsal ascent is the strong obturator internus muscle and the subjacent capsule. This is one of the more common dislocations. If the bone ruptures the obturator and the capsule, it rises to the pyriformis, and if this be broken, to the gluteus minimus, retaining the usual features of a dorsal displacement.[1]

If, however, the outer band of the ligament be ruptured, the limb is no longer necessarily inverted, but capable of eversion, and the dislocation is then the everted dorsal. The head of the bone, still suspended by the remaining inner band, can now be hooked over it above the spinous process; the dislocation is then supra-spinous, the limb being still

[1] See an account of the autopsy in Todd's case, No. XL. of Cooper.

straight. But if the femur has been hooked over the entire ligament, instead of the inner band only, the limb cannot hang straight; it assumes a very oblique attitude across the axis of the body. This I have called the anterior oblique dislocation. These three positions of the bone were described by Sir Astley Cooper as anomalous; but the explanation here given of their essential mechanism shows that they occur under prescribed conditions of the ilio-femoral ligament, and that they are therefore constant and regular. In short, all regular dislocations, including those upon the perinæum and the tuberosity, as well as the everted dorsal, the anterior-oblique, and the supra-spinous varieties, have constant and distinctive signs which they owe to the ilio-femoral ligament; and eversion in dorsal dislocation signifies that the outer band of this ligament has been severed.

Nothing can be more simple than the reduction of secondary dislocations from below the socket. If dorsal, and the flexed thigh has fallen to a horizontal position by a spiral movement downward and inward, reverse the movement and reduce the limb by a spiral upward and outward. If thyroid or pubic, and the knee has followed a spiral downward and outward, reduce it by a similar movement upward and inward. But the spirals of reduction practically amount to mere flexion; therefore, in either case, flex the limb and jerk it upward; and in the thyroid luxations it is well to aid the process by outward traction with a towel, or by a fulcrum in the groin. Finally, if the capsule offer resistance, sweep the flexed femur from side to side to separate its fibres and get the head below the socket, before jerking the bone up into place.

There is another point, which is now of less practical importance. By the now obsolete straight traction with pulleys reduction from the dorsum was sometimes difficult, or failed. Surgeons then called the dislocation "ischiatic." There was a superstition about the ischiatic notch. It was the maelstrom of the hip-bone. There was obviously in those days some real difficulty, which does not occur with the flexion method. Its most frequent source was the strong obturator internus muscle combined with an unusually sound and tense falciform edge of the subjacent capsule, interposed between the head of the bone and the socket, occluding the latter.

On this account I substituted for the term "ischiatic" the phrase "below the tendon," as explanatory of the manner of the displacement, the relations of the bone, and the general character of the difficulty of its reduction. The phrase "below the tendon" was desirable to distinguish this dislocation from those in which the head emerges above the tendon. In either case the head of the bone may reach and occupy a place "behind" the tendon (see "The Mechanism of Dislocation," etc., Fig. 15).[1]

When my paper was written, the bugbear of the ischiatic notch was still feared, because the practice of reduction by straight extension was still in vogue. In fact, surgical works are still illustrated with pulleys from Sir Astley Cooper. For more than fifteen years I have neither employed nor taught reduction by straight extension, and I have long

[1] The dorsal dislocation between the small rotator muscles, or any other which offered exceptional resistance, was no doubt sometimes mistaken for the "ischiatic" dislocation. I still incline to believe that my explanation of the old difficulty in "ischiatic" reduction is the correct one. The dislocation formerly called "dorsal" differs from the "ischiatic" in having the thick capsule which is behind the ilio-femoral ligament and beneath the obturator tendon, including the ischio-femoral band, so torn as to allow a greater shortening of the limb than used to be described as a sign of "ischiatic" displacement. During reduction by straight extension, the head of the bone could pass through the torn capsule to the socket as soon as it had slipped over the obturator tendon. The injury may be accompanied by the rupture of muscles, even of the obturator internus. In short, the classical dorsal and ischiatic dislocations differ from each other only in the extent of the laceration of the posterior capsule and muscles.

abandoned any especial description of the so-called ischiatic dislocation, whose chief and distinctive sign was that it resisted straight extension. For practical purposes this dislocation is dorsal, and may be called so. It is easily reduced by flexion.

So, also, it is useless to distinguish from the common dorsal dislocation those which lie between the small rotators; because, although interesting to the anatomist and the pathologist, it is very doubtful whether they will ever be diagnosticated with certainty during life. They exhibit, as I have shown, more inversion, more immobility, and more elasticity; but these signs are not pathognomonic. When these dislocations occur, the head of the bone is thrust directly backward through the capsule, and escapes this time, not below the tendon of the strong internal obturator, but above it, by the muscular interstice between this muscle and the pyriformis, or even higher, between the pyriformis and the gluteus minimus. The bone may possibly be reduced from these positions by vertical traction, or pried back through the interstice by the abduction method or by outward rotation; but I think such attempts will generally end in rupturing the muscles. The dislocation would then offer no distinctive features, and would belong to the common dorsal variety, in which we can only guess what rotators are ruptured. Indeed, it is the rule in dorsal dislocation that the quadratus or some of the rotators are torn, — which of them we need not know. Our business is to reduce the bone by flexion, — and by circumduction also, if that be necessary to rupture the capsule and muscles, and so to clear the way to a point below the socket, from which the femur can be lifted into place.

If, in accordance with these views, we suppress any distinct mention of the inter-rotator dislocations, — which indeed have never been separately classified (although, if it were possible always to identify them, they would deserve to be separately considered), — and of the obsolete ischiatic dislocation, by whatever name we call it, we have the following classification of regular dislocations, based on their direction from the socket: —

External to the socket, — the dorsal, and the everted dorsal.

Internal to the socket, — on the perinæum, the thyroid foramen, and the pubes.

Below the socket, — the dislocation toward the tuberosity.

Above the socket, — the sub-spinous, the supra-spinous, and the anterior oblique dislocations.

Of these, by far the more common are the dorsal, the thyroid, and the pubic, which offer the most convenient division for practical purposes. It leads to the following practical grouping of dislocations, based on the usual mechanism of their occurrence and of their reduction: —

Dorsal, — the dislocation on the tuberosity, the dorsal, the everted dorsal, the anterior oblique, and the supra-spinous.

Thyroid, — that on the perinæum, and on the thyroid foramen.

Pubic, — the pubic and the sub-spinous.[1]

The ilio-femoral ligament is unbroken in these regular dislocations, — excepting only the everted dorsal and supra-spinous varieties, in which its outer band is severed, while the inner band remains. All may be readily reduced after

[1] This is perhaps the best practical classification. Although the sub-spinous and the supra-spinous dislocations lie directly above the socket, the former is essentially a pubic dislocation, and after flexion needs only to be worked directly down into the socket. The supra-spinous dislocation on the contrary, like the anterior oblique, must be first unhooked from the ligament, and then circumducted to the socket by the way of the dorsum. It is essentially dorsal. In a regular dislocation the bone does not pass the ilio-femoral ligament, whether it approaches it from the inside or the outside.

flexion, with or without circumduction, — the thyroid and pubic with a towel or fulcrum in the groin if need be, in the one for outward, in the other for downward and outward traction. This method covers the reduction of the primary as well as the secondary forms of luxation.

It may here be added that a broken socket makes reduction difficult or impossible; and that if the femur tends to escape after being reduced, the flexed thigh should be abducted down to the bed, and confined there at right angles with the body, to take advantage of the tense ilio-femoral ligament in holding the bone in place, as in an instance before mentioned.

In illustration of some of these points, let me cite a few cases.

1. The classical case, No. XLIII. of Cooper. In this case, during straight thyroid reduction, the knee was raised, and the ligament, of course, relaxed. The head of the bone was thus unintentionally dropped from the thyroid foramen to a point below the socket. In this position it should have been jerked up into place; but unfortunately the limb was again straightened. The head of the bone rose, this time not to the thyroid foramen, but upon the dorsum, where it was engaged behind the close-fitting capsule, and probably the obturator muscle. From this position it could not afterward be drawn by straight extension, and was therefore pronounced irreducible. This case led Sir Astley Cooper to warn surgeons not to flex the thigh. In reality, flexion with an upward jerk was what the case required.

2. The similar case of Lisfranc,[1] — a dorsal dislocation, which that surgeon, with eight assistants, failed for an hour to reduce by straight extension. The patient then collapsed, and afterward died. The autopsy showed a state

[1] Malgaigne's "Traité," etc., tom. ii. pp. 818–829. Plate XXVI.

of things which doubtless existed in the case of Cooper. The neck of the bone was closely tied by the capsule; the head had emerged below the obturator internus, and was behind it. It was easily reducible by flexion.

3. Parmentier's case of dorsal dislocation between the rotators.[1] The posterior half of the capsule was largely torn. The head had escaped by a muscular buttonhole above the internal obturator, between that muscle and the pyriformis, which is next it.

4. The similar case of Servier, above the latter muscle.[2] Here the articular capsule was completely torn behind, the head of the bone having escaped by the "posterior notch of the acetabulum" (beneath the tendon of the pyriformis), emerging above the pyriformis, which closely confined it.

5. The case of Dr. Fenner, of New Orleans, quoted in Professor Hamilton's valuable and comprehensive treatise on "Fractures and Dislocations."[3] The head was on the dorsum. The limb was shortened an inch and a half, and the toes turned inward. The capsule was torn through one half its extent. Portions of the obturator externus, pyriformis, and gemelli were ruptured and lacerated. "Dr. Fenner now proceeded to cut away the muscles; and when all the external muscles about the joint had been removed, the thigh could not be brought down. The iliacus internus and psoas magnus were then severed, which permitted it to descend a little, but the head could not be replaced; the triceps adductor was then divided without effect; the ilio-femoral ligament was found tensely stretched. All the muscles between the pelvis and the thighs were then severed, and still it was impossible to reduce the dislocation;

[1] Bulletin de la Société Anatomique, p. 176. 1850.

[2] Bulletin de la Société de Chirurgie, p. 485. 1863.

[3] Fifth edition, p. 676.

the head of the femur could not be forced back through the rent in the capsule from which it had escaped, and it was not until the opening was enlarged from one half to three quarters of an inch that the reduction was accomplished. Dr. Fenner infers that the capsule possesses sufficient elasticity to allow the small head of the femur to pass out through a lacerated opening, which might at once contract so as to offer considerable resistance to its return, and that occasionally this is the true explanation of the difficulty in reduction." Although the existence of this degree of elasticity may be questioned, there can be no doubt that a close-fitting rent in the capsule is practically a "buttonhole," whether in the straight or flexed limb.

Among the details of these few cases will be found evidence of the efficacy of the flexion method, of its mode of action, and of the character of a difficulty which was sometimes insuperable by the old method of straight extension. They show that this difficulty may result from the interposition of capsule or muscle, or both, between the head of the bone and the socket, — or from a want of free aperture in the capsule; and that then the obvious resource of the surgeon is to enlarge the slit by circumduction. They show also the character of the intermuscular aperture between the rotators, which may require similar enlargement; and that it may sometimes be difficult to distinguish between these different impediments to reduction, — all of which yield to flexion, with circumduction if needed. All this is of the first interest to the surgeon, because it bears upon the question of reduction. The cases also contain evidence upon one or two points of minor interest and importance; namely, that dislocation may occur, not only with abduction as an element, as writers agree, but also by a direct thrust; and that in this case the socket need not be broken, as has been alleged.

Upon the ilio-femoral ligament I have based my theory of

hip dislocation, its classification, its mechanism and its reduction. Other bands of fascia, of capsule, and of muscle may indeed be incidentally concerned in confining the neck of the femur; but their action is a changing one, and secondary in importance. Divide the ilio-femoral ligament, leaving the rest of the tissues, and the mainstay of the characteristic deformity is gone. It is not difficult, indeed, still to work the limb into the semblance of a regular dislocation; but such displacements are exceptional, and their attitude is not constant. In short, they are irregular.

All that is most essential about hip dislocation and reduction may be learned from a pelvis and thigh-bone from which everything has been removed except the ilio-femoral ligament, with perhaps the obturator internus muscle and its subjacent capsule, although the last two can be spared.

The dissected capsule is a combination of membrane with fasciculi beautifully adjusted for universal motion, limited in all directions. The vessel-bearing and so called "ligamentum" teres within it is never strong, and is sometimes wanting; it is therefore unimportant in dislocation. Of the capsule itself the posterior part combines strength with great mobility, its pelvic insertion being far stronger than its femoral insertion. A general notion of the arrangement of the posterior part of the capsule may be had if we suppose that it is extended from the socket half way to the femur, being there reinforced by a thickened edge and tied to the trochanters by bands. The thick edge is represented by a fasciculus which is said to be "annular." It is parallel with the rim of the acetabulum, and midway of the capsule. It aids the pelvic half of the capsule in its effort to retain the head of the femur, and in the extended limb tightens it. It is tied to the trochanters by the ischio and pubo (or pectineo) femoral bands, which, as they pass from the pelvis to the trochanters, cross the annular ligament and are incorporated with it.[1] In these cross-bands lies the main strength of the femoral insertion of the posterior capsule. Between them, at a point between the trochanters, is its weakest part, — a mere membrane, supported by these fasciculi. It is often accidentally opened in dissection; and when torn along its margin, as sometimes happens in dislocation, after the bands are ruptured, the wide flap may occlude the socket as effectually as in Fenner's case.

But among these minor anatomical details connected with the posterior capsule, it is important not to lose sight of the main surgical facts. To these facts the ilio-femoral ligament is the key. It lies mostly in front. In an anterior view it is triangular, narrowest above. Its inner part, the ligament of Bertin, limits extension of the limb; its outer part limits eversion, while to the latter alone belongs the inversion of dorsal dislocation. The functions of its outer and inner portions are therefore largely distinct. The habitual action of the thigh tends to develop them separately. In fact, they can be easily distinguished by the direction of their fibres, some of the fibres of one branch being inserted into the other half way up. They are separated by a cribriform interval for vessels, corresponding to a frænum of soft capsule inside the joint, which adds to the thickness though little to the strength of the ligament. They vary in development in different subjects; the outer band is not unfrequently the more voluminous, and, as is stated in my paper, the whole ligament is sometimes of uniform thickness. In that case its margin acts as bands.

[1] The pubo and ischio femoral bands are best seen in extreme flexion, which in the recumbent subject brings the back and lower part of the capsule to the front, with the lesser trochanter above. Parallel lines then drawn from points on the pubes and the ischium, just above the socket and just below it, horizontally outward to the two trochanters respectively, will sufficiently indicate the two fasciculi, and the rectangular shape of the posterior capsule they enclose. In the extended limb they become oblique, and are no longer parallel.

In recent times the narrow ligament of Bertin has been generally described and recognized as the ilio-femoral ligament. It is but the inner part of it. Its outer band and even its triangular shape were scarcely known to modern anatomists, and were unknown in their surgical application to dislocation when I came across them in dissection.[1] I afterward found that while the Webers describe the ligament as simply triangular, the anatomist Winslow, and especially Weitbrecht, — still perhaps the highest authority on ligaments, — had described the "binæ divaricationes" a century and more ago. Thus much for the lower and sometimes distinctly forked insertion of the ilio-femoral ligament along the anterior intertrochanteric line of the femur.

The upper or pelvic insertion of this ligament is into the front of the inferior spinous process of the ilium, and also into the outside of this process, along a rough depression existing beneath the reflected tendon of the rectus, three-quarters of an inch or more in length.[2] All this part is thick, and arrests displacement directly upward. From this pelvic insertion the outer margin of the outer band runs to the trochanter major, and the inner margin of the inner band toward the trochanter minor. Together the two bands constitute the strongest ligament in the body. While it is not difficult by circumduction to tear the whole capsule on

[1] The only modern anatomy in which I find an allusion to the fan-shaped outline of the ilio-femoral ligament is that of Sappey, Paris, second edition, 1867. The first edition (1862) figures and describes only the ligament of Bertin. My photograph was taken in 1861 and published in 1869.

[2] This roughened surface, extending from the inferior spinous process outward, and in the normal oblique attitude of the pelvis a little upward, has been sometimes assigned by anatomists to the reflected tendon of the rectus. It belongs to the wide outside insertion of the powerful ilio-femoral ligament, to which the tendon is often attached by connective tissue only, having a comparatively small bony insertion beyond it.

either side up to the margin of the bands, these resist. In a strictly surgical point of view, the exact extent of their varying interval may have little importance; but in order to emphasize their separate normal functions, and especially the fact that the characteristic attitudes, the mechanism, and the reduction of hip dislocation are essentially dependent sometimes upon one of these sets of fibres and sometimes upon the other, I have given to the whole — as brief, and suggestive of its "binæ divaricationes" — the name (inverted) Y ligament.

THE MECHANISM OF FRACTURES OF THE NECK OF THE FEMUR.

FRACTURE OF THE NECK OF THE FEMUR.

IMPACTED FRACTURE OF THE BASE OF THE NECK, WITH EVERSION.

THE injury known as the "impacted fracture of the neck of the thigh-bone" has been well described by various writers. When it occurs, the neck, broken at or near its broad insertion into the head of the shaft, is driven into the loose cancellated tissue of the latter, and so fixed there that it sometimes requires a considerable force to withdraw it. That it may be a severe lesion, especially in the latter part of life, the numerous recent specimens to be found in museums sufficiently attest. In my own observation, while it is at least as frequent among elderly people as fracture of the neck within the capsule without impaction, the accident is comparatively common in middle life, and even later; and the bone is sometimes capable of uniting after a few months, with little deformity.

This fracture is characterized by shortening and eversion of the limb, sometimes so inconsiderable that we are obliged to accept a diagnosis based upon an almost imperceptible eversion, and a shortening of half an inch or less, by careful measurement.

The Museum of the Medical School of Harvard University contains a valuable collection of impacted fractures of the hip; and having through these specimens become familiar with the eversion exhibited by them in various degrees, I had my attention more carefully directed to the subject by the following not unusual case.

A gentleman slipped upon the ice before his door, and fell upon his hip. He walked up stairs with assistance, and was placed upon his bed. His attending physician, in the absence of any obvious shortening or eversion of the limb, entertained some doubt in regard to the nature of the injury, but after ten days, finding no improvement in the symptoms, — the pain and soreness having in fact increased, — requested me to see him. The local tenderness and pain on motion, together with a very slight eversion, — best seen on attempting to invert comparatively the two feet, — and a shortening of less than half an inch, led me to the conviction that the bone was slightly impacted; and I conceive this view to have been corroborated by callus subsequently felt about the trochanter, and by the length of time required for the recovery, — the patient having been confined to his bed a little more than two months, and unable to walk without crutches until after the lapse of four months.

Since that time I have had sufficient opportunities to satisfy myself that though this accident may be serious when it occurs late in life, it is by no means so to a middle-aged and healthy subject; that the impaction is sometimes slight, and its indications proportionably so; and that the following signs may be relied on as generally pathognomonic, — disability; pain and tenderness resulting from local violence, especially when applied laterally, as in a fall upon the hip; shortening and eversion, however slight; absence of crepitus; and lastly, the rotation of the trochanter through an arc of a circle of which the head of the bone is the centre, instead of upon the axis of the shaft, as in detached fracture of the neck.

The practical importance of readily identifying this fracture lies in the fact that its progress, as regards both time and good union, is in general more favorable than that of the unimpacted fractures; that though it is a comparatively common and disabling accident, it may exhibit little deformity; and lastly, that the object of extension in its treatment is to steady the limb, and not to draw it down.

The following details of the anatomical structure of the femur sustain the foregoing statements in respect to the shortening and eversion incident to this lesion.

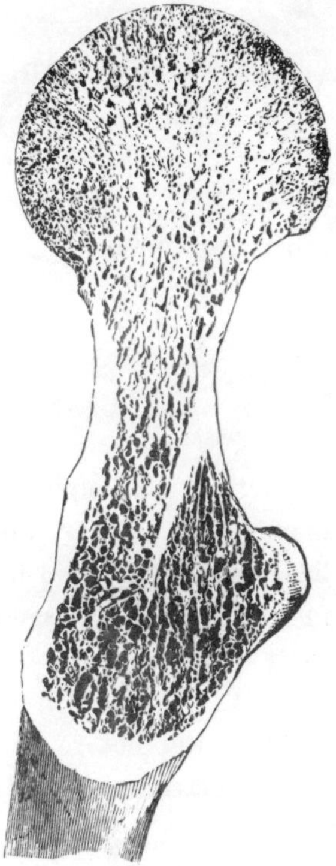

FIG. 1.[2]

ANATOMICAL STRUCTURE OF THE NECK OF THE FEMUR.

Let a well-developed femur be placed in a vice with its back toward the observer, in its natural upright position, but obliquely, as if the legs were widely separated, the shaft being so far inclined that the neck is horizontal. Let a first slice be now removed from the top of the head, neck, and trochanter by a saw carried horizontally through the neck. Let a second and third slice be removed in the same way, so that the neck shall be divided into four horizontal slices of equal thickness.[1]

It will be found that the upper section exhibits the anterior and posterior walls of nearly equal thickness; but that as we

[1] If the head of the bone be now vertically transfixed by a wire, the sections may be spread for examination like a fan.

[2] Fig. 1 exhibits a bird's-eye view of a horizontal section of the neck of the femur, showing the posterior wall plunging beneath the intertrochanteric ridge, at the angle where the neck joins the shaft. The posterior wall is of the thinness of paper, and here impaction occurs. The anterior wall, on the contrary, is seen to be quite thick, and forms by its fracture a hinge which is very rarely impacted.

approach the lower surface of the neck the anterior wall becomes of great thickness and strength, while the posterior wall remains thin, especially at its insertion beneath the posterior intertrochanteric ridge, where it is of the thinness of paper.

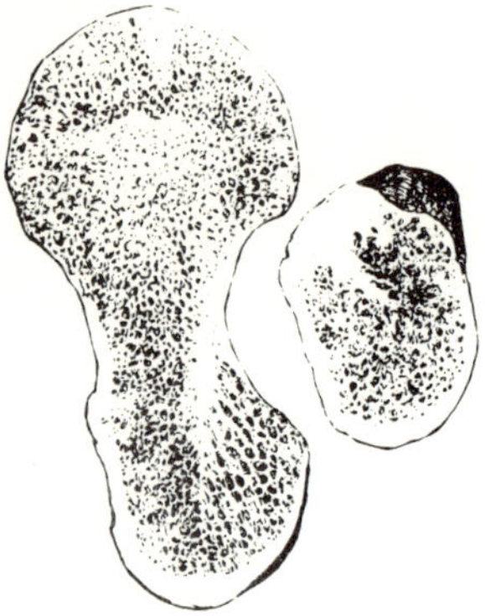

FIG. 2.[1]

ROTATION.

The result of this conformation is obvious. In impacted fracture, the thin posterior wall is alone impacted, while the thick anterior wall, refusing to be driven in, yields only as a hinge upon which the shaft rotates to allow the posterior impaction. This phenomenon, varying a little with the injury, is constant in every specimen of simple impacted fracture I have examined; and in fact it must be so from the arrangement of the bony tissues, which at once invites and explains the eversion.[2]

SHORTENING.

The hinge before alluded to is oblique, following the anterior intertrochanteric line. Were it vertical, by bending this

[1] The same as Fig. 1. The section of the shaft near the lesser trochanter shows the lower extremity of the septum, where the wall is thicker and changes its direction. (From a photograph taken in 1861.)

[2] M. Robert, in a memoir upon impacted fractures of the neck of the femur, attributes the posterior impaction to the supposed fact that the tangential plane of the external surface of the trochanter is inclined obliquely backward to the axis of the neck, and that a force applied to its centre would tend to increase the obliquity of this angle, and thus to produce outward rotation of the shaft. The shortening of the limb he attributes to the fact that the impaction is greatest at its lowest part. (Mémoire sur les Fractures du Col du Fémur accompagnées de Pénétration dans le Tissu Spongieux du Trochanter. Par Alphonse Robert, Professeur Agrégé, etc. Mémoires de l'Académie de Médecine, tom. xiii. p. 487.)

hinge we should produce rotation without shortening. On the other hand, if it were horizontal and transverse, bending it would produce shortening without rotation; but as it stands at an angle of 45°, the shaft rotating upon this broken interval is shortened in proportion to its rotation,—or, what is the same thing, the neck is reflected upon its hinge downward and backward till its axis normally oblique may become even transverse, with great outward rotation of the shaft and a shortening of perhaps two inches. This is probably the most common cause of shortening, although the head of the bone may be otherwise depressed.[1]

TRUE NECK.

Upon examining the lower of the above sections in a well-marked bone, the posterior or papery wall of the neck will be seen to be prolonged by radiating plates into the cancellous structure beneath the intertrochanteric ridge. That the thickest of these (Fig. 1) is a continuation of the true neck may be shown in another way. Let the whole of the posterior intertrochanteric ridge, including the back part of both trochanters, be removed by a narrow, thin saw. (Fig. 3.) The bone being now laid upon a table, let a chisel, or what is better a gouge, be held perpendicularly upon the cancellous structure thus exposed, and lightly twirled until the friable and spongy tissue is removed and the instrument arrested by the septum, or wall, alluded to. To expose its inner surface, the shaft should be split by a vertical and curved section behind this wall, and the cancellous structure removed in the same way.

The septum will then be distinctly seen as a thin, dense plate of bone continuous with the back of the neck and reinforcing it, plunging beneath the intertrochanteric ridge in an endeavor to reach the opposite and outer side of the shaft. At its lower

[1] See pp. 157, 161, 163.

extremity it curves a little forward, so as to take its origin when on a level with the lesser trochanter from the centre, instead of the back, of the cylindrical cavity, — a disposition easily seen in a transverse section of the shaft just above the trochanter minor. (Fig. 2.) Or it may be said that the posterior wall of the neck forks before reaching the intertrochanteric line, one layer being seen upon the surface, while the other dives beneath the intertrochanteric ridge in a vain

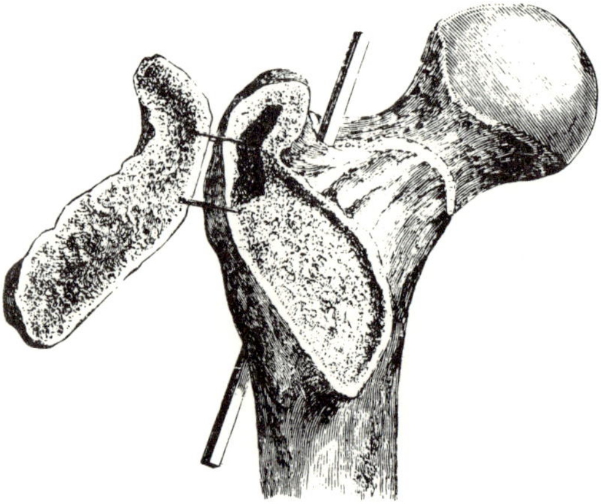

FIG. 3.[1]

attempt to reach the outer wall of the shaft. If these views be correct, the intertrochanteric ridge is simply a buttress erected for the insertion of muscles upon and over the true neck, by the impaction of which it is in fact often split off and detached in a mass,—the force exerted by the true neck, though slight, being nevertheless an effort to resist such impaction.

[1] Anatomy of impacted fracture. The intertrochanteric ridge has been removed, and the cancellous structure so excavated as to exhibit the true neck beneath. The rod is placed in a longitudinal fissure by which the shaft of the bone has been split, in order to exhibit the true neck from within. (From a photograph taken in 1861.)

REMARKS.

Surgical writers have been at some pains to indicate the distinguishing marks and tendencies of the so-called fractures "within" and "without the capsular ligament," — names which have but little practical significance. While the impacted fracture of the base of the femoral neck unites by bone, if at all, there seems to be a decreasing tendency to osseous union as we approach the smaller portion of the neck near its head, — a circumstance probably due in part to the feeble nutrition of the detached extremity, and in part to its mobility. The fact, which Sir Astley Cooper did not deny, that bony union is possible "within the capsular ligament"[1] and at the slenderer portions of the neck, is now sufficiently attested by existing specimens, our University Museum possessing two of these. But in examining specimens of such bony union it is often difficult to say just how far the fracture was originally within or without the capsule, because the exact position and limit of the capsule itself are variable;[2] and if we except the impacted fracture at the base, it is impossible during life, by any justifiable examination, to decide what part of the neck is broken, or whether the fracture has occurred within or without the capsule. Nor is it a matter of importance in the treatment, which is one and the same in both cases, or in prognosis, if the so-called varieties cannot be distinguished. In lecturing upon this subject, I have been in the habit of dividing the injuries of the neck of the femur into the impacted fracture of the base of the neck and the unimpacted fracture of the rest of the neck, without regard to the capsule, — a practical classification embracing a majority of cases, and to which the other lesions may be regarded as exceptional.

[1] Treatise, etc., pp. 137, 138.

[2] The Insertion of the Capsular Ligament of the Hip-Joint, and its Relation to Intra-Capsular Fracture. By George K. Smith, M.D., Demonstrator of Anatomy, etc. New York, 1862.

It is indeed possible for the small extremity of the neck to be impacted into the detached head, and so steadied by it as to favor union. Such was the injury in the specimens in our Museum described below. It is also possible for the base of the neck to be impacted with inversion; but in the large majority of cases, if there is a serious injury to the neck of the bone, it is either a common impacted fracture of the base of the neck, easily diagnosticated by the signs already described, or some other fracture, about which it is of no practical consequence in its treatment to know anything, except that it exists and needs extension.

In brief, the presence of excessive pain on motion leads to the suspicion of severe injury. The age of the patient; the shortened, everted, loosely hanging, and uncontrollable limb; crepitus, which when once felt is as satisfactory as if felt, to the detriment of the patient, many times, — and, lastly, the head of the trochanter rotating on the axis of the shaft and not through an arc, readily and quickly identify the unimpacted fracture. On the other hand, the impacted fracture of the base, which occurs in the adult at all ages, though more frequently in the latter half of life, is characterized by less local pain and disability, by shortening and eversion[1] (which may be slight), and by the absence of crepitus, while the trochanter rotates through an arc upon the articulation as a centre.

The importance of distinguishing between the different fractures of the neck of the femur is not so great as to justify any protracted or considerable examination. Flexion of the thigh, its repeated rotation, or other unscrupulous or unskilful handling, is liable to lacerate the remaining capsule, to displace the bony fragments, or, by loosening and detaching an impacted fracture, to render its union more difficult, — adding, perhaps,

[1] As before stated, a slight eversion is perhaps best indicated by a comparison of the extent to which the two limbs can be inverted.

to the accuracy of the diagnosis, but directly diminishing the chances of the patient.

The treatment of all these fractures is similar, — the unimpacted fracture obviously requiring extension, the purpose of which in the impacted fracture is to steady, not to elongate, the limb. Among the many expedients presented to the choice of the surgeon, I have for my own part found as good results, even in bad cases, from a flat bed, with a book or other weight attached to the foot for extension, and perhaps a broad band about the hips to steady the parts, and a cushion or pillow under the broken hip to prevent its eversion, as from more complicated and less comfortable apparatus. The prognosis of these fractures it is difficult to give. Elderly people may die of them at the end of a few weeks, or may linger many months. On the other hand, when the fracture is near the base of the neck, cases occur of recovery, with little lameness, both from the impacted and the unimpacted varieties, especially the former.

To facilitate a differential diagnosis, the principal lesions of this region will now be described.

IMPACTED FRACTURE OF THE BASE OF THE NECK WITH INVERSION.

This accident is of rare occurrence. Smith and Hamilton each cite but one case. Indeed, the structure of the bone, as has been shown, is such as to insure an almost uniform eversion of the shaft. A specimen from a dissecting-room has enabled me to examine this rare lesion, and to identify the conditions under which it probably occurred. In this subject (an old woman) the limb was flexed a little, shortened to the extent of three inches, and inverted so that the patella faced inward; the limb was in slight abduction, and could neither be everted nor brought to the median line. The trochanter was felt to be much thickened. Upon examination of this exceptional specimen, the neck of the bone was found to be firmly united at right angles with the shaft, which was split open and spread so widely as to receive the whole impacted neck, leaving a fissure an inch or more long and a quarter of an inch wide between the anterior wall and the neck, and extending nearly to the outer wall of the shaft, while another similar fissure existed behind the neck. The principal posterior fragment comprised the two trochanters with the intertrochanteric ridge, and also a large fragment of the external portion of the shaft, — while above, the region of the great trochanter seemed to have been comminuted and driven downward and inward. Anteriorly the fracture had occurred, as usual in impacted fracture, along the oblique spiral line, although differing from that injury, the neck being deeply driven in behind this wall, from which it had slipped instead of turning upon it as a hinge. The whole upper part of the bone above the trochanter minor seemed to have been bent inward, so that the posterior intertrochanteric line, instead of inclining obliquely to the axis of the shaft, was vertical. The inversion was due to the extent

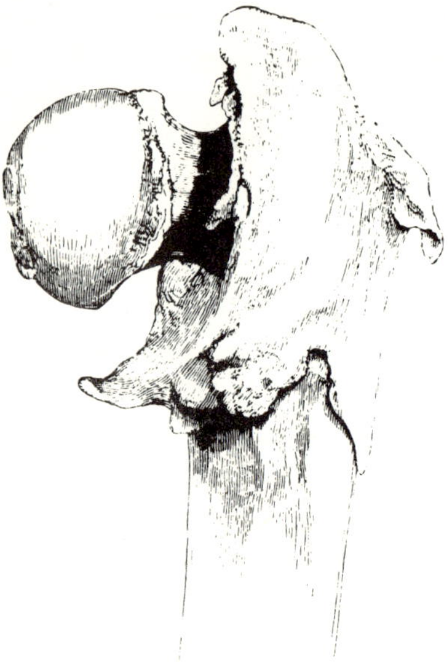

FIG. 4.[1]

[1] Figs. 4 and 5. — impacted fracture with inversion. Fig. 4, posterior view; Fig. 5, anterior view. The foreshortening fails to show the length of the tapering prolongation of the trochanter minor.

of the comminution, which had separated the walls of the shaft so as to receive in the interval the whole neck instead of the posterior wall only, as commonly occurs, — thus producing an anterior as well as a posterior impaction. The shortening resulted both from the horizontal position of the neck and from an additional upward displacement of the shaft caused by the comminution. A good deal of callus had been thrown out in various directions, and the movements of the limb must have been quite restricted. A curious spicula stood at right angles with the shaft near the lesser trochanter, and may have been a displaced fragment or the ossified insertion of the psoas tendon. The same bony spicula exists in another specimen before me, and is not uncommon.

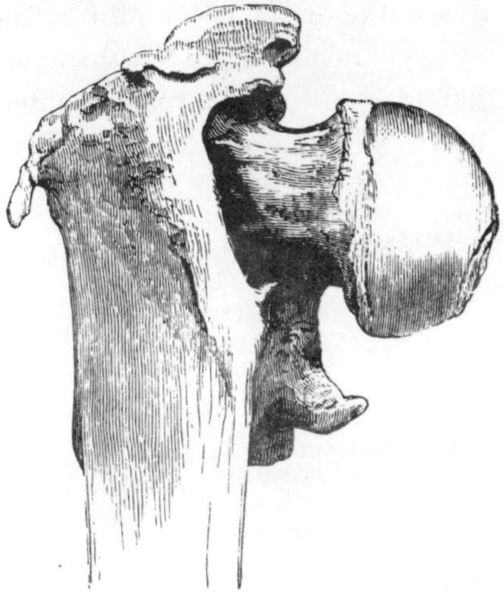

FIG. 5.

In examining the accompanying illustrations, it will be seen that the intertrochanteric ridge is split off, as often happens; but in this case it has carried with it the outer and posterior walls of the shaft, with the two trochanters.

Smith[1] (Case XLVI.) cites a similar case of inversion, which the accompanying figure shows to have resulted from a similar cause. The posterior intertrochanteric ridge, with the greater part of the two trochanters, has been detached in a

[1] A Treatise on Fractures in the Vicinity of Joints, etc. By Robert William Smith, M.D., M.R.I.A., etc. Philadelphia and Dublin, 1850. (See also Case XXXVII.)

mass, and so widely that the neck of the bone has slipped from its anterior hinge. In both specimens the impaction is arrested near the outer wall of the shaft. The entire neck in my specimen can be seen through the lateral fissures, while in that of Smith its extremity is detected through an interval of the fragments near the great trochanter. A similar specimen, numbered 248, in the Mütter Museum in Philadelphia, shows neither inversion nor eversion.

IMPACTED FRACTURE OF THE NECK OF THE FEMUR NEAR THE HEAD.

The following cases of impacted fracture of the femur near the head, — one resulting fatally, the other in complete recovery, with the exception of persistent pain, — may be regarded as instances of fracture fairly within the capsule. They illustrate not only the possibility of bony union of the detached articular extremity, but also the circumstances which contribute most frequently to its occurrence, — if, indeed, they are not essential to it. In two specimens (Nos. 2111 and 1540) in the Museum of the Medical School of Harvard University, of undoubted bony union after fracture of the femoral neck, the line of separation is near the head, which is tilted obliquely downward toward the lesser trochanter, as in the following cases.

A man aged seventy-six entered the Massachusetts General Hospital, March 9, 1863, under the charge of Dr. Gay, who has kindly furnished me with a record of this interesting case. The patient fell in the evening upon the sidewalk, striking the right trochanter. Feeling only that he had received a severe bruise, he crawled upstairs alone, and sat in his chair long enough to read his newspaper before going to bed. Two days after, he entered the Hospital. Upon examination, it appeared that the right leg was shortened half an inch; the foot was everted, and could not be inverted beyond the perpendicular; the thigh could be flexed and extended without difficulty, but with pain; the trochanter was less prominent than that of the other side. At the end of two weeks he died of pneumonia, at two o'clock in the afternoon; but at half past ten in the morning of that very day he had asked to have the splints removed, saying that the leg felt well, and at the same time lifting the whole limb several inches from the bed without assistance.

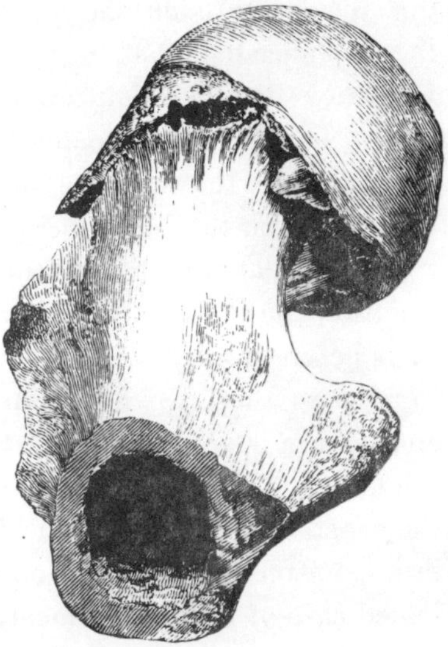

FIG. 6.[1]

In this interesting case, of which an excellent illustration is here given, the head was found to be broken from the articular extremity of the neck, which was short and thick, the fracture behind being almost at the line of junction of the articular cartilage and the bone, while in front it ran irregularly across the neck,

[1] Dr. Gay's case of impacted fracture near the head. In this specimen the neck of the bone was originally short and stout. Below and behind it the fracture follows, as nearly as may be, the line of the articular cartilage, while anteriorly and above it is about half an inch distant from this line. The impaction in the recent state was firm, the thin surface of the neck at its lower and posterior part having been driven into the cancellous structure of the head to the depth of about half an inch, while the cancellous structure of the head of the bone has penetrated to the depth of three quarters of an inch into that of the neck, this mutual impaction being very firm. The head rests obliquely upon the lower fragment, as if the shaft had been rotated outward, opening the anterior part of the fracture to the width of nearly a quarter of an inch.

from a quarter to half an inch below this line. The head was bent on the neck obliquely backward and downward toward the lesser trochanter,—the tilting of the head opening the fracture on the outside of the neck,— and was so firmly impacted that considerable force was required to withdraw it. The impaction was double, the shell of the neck being driven to the depth of half an inch into the head behind, while the centre of the head had entered the cancellous tissue of the shaft, being much the more dense of the two. The patient was evidently not aware of the existence of fracture, and it would have been impossible for the surgeon to infer before death the exact nature of the injury. It is fair to suppose that two bony fragments thus mutually impacted and held in apposition would have united by bony union had the patient lived, and in this case it cannot be doubted that the fracture was wholly within the capsule. An additional interest attaches to this specimen in connection with the subjoined case of fracture, almost identical with it in character, and presenting unequivocal bony union.[1]

The following case of bony union, in a fracture curiously resembling the preceding, occurred in the practice of Dr. Cushing, of Dorchester, Mass.,—a practitioner of large experience, whose opinion in respect to the general character of an injury of this sort would be entitled to weight, even were it not corroborated by the specimen here represented, the section of which shows unequivocal evidence of fracture. A woman seventy years of age, while reaching to wind up a clock, fell upon her side. Dr. Cushing, being called at once, found that although the limb was not obviously displaced, it was so dis-

[1] For a case of mutual impaction of the neck and head, but complicated with a second impaction, old or recent, of the base of the neck, see a paper by Thomas Bryant, F. R. C. S., etc., in the Medical Times and Gazette, May 1, 1869. As the result of this double impaction, there was "some shortening of the limb, but no eversion of the foot."

abled as to leave no doubt of the existence of a fracture. The patient was laid upon her back, with the knee flexed and two pillows beneath it. For two and a half or three months she kept her bed, and then began to sit up with the limb extended. Crutches were used for six months longer; then a crutch and a cane; but for the last two and a half years neither, the patient being able to go about the house and a little way out of doors. There was little, if any, shortening, and she limped but slightly. During the first few weeks she had much pain at the seat of the injury and in the limb, which was gradually atrophied. Her health was generally good until near her death, four years and eleven months after the accident, from internal disease.

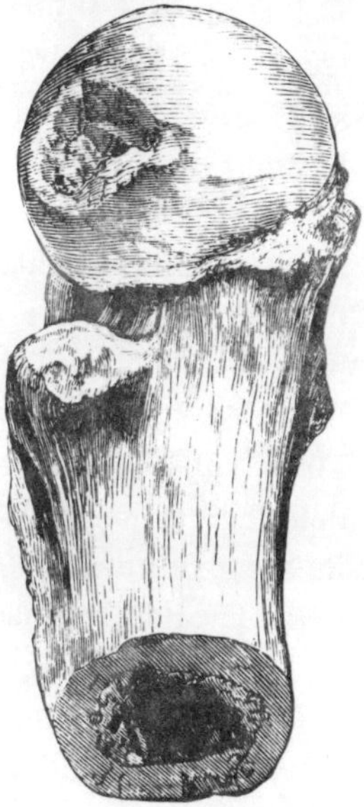

FIG. 7.[1]

In this instance, also, the neck of the femur is short and thick, — the line of fracture corresponding very nearly with that of the articular cartilage. The head of the bone has been depressed so that the neck is now nearly transverse, — the head being also bent obliquely backward and downward toward the lesser trochanter, and the shaft rotated outward. In front the neck of the bone projects beyond the articular cartilage, while behind it is buried beneath it, as in the preceding specimen. The neck is thus posteriorly impacted into the head, which in bending backward opens a fissure in front, filled with an irregular bony callus.

It was not observed in this case that the limb was everted, as the specimen implies. At the time of death the foot was

[1] Dr. Cushing's case of impacted fracture near the head, with bony union.

straight. Smith records a case (No. LVIII.) in which there was slight inversion.

COMMINUTED FRACTURE OF THE TROCHANTERS WITHOUT IMPACTION.

The alleged injury thus described detaches the entire neck from the shaft, and is generally represented in museums by specimens, the comminuted fragments of which are reunited in their normal position. Museum specimens of this fracture are less frequent than those of the common impacted fracture, and might be still more rare were it not that the impaction, which I conceive to be the rule in fracture at the base of the neck, does not always persist, being sometimes liberated by the extensive comminution of the bone, or by force subsequently applied. The impacted bones are undoubtedly separated, in many cases from want of care both in the examination and in the subsequent treatment of the patient, and likewise in the process of their preparation as specimens.

It is fair to suppose that local crepitus can be felt in the trochanteric region, so extensively comminuted. The lines of fracture present great variety. The anterior and posterior trochanteric walls, or either of them, may be detached entire or in fragments. The posterior intertrochanteric ridge may be split off partially or wholly, and the trochanter minor broken off by itself. The summit of the outer trochanter, and in fact the whole upper region of the shaft, may be comminuted and driven in as by a blow from above.

As in other fractures of this part, inversion of the limb is here the rare exception, and eversion the rule. Smith cites twenty-eight cases of extra-capsular fracture, of which four only were inverted. Assuming that anterior impaction is essential to inversion, we may seek the cause of the latter both in the direction of the blow received and in the action of the muscles. The influence of these is well illustrated in the case already detailed (Figs. 4, 5), where the mass of large and small rotators evert the upper fragment only, leaving the shaft to be inverted by the anterior fibres of the gluteus medius, and especially of the gluteus minimus, which is inserted lower down. This occurs when both the trochanters are detached, whether separately or (as in this specimen) in a single piece. Smith's four cases of inversion[1] sufficiently illustrate these points, as does also a specimen in the Chatham Museum,[2] where, in addition, "an arch of new osseous matter . . . extends from the anterior inferior spinous process of the haunch-bone across the joint to the upper part of the shaft of the thigh-bone," and which, it may be inferred from its insertions, was the Y ligament and the neighboring fibres (see Fig. 22, page 74 of this volume). Shortening not unfrequently results from mere depression of the neck without corresponding rotation of the shaft, as in the regular impacted fracture; and the transverse neck may then be displaced outward upon the shaft, so as to resemble a hammer upon its handle.

FRACTURE OF THE NECK OF THE FEMUR RESULTING IN FALSE JOINT.

The frequency of this lesion is attested by the common museum preparations, showing the hemispherical head of the bone slipping upon the absorbed and shortened neck, or upon a broader surface with more restricted motion nearer the shaft. In the latter case the lower surface of the neck

[1] A Treatise on Fractures in the Vicinity of Joints, etc. Cases XXIX., XXXVII., XXXIX., XLVI.

[2] See the third Fasciculus of Anatomical Drawings, etc., Army Medical Museum of Chatham; also, A Case of Fracture of the Neck and Trochanter of the Thigh-bone with Inversion, etc. By George Gulliver. Edinburgh Medical and Surgical Journal, vol. xlvi. p. 312. 1836.

not unfrequently rests upon a bony projection near the lesser trochanter. False joint is a frequent result of unimpacted fracture, and is not to be averted by any special form of apparatus.

CRACK IN THE NECK OF THE FEMUR.

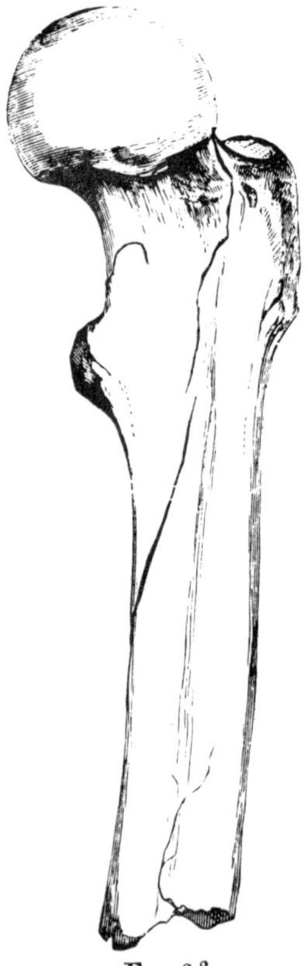

FIG. 8.[2]

It is obvious that while a simple crack or fissure of the femur would produce no immediate deformity, it might yet give rise, as in the radius at the wrist, to lameness and inflammation of long duration, with corresponding obscurity of diagnosis. The tendency of glass tubes and other brittle cylinders to crack in a spiral line is well known; and M. Gerdy has remarked upon the occurrence of oblique or spiral fissures in the long bones, producing at their intersection acute angles like the letter V. Those of the tibia sometimes exhibit a singular symmetry and mutual resemblance.[1] The annexed woodcut (Fig. 8) represents a portion of a left femur from a patient who died under my care at the Massachusetts General Hospital, of fracture and internal injuries. The specimen is now in the Museum of the Medical School of Harvard University, and has been described by

[1] See Pratique Journalière de la Chirurgie, p. 67. Par Adolphe Richard, Chirurgien de l'Hôpital Beaujon, etc. Paris, 1868.

[2] Crack of the femoral neck. Near the lesser trochanter is seen the hook-like extremity of the fissure, separated by a narrow interval of bone from the main line of fracture.

Dr. J. B. S. Jackson, Dr. Mussey, and Dr. Hamilton. The femur is large and well marked. A spiral fracture ascends the shaft and winds round the neck, completely detaching it, except at a narrow isthmus in front half an inch wide.

The shaft is broken transversely, eight inches below the trochanter. Here a spiral fissure begins, near the linea aspera, and winds upward and inward to the front of the bone, crossing the anterior intertrochanteric line midway between the trochanters; thence vertically upward to the outer edge of the cartilage; thence transversely across the top of the neck to its posterior surface, here touching the cartilage again; thence vertically down behind the neck to a point half an inch from the lesser trochanter, terminating on the under side of the neck in an S-shaped extremity, half an inch from the point where the fissure crosses the intertrochanteric line in front. The elastic bony pedicle thus formed allows a slight springing motion of the head, but maintains it firmly in place.

THE TRUE NECK OF THE FEMUR: ITS STRUCTURE AND PATHOLOGY.[1]

I. STRUCTURE.

SOME of the later numbers of Virchow's Archives contain a protracted yet interesting discussion upon the interior structure of bones, notably of the head of the femur. According to Merkel,[2] G. H. Meyer, in 1867, pointed out certain arching fibres in their cancellated structure as "a well-marked architecture, which stands in the closest relation to the static and dynamic forces of the bones."

In 1870,[3] Wolff made further investigation of this subject; and in addition, this writer incorporated into his paper certain elaborate mathematical calculations of Culmann, of Zurich, showing that interior braces intended to aid in supporting a weight upon the end of a cylinder, curved like the thigh-bone, or like a crane or derrick, should be placed, in order to act to best advantage, precisely where the trabeculæ of the spongy tissue of this bone actually exist. "Nature," says Wolff, "has built the spongy bones as an engineer would construct a truss bridge, mathematically."

This recent German investigation, apart from the mathematical calculation which Merkel avows his inability to follow, was anticipated, so long ago as 1850, by the late Professor

1 The Boston Medical and Surgical Journal, Jan. 7, 1875.

2 Virchow's Archives, 1874; vol. lix. p. 237.

3 Ibid., 1870; vol. l. p. 389.

Jeffries Wyman, who, in a comprehensive article upon this subject,[1] reached the following conclusions: —

"1. The cancelli of such bones as assist in supporting the weight of the body are arranged either in the direction of that weight, or in such a manner as to support and brace those cancelli which are in that direction. In a mechanical point of view, they may be regarded in nearly all these bones as a series of 'studs' and 'braces.'

"2. The direction of the fibres in some of the bones of the human skeleton is characteristic, and, it is believed, has a definite relation to the erect position, which is naturally assumed by man alone.

"These structures are most clearly defined in adult and middle-aged skeletons."

Dr. Wyman illustrates his paper by diagrams alone sufficient to demonstrate, even to a common mechanic, an advantageous adaptation of means to end. An internal structure, shown to be rectangular in the vertebræ, radiating in the tarsal bones, and arched in the neck of the femur, obviously offers economical resistance to the weight it is designed to carry. But if doubt be still entertained, the laborious calculations of Culmann, assumed to be correct, establish the fact absolutely, so far as the femoral neck is concerned.

Thus much for the spongy structure of the bones in general (Fig. 1). We are now to consider an arrangement peculiar to the interior of the neck of the thigh-bone. According to Merkel, a section of this may be seen in an illustration designed for another purpose, many years ago, by Pirogoff, who, however, does not allude to it. In 1870,[2] Wolff speaks of it as "a compact tissue beneath the trochanter minor."

In 1874, in an able paper largely devoted to its description,

[1] Boston Journal of Natural History, 1850; vol. vi. No. 1, p. 125. Report of the Committee on Medical Sciences; Transactions of the American Medical Association, 1850.

[2] Virchow's Archives, 1870; vol. l. p. 389.

Merkel[1] calls this compact tissue the "calcar femorale," "schenkelsporn," or thigh-spur. The special object of Merkel's paper is to prove the predominant importance of this tissue in sustaining the weight of the body, and to show that the strength of the neck of the femur is mainly due to this dense tissue, and not to the braces of Wolff and Culmann. Although a little embarrassed by variations of the "spur," as it appears in different preparations, "being in some straight, in others curved," he insists strongly

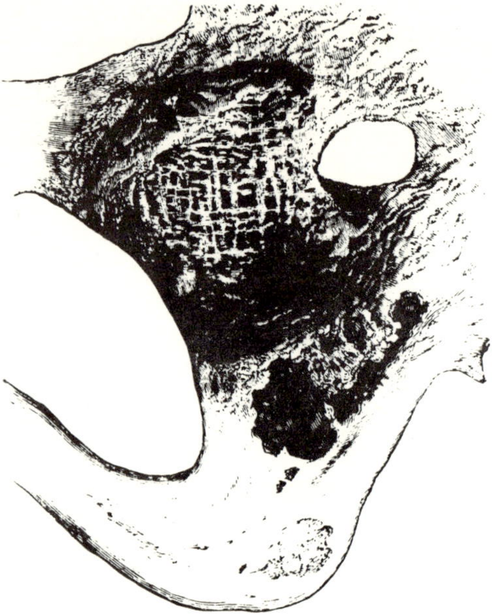

FIG. 1.[2]

1 Virchow's Archives, 1874; vol. lix. p. 237.

2 A specimen showing repair of the acetabulum after hip disease is here figured. The subject in which it was found, a boy of a dozen years, was from the dissecting-room. Large sinuses still remained open. The head and neck of the femur had disappeared, and the trochanters were united to the ilium by a narrow isthmus of bone, an inch above and behind the socket. The latter is filled with a curious right-angled net-work, extending to some depth, the explanation of which is not obvious; and whether it be sought in the influence of a neighboring rectangular spongy tissue toward the spine of the ischium, or in prolonged fibres of the vertical ramus of the ischium and the horizontal one of the pubes interlaced beyond their normal boundary in the healthy socket, or lastly in some accidental traction upon tissue afterward ossified, the interpretation is equally unsatisfactory. At the bottom of the figure is the tuberosity. A perforation near the socket was in the track of a sinus.

upon its teleological importance; doubting whether the arrangement of the spongy tissue possesses the same significance, because the calcaneum of man and that of the ox, as shown by Wolfermann, really perform very different functions, although they offer a similar internal structure, — a statement equally true of the spongy system generally. On the other hand, Wolff, in a second paper,[1] replies that "the calculations of Culmann prove that the 'spur' is not at the point of greatest strain, nor yet where strength is most needed;" that "Merkel's theory in no way agrees with Culmann's calculations, which may be accepted as beyond controversy;" and that "Merkel has ascribed to the 'spur' a wholly erroneous importance."

In the following foot-note,[2] Merkel again insists upon his views: —

> "While these sheets are being printed, I have received the work of Bigelow upon the Mechanism of Dislocation and Fracture of the Hip, translated by Pochhammer (Berlin, Hirschwald), in which the *schenkelsporn* is both described and figured; he does not, however, follow out the significance of the structure."

Before again expressing my own opinion of the purpose of the bony plate in question, it may not be amiss to cite here the description alluded to by Merkel, especially as I do not discover that anything of importance has been added to it since its publication in 1869: —

ANATOMICAL STRUCTURE OF THE NECK OF THE FEMUR.[3]

Let a well-developed femur be placed in a vice with its back toward the observer, in its natural upright position, but obliquely, as if the legs were widely separated, the shaft being so far inclined

1 Virchow's Archives, 1874; vol. lxi. p. 417.

2 Ibid., 1874; vol. lix. p. 251.

3 Mechanism of Dislocation and Fracture, etc., p. 120. Philadelphia, Henry C. Lea. 1869. (See p. 141 of this volume.)

that the neck is horizontal. Let a first slice be now removed from the top of the head, neck, and trochanter, by a saw carried horizontally through the neck. Let a second and third slice be removed in the same way, so that the neck shall be divided into four horizontal slices of equal thickness.[1]

It will be found that the upper section exhibits the anterior and posterior walls of nearly equal thickness, but that, as we approach the lower surface of the neck, the anterior wall becomes of great thickness and strength, while the posterior wall remains thin, especially at its insertion beneath the posterior intertrochanteric ridge, where it is of the thinness of paper (Fig. 2).

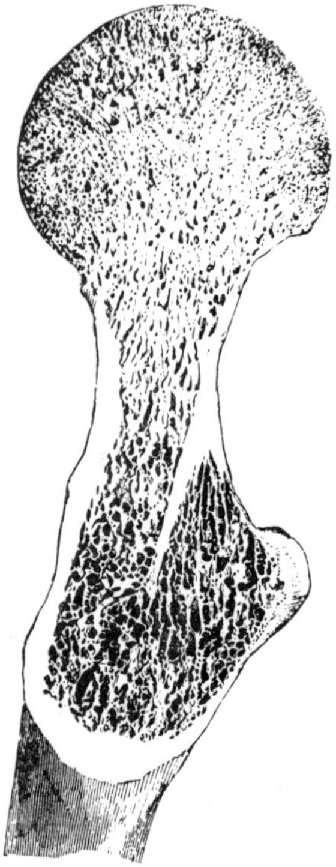

Fig. 2.[2]

TRUE NECK.

Upon examining the lower of the above sections in a well-marked bone, the posterior or papery wall of the neck will be seen to be prolonged by radiating plates into the cancellous structure beneath the intertrochanteric ridge. That the thickest of these is a continuation of the true neck may be shown in another way. Let the whole of the posterior intertrochanteric ridge, including the back part of both trochanters, be removed by a narrow, thin saw. The bone being now laid upon a table, let a chisel, or what is better a gouge, be

[1] If the head of the bone be now vertically transfixed by a wire, the sections may be spread for examination, like a fan.

[2] Exhibits a bird's-eye view of a horizontal section of the neck of the femur, showing the posterior wall plunging beneath the intertrochanteric ridge, at the angle where the neck joins the shaft. The posterior wall is of the thinness of paper, and here impaction occurs. The anterior wall, on the contrary, is seen to be quite thick, and forms by its fracture a hinge which is very rarely impacted.

held perpendicularly upon the cancellous structure thus exposed, and lightly twirled until the friable and spongy tissue is removed, and the instrument arrested by the septum, or wall, alluded to. To expose its inner surface, the shaft should be split by a vertical and curved section behind this wall, and the cancellous structure removed in the same way (Fig. 4).

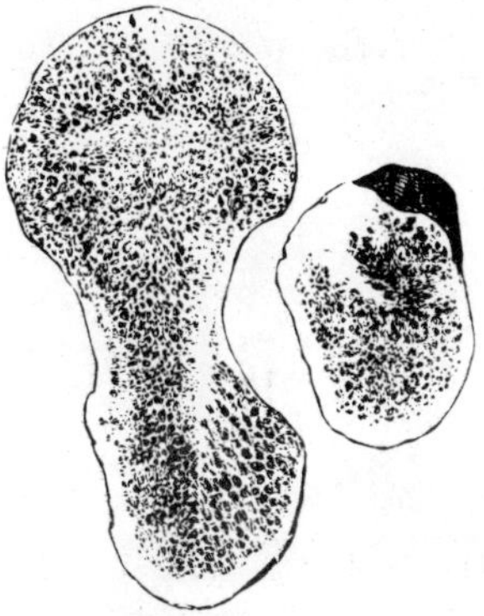

FIG. 3.[1]

The septum will then be distinctly seen as a thin, dense plate of bone continuous with the back of the neck, and reinforcing it, plunging beneath the intertrochanteric ridge in an endeavor to reach the opposite and outer side of the shaft. At its lower extremity it curves a little forward, so as to take its origin, when on a level with the lesser trochanter, from the centre, instead of the back, of the cylindrical cavity, — a disposition easily seen in a transverse section of the shaft just above the trochanter minor (Fig. 3). Or it may be said that the posterior wall of the neck forks before reaching the intertrochanteric line,— one layer being seen upon the surface, while the other dives beneath the intertrochanteric ridge in a vain attempt to reach the outer wall of the shaft. If these views be correct, the intertrochanteric ridge is simply a buttress erected for the insertion of muscles upon and over the true neck, by the impaction of which it is in fact often split off and detached in a mass, — the force exerted by the true neck, though slight, being nevertheless an effort to resist such impaction.

As regards ordinary spongy tissue, the teleological question is satisfactorily answered in either of two ways. We may attribute its architecture to that immediate necessity which in pathology builds a buttress to support a bone curved by

[1] The same. A section of the shaft near the lesser trochanter shows the lower extremity of the septum, where the wall is thicker and changes its direction. (From a photograph taken in 1861.)

rickets or weakened by fracture, or explain it by a general principle of conformation, in a measure automatic, developed in the lapse of generations by a frequently recurring necessity, and still continuing to act without immediate stimulus.

But the purpose of the osseous plate, whose structure and pathology it is the main object of this paper to discuss, may be at first a little less obvious. It plainly adds a certain strength to the bone; and yet in most bones it terminates beneath the trochanters in papery lamellæ wholly inadequate to lend it material support. It is usually united, even to the trochanters, only by a delicate wall and spongy tissue. It obeys the laws of similar bony structure, being feebly developed in childhood; while later in life, its absence in the femoral neck impresses us, as do bone-sections generally, with the truth of the observation of Henle, — that the so-called brittleness of age depends not so much on the loss of animal substance as upon the atrophy of the bony walls and anterior structure.

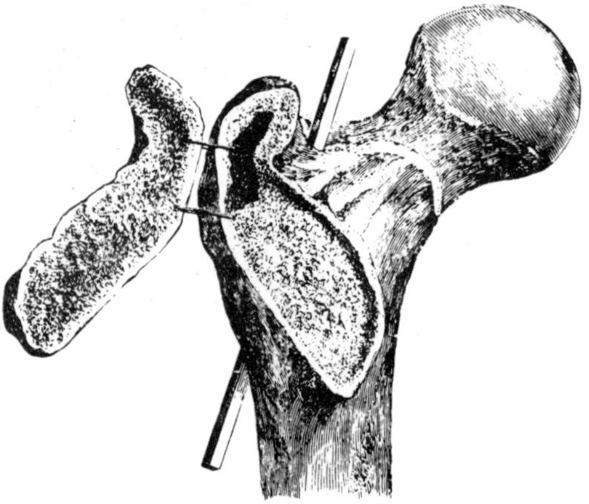

FIG. 4.[1]

These varying appearances might well leave us in doubt as to the purpose of this osseous plate; but no doubt can exist

[1] Anatomy of impacted fracture. The intertrochanteric ridge has been removed, and the cancellous structure so excavated as to exhibit the true neck beneath. The rod is placed in a longitudinal fissure by which the shaft of the bone has been split, in order to exhibit the true neck from within. (From a photograph taken in 1861.)

in the mind of one who examines an exceptionally well-marked adult bone. Such a bone fell under my observation in 1861 (Fig. 4). The dense plate is there a continuation of the neck, completing the interval everywhere except at its upper part. In this form it adds greatly to the strength of this part of the femur, while the trochanters and their ridge erected upon it both reinforce it and give attachment to the muscles.

This may be again shown. In a back view of the femur (Fig. 5) the neck appears as a pyramid, with its base to the trochanters.

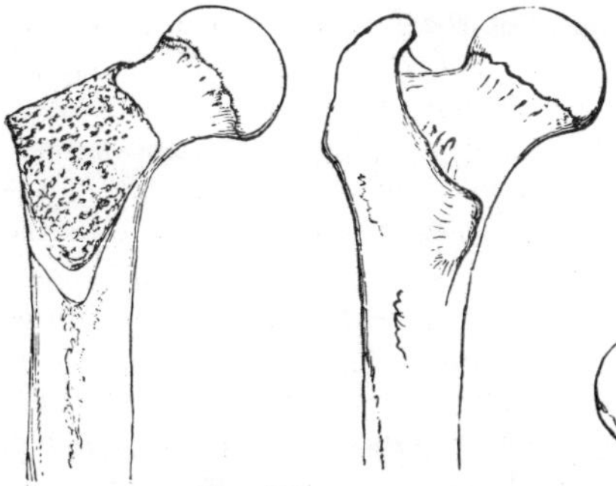

FIG. 5.[1]

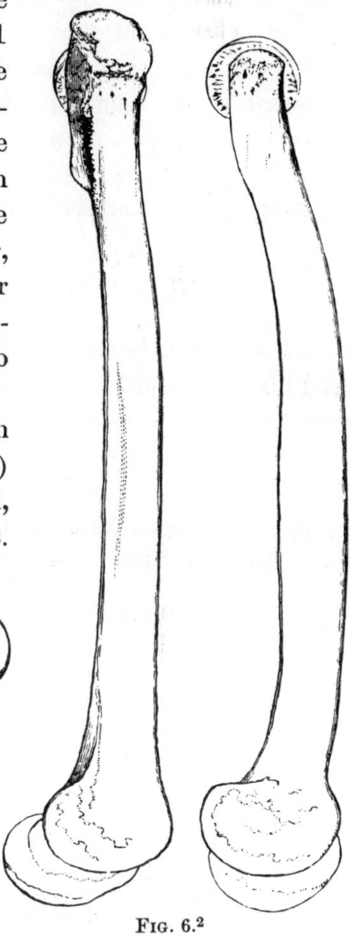

FIG. 6.[2]

[1] Rear view of left femur with and without the trochanters. The removal of these, in the left-hand figure, exposes the true neck.

[2] Side view of the same. While these views are designed to exhibit the true neck, it is not denied that the trochanteric shell helps to stiffen the curving shaft and to sustain any weight resting upon the head of the bone; especially through the intervention of the upper and horizontal part of the neck.

The cylindrical shaft also spreads as it rises to meet the trochanters. In a side view (Fig. 6) it is seen that both these cylinders, joined at their bases, are flattened from front to back, and are continuous in shape and direction, although surmounted at their junction by the trochanteric prominences. If we now remove the trochanters with their connecting ridge (Figs. 5 and 6), it may be again observed that what we have called the true neck maintains the continuity of the shaft. It no longer resembles a "spur," with its edge exposed by excavating the wall, as in Merkel's preparations. Thus denuded, the shaft has an air of symmetrical strength. It is flattened to resist weight, like a bone curved by disease, while the trochanters seem to have been added for a different purpose (Fig. 7).[1]

Unfortunately, bones like that above alluded to are rare. The true neck is often at best but an ineffectual attempt to bridge the interval beneath the trochanters, as seen in Merkel's figures; while in the latter half of life it degenerates

[1] Diagram of a section of the head of the femur of a sheep, showing a deep trochanteric fossa. If this fossa were filled with spongy tissue (as seen beneath the dotted line), the posterior neck would be partially concealed, as in the human femur. The analogy, whether true or not, is too striking to be overlooked. A deeper fossa exists in certain animals, especially South African ruminants, of which I examined sections in the Hunterian Museum in 1868. In this specimen the tendon inserted at the bottom of the fossa is prolonged into the spongy tissue by radiating lamellæ, which intersect concentric arches as represented in the diagram, and resist traction to great advantage.

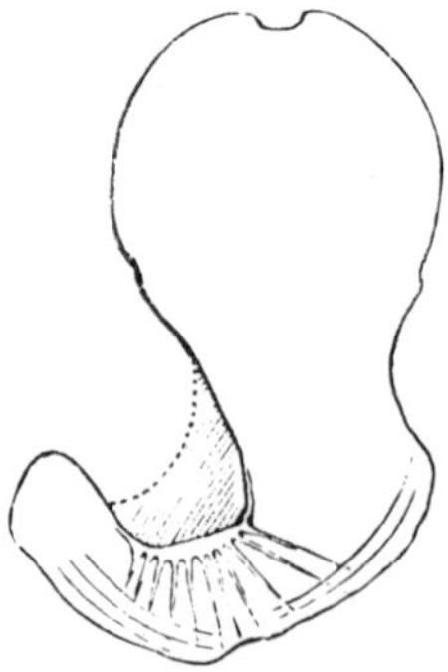

FIG. 7.

In examining a number of preparations lately made by my friend Dr. Dwight, I am satisfied that the tendency of what I have called the true neck is to attach itself below, where it becomes thin, as a tangent to the inside of the cylinder of the shaft; and also that it may be tolerably well pronounced in a subject six or eight years of age.

into papery plates, radiating downward from a point near the lesser trochanter.

Weakened in this way both by its own tenuity and by its slender union to the trochanteric ridge, the true neck has great practical interest for the surgeon. Even the adult femur is generally defective in construction at this point; and here occurs the most common form of fracture,—namely, the posterior impacted fracture of the base of the neck.

II.—PATHOLOGY.

IMPACTED FRACTURES.

POSTERIOR IMPACTED FRACTURE OF THE BASE OF THE CERVIX.

THE posterior impacted fracture of the base of the cervix often occurs in old people. I have met with it also in middle life, and do not hesitate to express the belief that it is the most common of the fractures of the neck of the thigh-bone. That

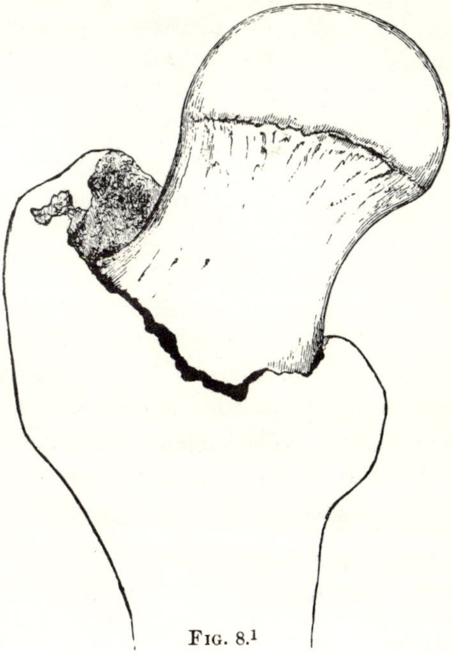

FIG. 8.[1]

[1] Front view of right femur, showing the fractured cervix bending like a hinge at the anterior intertrochanteric line, to allow the posterior impaction. The head of the bone leans more distinctly from the observer than the perspective indicates.

it has not been so considered may be explained by the following considerations: —

1. It has been generally recognized only of late years.
2. The injury may be a comparatively slight one.

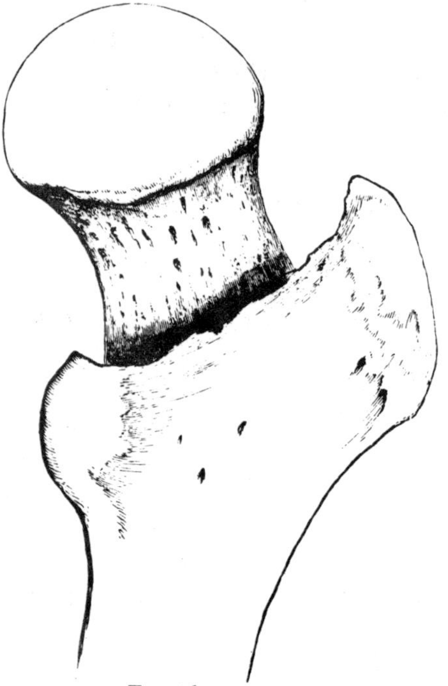

Fig. 9.[1]

3. Its signs are in some cases a shortening and eversion hardly perceptible.
4. When it unites, there may be no lameness to attract subsequent attention.
5. When it proves fatal before union, the impaction may have been disengaged by manipulation or otherwise, during life or after death,—especially by macerating the specimen for preservation.
6. On the other hand, unimpacted fracture of the small part of the neck, usually supposed to be most common, is marked by prominent symptoms. It entails great and persistent lameness, inviting attention and examination after death, however remote, and the specimen when obtained is unmistakable.

The displacement varies greatly in degree. One wall only — the posterior one — is impacted at the intertrochanteric

[1] Rear view of same, showing the cervix impacted beneath the posterior intertrochanteric line. The head of the bone leans toward the observer.

line, where the bone is a mere shell, driving the true neck, or the remains of it, farther beneath the trochanters, and sometimes detaching the latter. The firm anterior wall resists impaction, but bends at the line of fracture as a hinge. If this hinge were vertical, the shaft would be only everted; while if it were transverse, the neck would be only bent and the leg shortened. But as the hinge stands at an angle of about 45°, shortening and eversion are nearly equal (Figs. 8, 9, 10). Impaction, when slight, is detected by a difficulty of inverting the foot rather than by actual eversion; and the shortening may seem doubtful.

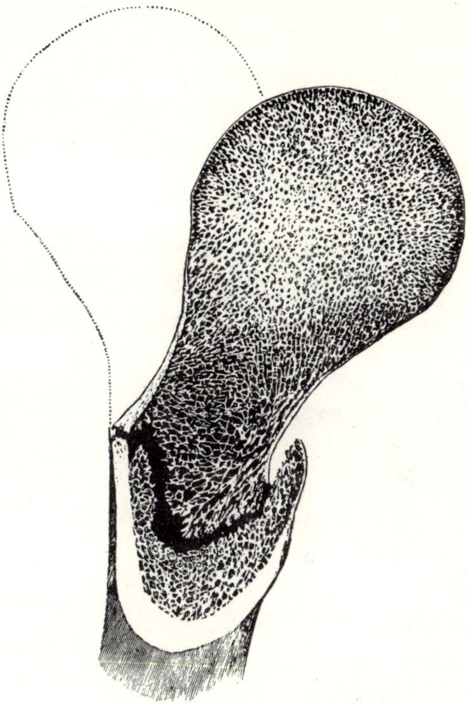

FIG. 10.[1]

It is needless to say that the rotated trochanter still sweeps through an arc of which the head of the femur is the centre, and that there is no crepitation.

[1] Horizontal section of the same, showing the anterior hinge and the posterior impaction. The dotted line shows the normal position of the head. The patient who furnished the specimen from which these figures were taken was seventy-two years of age. It will be seen that the prolongation of the true neck has disappeared by senile atrophy, leaving only a few radiating lamellæ. The specimen is of exceptional interest as showing this form of impaction with little comminution or other injury of the bone.

Shortening and eversion, however inconsiderable, point directly to this lesion. A large number both of cases and of specimens are referrible to this type, — impaction behind, with a hinge in front, each at its respective intertrochanteric line. In some of these specimens the neck is bent down nearly to a right angle with the shaft.

The remaining varieties of fracture of the femoral neck are susceptible of classification, and deserve, for the purpose of comparison, to be mentioned in this connection.

IMPACTED FRACTURE OF THE HEAD OF THE FEMUR.

The impacted fracture of the head of the femur is rare, and I do not believe it possible to distinguish it from that just described, even if it were desirable to do so. In three cases I have known there was the same shortening and eversion, and the same comparative ability to move the limb. A woman who died of the injury was able at all times to get into and out of bed with but little assistance, and the trochanter, when rotated, swept through its arc. There was no union. The small extremity of the cervix was rather "rebated" than impacted with the head of the femur, and the fracture was "within the capsular ligament"[2] (Fig. 11).

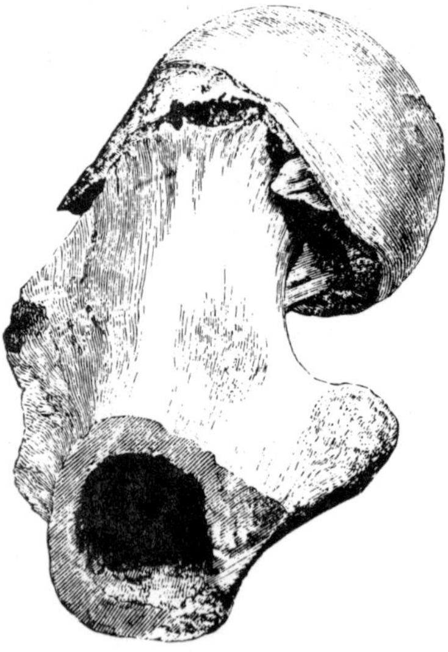

FIG. 11.[1]

[1] Impacted fracture of the head of the femur. The patient who furnished this specimen died of pneumonia in two weeks.

[2] See extracts from the Proceedings of the Society for Medical Improvement; Boston Medical and Surgical Journal, No. 1 (1875), p. 20.

The firmness of the fragments in such a case is chiefly due to the dense central cone of spongy tissue which projects from the head of the bone and impacts itself in the friable cavity of the cervix. If the cylinder of the cervical portion is simultaneously impacted into the head of the femur, around the base of the cone, immobility is doubly insured.

I have elsewhere expressed the opinion that these conditions are essential to the very exceptional occurrence of bony union of the small part of the cervix. In default of anchylosis the neck is doubtless absorbed, presenting after a time the familiar conditions of an old "ununited fracture." So that permanent lameness may result from a fracture which, by simulating impaction of the base, promises, at first, bony union, with comparatively little deformity.

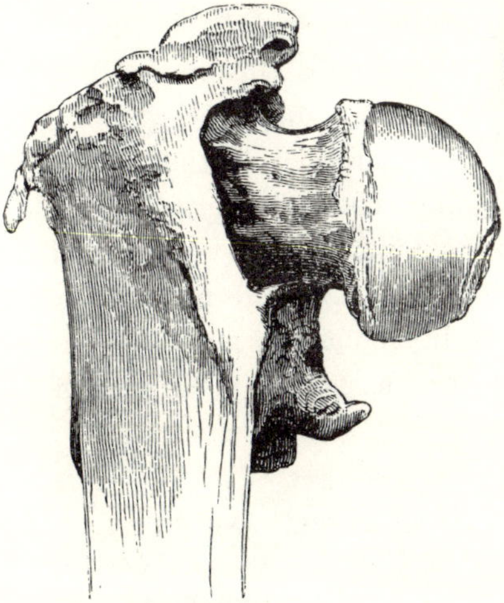

Fig. 12.[1]

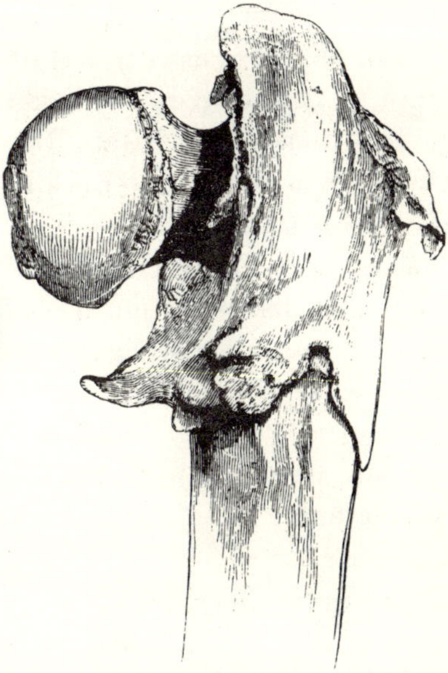

Fig. 13.

[1] Figs. 12 and 13, — impacted fracture of the base with inversion. The anterior view (Fig. 12) shows the neck slipped off its thick hinge, into the cavity of the shaft. To allow this, the whole trochanteric mass must have been detached, as seen in the rear view (Fig. 13).

IMPACTED FRACTURE OF THE WHOLE BASE OF THE CERVIX, WITH INVERSION.

The very rare impacted fracture of the neck with inversion, instead of eversion which is the rule, occurs when the neck in front slips off its hinge into the cavity of the shaft. This is hardly possible, as I have elsewhere shown, unless the whole posterior intertrochanteric mass, including the trochanters, is fairly detached (Figs. 12, 13).

UNIMPACTED FRACTURES.

FRACTURE OF THE SMALL PART OF THE CERVIX OF THE FEMUR.

THE fracture of the small part of the cervix of the femur, which has been usually described as the most common fracture of elderly persons, and erroneously as deriving importance from being within the capsular ligament, is a loose fracture, with no interlocking to maintain the immobility of the small extremities, even were they disposed to bony union. Familiarly characterized by increased motion, great pain and disability, much shortening, marked eversion, and the rotation of the shaft upon its axis instead of through an arc, it is not likely to be mistaken even at first sight. But its relations to the capsular ligament are probably uncertain, owing to differences in the size and insertions of the latter.

COMMINUTED FRACTURE OF THE TROCHANTERS AND SHAFT.

Lastly, when the trochanteric portion of the femur is comminuted, the detached neck and head of the bone may be very variously placed in bony union, both as to angle and as to the part which becomes subsequently attached to the shaft.

In completing the list of injuries to be borne in mind while examining a hip with reference to impacted fracture, we may enumerate dislocation, sprain, crack, the rare separation of the epiphyses, and the fracture of the acetabulum into the pelvis.

TREATMENT.

A few words of a practical character may be added here. Apart from dislocation, the main object of examination is to decide, with reference to treatment, whether a fracture is loose or impacted. I have demonstrated here and elsewhere the following points, illustrating the difficulty of further diagnosis: —

1. The common impacted fracture of the base of the neck and the rare one of the head may be indistinguishable from each other.

2. A fracture seemingly impacted and promising bony union may yet result in ligamentous union with corresponding lameness.

3. In loose fractures with great shortening, it may be sometimes difficult to distinguish a fracture of the small part of the neck, which does not promise bony union, from that of the trochanters, which does.

But while an accurate diagnosis of such cases is sometimes absolutely impossible, no embarrassment need be felt in the treatment of these injuries. Their treatment is simple.

If to extend a limb means to draw it down, impacted fracture and whatever resembles it should never be extended, but only steadied by weight or splint. On the other hand, a loose fracture with decided shortening should be first drawn down to something like its normal length. Or, more briefly, treatment consists in immobility, with the previous extension of a loose fracture.

A careful review of these injuries thus leads back to a practical rule already usually adopted. But it leads further, and demonstrates conclusively that prolonged and active flexion and rotation of the hip, in search of positive signs, is more than superfluous. Without anæsthesia it entails needless suffering; and with or without it, by loosening impaction or lacerating tissues, it may be disastrous.

The question of dislocation settled, a very brief and gentle examination is alone admissible, — chiefly to determine (1) the degree of shortening; (2) whether the shaft rotates through an arc or on its axis. The most useless and damaging examination is that by quick and persistent rotation, and by flexion of the thigh as far as a right angle.

The prognosis, if the patient lives, is favorable for bony union, except in the case of loose fracture of the small part of the cervix, which, if not readily distinguished, should be disturbed as little as possible.

Familiarity with the posterior impacted fracture of the base of the neck will remove the most frequent source of doubt in the diagnosis of injuries of this region; and the sooner the old classification of "intra and extra capsular fractures" is abandoned, the better it will be for science, for diagnosis, and for treatment. In the interest of the patient and of treatment the question should be, "Is the fracture loose or impacted?" and science is often compelled to rest satisfied when this is settled.

FRACTURE OF THE NECK OF THE THIGH-BONE.[1]

Few accidents are more common or more important than this; and few give rise to greater doubt in diagnosis. I aim in this lecture at such a general view of the subject as will be useful to you in practice.

The fractures of the head of the femur, or, as they are usually called, of "the hip," are tolerably well recited in the books. The principal ones are three in number. First, the so-called fracture within the capsular ligament, which I call fracture of the middle of the neck; and, second, two others,—the impacted fracture of the base of the neck, and the impacted fracture of the upper end of the neck; the one being an impaction of the neck into the trochanters, the other an impaction of the neck into the head of the bone.

This leaves for further consideration only the irregular fractures, or set of fractures, about the trochanters, which though not susceptible of classification fortunately do not need to be classified in treatment; they may be considered as one.

Contrary to the usual belief, I regard the impacted fracture of the base of the neck into the trochanters as the most frequent fracture of the head of the femur. Let us first, however, consider the one usually known as "the fracture of old people,"—that "within the capsular ligament" as it has been usually called,—or, as I term it, "the fracture of the middle of the neck."

We have in the hospital wards four cases of injury to the hip; three are the usual impacted fracture, and one the frac-

[1] A Clinical Lecture. January, 1880. Now first published.

ture I am now about to speak of. It usually occurs in late life, when the outline of the neck of the femur is no longer what it was in the young adult. In the perfect femur the neck is a flat pyramid, with its apex above, and its base spreading from one trochanter to the other. Its smallest part is next the head. Later in life the neck changes in shape, and is smallest at the middle, where it breaks. Its texture does not become more brittle, as usually stated, but there is less bone. Its interior is so changed that the neck is but a thin and almost papery shell, which may yield to slight injury. Sometimes the patient is even supposed to have broken his, or rather her, hip (for the injury occurs more frequently in women) before falling. The neck yielding near its middle, the limb is left at the mercy of the muscles, hangs loose, and, in an erect posture, swings. The muscles of the haunch evert the trochanter, and of course the toe. There may be a considerable shortening, — two inches and more.

I have often mentioned a patient I once saw in the street,— a lady who fell, and when raised and supported by the bystanders had a swinging leg, everted toe, and the limb so shortened that I diagnosticated a fracture of the neck of the thigh-bone across the street. Such a patient placed upon a bed is usually in great pain, because the muscles are nipped by the displaced fragments, the pinching of the soft parts being the usual cause of pain in a fracture. So great is the eversion that the foot generally lies upon its outside. Under these circumstances it is useless to try to get crepitus; the effort is not only productive of pain, but also damages the part. The evidence is sufficient without it. Crepitus can be got, however, by drawing the limb down until the fragments rub together in apposition.

The prognosis of this fracture is unfavorable as to union, perhaps in proportion to the displacement; also to the age of the patient and her health. The accident is sometimes grave, and may be a fatal one. The patient may die in a period varying from a few days to a year after the accident, gradually worn out. On the other hand, the bone generally unites by ligament, and the patient is able to walk with crutches, or a crutch and a cane. If such a patient is finally able to walk with a cane, the accident was probably not the one we are considering, but rather one of the impacted fractures, or a fracture of the trochanter. The ligament which unites the bone may be longer or shorter, and the mobility greater or less. The neck will eventually become absorbed, and the head of the bone may after a while rest directly upon the shaft of the femur. The explanation of non-union is to be found in the mobility of the fragments and the impossibility of keeping them in apposition; and there is also something in the fact that the upper fragment does not contribute its share to the mutual union, being suspended from the pelvis by the capsular ligament only, for the ligamentum teres is not a true ligament, but merely a fasciculus for the passage of vessels.

I have already said that the fracture of the middle of the neck is not the most common one. It is, however, the most striking and the most persistent in consecutive results. This subsequent persistence of deformity or lameness directs attention to the hip bone at an autopsy, and the specimen is saved; while other fractures resulting in bony union are forgotten, or if the head of the bone is procured it is so repaired as to leave the exact character of the injury in doubt. Consequently fractures of the middle of the neck are, or have been, the most familiar by reason of their frequency as museum specimens. It is also the fracture most easily diagnosticated. In fact it can hardly be mistaken even when seen for the first time.

The most common fracture is the impaction of the base of the neck into the trochanters. It deserves to be thoroughly considered, because its signs are sometimes not at all satisfactory to the surgeon who is unfamiliar with them. They depend upon an anatomy comparatively new, and which was first described by myself. We have seen that the neck of the femur is seated upon the oblique line of the trochanters. When the fracture is impacted the neck is driven into the trochanters. But there is a rule about this; and that is, the neck is always impacted more behind than in front; and the head of the bone is in this way bent backward, or — which is the same thing — the shaft of the femur is rotated outward. From this results the eversion which belongs to the accident. The cause of the unequal impaction is a difference in the thickness of the walls of the neck in front and behind. In front the bone is thick; behind it is exceedingly thin; and it is behind that it yields. The bone has a thickness of perhaps an eighth of an inch along the front of the neck, and in some cases more; behind it has only the thickness of paper.

The head and neck of the femur have been repeatedly sawed longitudinally and vertically; and anatomists (notably the late Jeffries Wyman) have given details of the very beautiful cancellous structure, whose fibres are arranged in radii, arches and stringers, to support and suspend the head of the bone from the trochanter. But a transverse section of the head remained to be made. For this purpose the femur should be placed with its back toward you, upright, but as if the patient were straddling, so as to bring the neck of the femur to a horizontal position. Now, if you slice off the top of the femur, neck, and trochanters, and then take a second, a third, and perhaps a fourth horizontal slice, you will find as you get toward the bottom of the neck that the anterior wall is so thick, and the posterior wall so thin, as to leave no doubt of the facts I have mentioned. The posterior wall which yields actually starts thick from the head; but instead of being inserted thick into the trochanters, it plunges beneath them in the direction of the shaft of the femur. If it were inserted there, it would be strong; but in an attempt to gain the shaft of the femur it becomes more and more attenuated until it loses itself and disappears in a series of radiating papery plates. This construction was first pointed out in my paper on "The Mechanism of Dislocation and Fracture of the Hip," and was some years afterward again described by Merkel, as the "Schenkelsporn," in a paper in Virchow's Archives; and since by Dr. Dwight, of Boston.

The anatomy of this part of the femur illustrates and explains the important signs which enable us to identify the impacted fracture of the base of the neck. The anterior wall of the neck being thick is not impacted; the posterior wall being thin is crushed and driven together. The thick anterior wall rocks upon its broken edges as a hinge, but is rarely otherwise displaced. You see this in these museum specimens, of which ours has a dozen or twenty. Specimens in other museums also show that this impacted fracture obeys a constant law. The neck bends only at its anterior hinge, while it is impacted posteriorly. This explains eversion. The whole limb is everted.

A word as to shortening. If we hold a common hinge horizontally, a femur attached to the lower part of the hinge would be shortened by just so much as we shut the latter. If on the other hand the hinge-joint were vertical, there would be no shortening, but the shaft of the femur would be everted when the hinge was bent. Now, as the inter-trochanteric line is neither vertical nor horizontal, but oblique at an angle of forty-five degrees, the hinge which it represents is half vertical and half horizontal. Its movement is one of half eversion and half shortening, — of shortening in proportion to the eversion, and eversion in proportion to the shortening. A limb much everted is a good deal shortened, and when it is little everted it is but little shortened.

Suppose the impaction is great. There is no difficulty in determining its existence; the eversion and the shortening both announce it. But suppose that the impaction is slight.

In this case you have hardly any eversion and hardly any shortening; so that in fact you may be in doubt whether the limb is shortened or not. Now, here is a rule for determining the existence of an impacted fracture where the impaction is slight. Let the patient be directed to evert the feet, — first the sound one, and then the other. One is everted as easily as the other. But let him be directed to invert them, and you will find that while he can invert the sound one, the affected limb, by reason of its impaction behind, cannot be inverted quite as much. So that in the very common accident of a slight impaction of the base of the neck of the femur you may accept as its pathognomonic sign an undemonstrable or hardly perceptible shortening, with only a diminution of the power of inversion. In other words, *inability to invert is eversion.*

This throws light upon many cases of injury to the hip, about which even good surgeons not unfrequently differ. Cases we have now in the hospital illustrate these fractures. A patient upstairs, a female, whom you saw on Saturday, sixty-five years of age, fell upon her hip on a slanting, icy sidewalk. She came in here five hours afterward. She had pain at the trochanter, increased by motion, and tenderness on pressure. She was disabled so far as the use of the limb goes. The eversion was in this case obvious, the foot standing at an angle of about forty-five degrees, and the shortening being three-quarters of an inch. There was no crepitus. These signs indicated impaction.

In another case the injury is less marked. It illustrates better what I have said of slight impaction. The patient, also a woman, is twenty-nine years old. She fell upon the sidewalk, upon her hip, two days before coming here. There was pain over the great trochanter and its neighborhood, much increased by motion, and of course tenderness on pressure, and disability. There was an inability to invert the foot beyond the perpendicular, — which was as pathognomonic as if the patient had an everted foot. There was little or no shortening, because there was little or no eversion. But I have no doubt that it was a case of impacted fracture.

A third patient, thirty-eight years old, fell a distance of five feet upon his right hip. There were the usual pain and tenderness over the great trochanter. The disability was not very great; he could move his limb. The eversion was only shown by the absence of power to invert. There was little or no shortening, and no crepitus. You will anticipate me in the diagnosis.

We may contrast these cases with another, — a male patient, sixty-one years of age, whom you saw in the large ward. There was well-marked crepitus; the shortening was nearly an inch, and the eversion was very pronounced. Here the injury was doubtless a fracture of the small part of the neck of the bone, leaving only a doubt whether it was not originally an impacted fracture in which the fragments had been detached and drawn apart by unjustifiable examination, — which is a matter we shall come to.

So that the point important to remember is, when a patient meets with an injury, however slight, about the hip, as indicated by pain and disability there, and upon examination has no crepitus, next to no shortening, and but little apparent eversion, and you ask yourself, Is this only a sprain; can he have a fracture of the hip? — the answer is, Unquestionably he can. He may have a very slight impaction of the base of the neck into the base of the trochanter, which may disable him for two or three months, which may heal without difficulty, and leave little or no traces in the bone of its existence; or, on the other hand, the impaction may be such — the parts so firmly locked together — that if you had the specimen in your hands, you could not draw the neck of the bone out of the trochanters. Do not forget, however, that it may be quite the reverse when you resort to the powerful leverage of the bent leg held at the knee and ankle in a futile search for crepitus. You may then twist the fragments apart, doing the patient a serious damage, which he would have escaped had you been more familiar with the signs of the accident and avoided an unnecessary examination.

The impaction of its base being the most frequent accident to the neck of the femur, there is, on the other hand, an impaction at the other end of the neck, which, so far as specimens testify, is very rare; namely, that in which the neck is driven into the head. An illustration of this is seen in a specimen I show you from a case of the late Dr. Gay, obtained from a patient who died in the hospital,—a case I have mentioned in my paper on this subject. This man slipped at the foot of his steps on the sidewalk, but nevertheless got into his door, climbed one flight of stairs, went to bed without assistance, and only sent for Dr. Gay on the next day. He was removed to the hospital, where about ten days after he died of pneumonia. A few hours before his death he said, "Doctor, I am getting along well with my leg," lifting it off the bed, without help, to justify the assertion. There is no reason why he should not have been able to lift his broken leg if the parts were firmly impacted. A man can walk with a dislocated hip where the bone is firmly supported by the ligaments, and he can also sometimes bear weight on the common impacted fracture. In this case the fact of the fracture was established by the specimen. The neck was driven into the head, and the head was bent backward toward the trochanter minor,—which I believe to be the rule, although a case is recorded where the head was tilted a little the other way. In this remarkable and interesting case, cited by Pirrie,[1] the limb was flexed and inverted across the abdomen, as in the

[1] The Lancet, 1879, p. 5.

first stage of dorsal dislocation. Here the capsular ligament proved to be sound; and it probably aided in maintaining the deformity, the neck being broken near the head. These cases explain others. Dr. Cushing, of Dorchester, had a patient, an elderly lady, who fell while winding up a clock. He was sure from all the signs that she had a fracture of the neck of the thigh-bone. She lived a number of years, and got about, walking pretty well. The articulating surface, as you see, was broken off like a watch crystal, tilted back, as in Dr. Gay's case, and united by bone in its new position. We have a third specimen of this same sort.

This last named fracture, far rarer than the impaction of the base, cannot be distinguished from it. Indeed, there is no advantage in making such a distinction. If a patient has an impaction of the neck of the bone you need not know any more; the chances are that he will have bony union. I believe that all the specimens of bony union of the neck of the thigh-bone within the capsular ligament — as they were called in old times — are cases where the summit of the neck was impacted into the head of the bone, and the parts were fixed and at rest. If mobility is one great obstacle to union, it should follow that where the fragments are kept at rest by impaction there will be a tendency to union; and we find this to be the fact.

In corroboration of this you will observe that in the vertical section of almost all specimens of intra-capsular fracture with osseous union, such as the books usually figure, there is a dense white line of bone. This is the posterior wall of the lower fragment imbedded in new material, and is usually long enough to show that the fracture was at the upper part of the neck.

Here, then, are three lesions, — the most common being the impacted fracture of the base of the neck; the least common the impacted fracture of the other end of the neck, which need not and cannot be distinguished from it; the third and familiar one being the fracture at the small part of the neck, — the fracture of old people.

Let me now suppose another state of things. I have said that the impacted fracture of the base of the neck is attended with eversion, due to the bending of the neck upon an anterior hinge. Let us suppose that impaction has been so great that the neck is displaced from this hinge, and driven squarely in between the walls of the trochanter. When this happens the whole inter-trochanteric mass, including the greater and the lesser trochanter, is split off. The anterior hinge no longer exists. There is no longer any cause for eversion, and there may be actual inversion instead of the usual eversion. This injury is a rare one.

A subject in the dissecting-room was transferred to me a dozen years ago as a case of unreduced dislocation upon the dorsum, the knee being greatly inverted. Upon examination I found that instead of a dislocation there was an impacted fracture of the neck, with inversion. In this instance the neck had penetrated between the anterior and the posterior walls of the inter-trochanteric mass, splitting them apart, and had finally united, presenting a specimen of the very rare fracture of impaction of the neck with inversion. I have seen very few such specimens, and I have looked over many museums. Smith, of Dublin, mentions their exceptional occurrence.

It only remains for us to consider the group of fractures that occur about the head of the shaft. We may class them together as fractures of the trochanters.

There is here no rule for the position of the limb. It is generally everted. There is no rule for the line of the fracture, nor advantage in knowing it; there is no limit to the extent of the comminution. The neck of the bone may lie transversely instead of obliquely, and may be displaced so far outward that it becomes united by its middle to the shaft, as in the letter T, and the femur looks like the handle of an old man's cane. Of course you get crepitus; you find a certain mobility; you detect shortening, and in its treatment you would instinctively draw the limb down and keep it there.

I cannot see how you should mistake such a loose fracture for an impacted fracture. But you might mistake it for fracture of the middle part of the neck, — fracture of old people, — and so err, not in treatment, but in prognosis; inasmuch as the former usually unites by bone, — the latter, so far as I know, never.

And now as regards treatment and its results. If the injury is not a dislocation, — which you ought to be able to determine, — you can do nothing better than to draw the limb down and keep it steady. But if there is no great shortening, — as in the case of an impacted fracture, — then obviously you need not draw the limb down, because it is not much drawn up. In fact, if you try to draw it down you may do great damage by separating the impacted fragments. So that the treatment reduces itself to a very simple matter. If there is much shortening and mobility, draw the limb down, correcting as far as you can the usual tendency to eversion; if not, only steady it.

I again repeat, in impacted fracture you should be careful not to draw or twist the fragments apart. You saw the case in the wards where a surgeon had probably detached the fragments, and I have said that you get great leverage by taking hold of the ankle and the bent knee. In this way you can almost break a sound bone. No surgeon is justified in twisting such an injured limb about — especially if, employing ether, he is unrestricted by the pain he gives the patient — in persistent attempts to get crepitus. Much less is it desirable that a number of surgeons, one after the other, should do so.

In a person of an age liable to "the fracture of old people," great shortening, eversion, and mobility usually mean fracture of the middle of the neck, and you can say to the patient, "You will probably be lame;" and yet a case of this sort occasionally happens which you cannot distinguish from one of fracture of the trochanters, likely to result in bony union with some lameness, — perhaps only that which follows from a shortening which the spine cannot compensate, or from bony callus about the joint. Late in life shortening of the femur is not, however, readily corrected by a spinal curve. In a robust or young subject a fracture about the head of the bone, not attended with great shortening or eversion, is probably impacted, and will in all likelihood unite by bone, leaving the patient not very lame. An inch and a half shortening after a fracture in the region under consideration is no great matter; a man may walk nearly as well with it as without it. After a while the pelvis tilts, and you may not be able to determine by the gait which limb is the shortest.

I have just intimated that a comminuted fracture of the trochanters sometimes leaves a mass of bony callus, productive of lameness; and as this fracture cannot always be distinguished from loose fracture of the small part of the neck by any justifiable examination, it is safest, where there is much shortening, eversion, and mobility, to give a guarded prognosis. If the patient ultimately walks better than you predicted, he will not object.

You should always see that an effort is made to correct eversion in every case of fractured femur. I do not know any more effective means to this end than long sandbags packed under the trochanter from the outset, — in fact, outside the whole limb; indeed, you had better put sandbags on both sides of it. And you must watch the patient, who is always trying to ease his limb. The patella and the great toe should look directly upward. A sole-piece and splint may be attached to the foot and leg, which can so be kept vertical.

Extension, whether for the purpose of drawing down a loose fracture or of merely steadying an impacted one, is best applied by the familiar expedient of adhesive straps, a pulley, and a weight of five to eight pounds, upon a bed without a foot-board, — its lower end being raised six inches, if necessary, to secure counter-extension.

PART II.

RAPID LITHOTRITY, WITH EVACUATION.

RAPID LITHOTRITY.

WHEN Sydney Smith asked, "What human plan, device, or invention two hundred and seventy years old does not require reconsideration?" he would no doubt have regarded with favor an occasional reconsideration of the theory and practice of medicine and surgery, — especially in view of the current belief that their traditions had been kept alive and their rules prescribed in part by authority. The surgical literature of Lithotomy, both French and English, so long showed the influence of the early specialists, that we have hardly now escaped from its exaggerated circumstance and detail; and yet, with attention to a few precise rules, the operation of lithotomy is quite a simple one, — much less difficult, for example, than the dissection of tumors. It is not impossible that convictions in some degree traditionary may prevail in regard to certain points connected with the practice of the more recent art of Lithotrity.

Civiale was among the first to inculcate the excessive susceptibility of the bladder under instruments. Later surgeons, perhaps influenced in part by his teaching, have continued to invest the operation of lithotrity with precautions which though by no means groundless, because under certain conditions both the bladder and urethra actively resent even slight interference, are nevertheless greater than this operation generally requires. As a rule, there is little mechanical difficulty in its performance. The stone is readily caught and broken into fragments, of which a few are pulverized; a large-eyed catheter is then sometimes introduced; a little sand and a few bits of stone are washed out; after which the patient is kept quiet, to discharge the remainder and to await another "sitting." Under favorable circumstances such an operation, lasting a few minutes, is not only simple, but, if skilfully performed, safe.

On the other hand, it is not always safe. This is the fact that seems to have arrested so strongly the attention of surgeons. It may happen that during the night succeeding the operation the patient has a chill, — not the chill of so-called "urethral fever," which sometimes follows the mere passage of a bougie, and which is of little consequence; but one followed by other symptoms, such as tenderness in the region of the bladder, a quickened pulse, an increasing temperature, and the frequent and painful passage of urine. These symptoms may insidiously persist rather than abate. Others may supervene. The surgeon vainly waits for a favorable moment to repeat his operation; it becomes too evident that the patient is seriously ill, and it is quite within the range of possibilities that in the course of days or weeks he may quietly succumb. An autopsy discloses a variety of lesions, some of them remote or obscure, others of more obvious origin,— and among them, not the least common, an inflamed bladder, upon the floor of which angular fragments and chips of stone are resting. It is then evident that during a certain interval before death the bladder was not in a condition for further instrumental interference; and although, in view of the fatal result of delay, lithotomy or active lithotrity, to both of which I have resorted, might have been deemed on the whole the less dangerous, still it is plain that either operation would have furnished in itself an additional cause of progressive inflammation.

Such cases have been supposed to point to the necessity of extreme precaution, as well as of extreme remedies. It is evident that the purpose of interference at an unfavorable moment is the removal of the offending fragments as a last resource. But if at the first operation the bladder could have been completely disembarrassed of every particle of stone, even with the risk of irritating its lining membrane, we can hardly doubt that the relief would then have been followed by comparatively ready repair. In short, it is difficult to avoid the conviction that in an average case damage to the mucous membrane is as likely to result from irritation by angular fragments, added to the injury inflicted by an operation, as from the use of instruments protracted beyond the usual time for the entire removal of a stone, if this result can be accomplished.

It is probable that injury from the use of instruments has been confounded with that resulting from the presence of fragments in the bladder. That the average bladder and urethra have no extreme susceptibility is attested by the generally favorable results of lithotrity, and even of catheterism, which are practised with very varying skill everywhere; also by the singularly innocuous results of laceration of the contracted urethra, by an instrument like that of Voillemier, for example; so, too, by the recovery of these organs from the considerable injury inflicted during the extraction of a large and rough stone in lithotomy. The bladder is often also to an extraordinary degree tolerant of the presence even of a mulberry calculus. If we remember that in this case it clasps the stone at every micturition, often with a persistent gripe, the comparative immunity of its tender mucous membrane is quite remarkable. But when after an operation sharp fragments are thus embraced, presenting acute angles, which do not soon become blunted, and to which the bladder is unaccustomed, it is still more remarkable that serious consequences are the exception and not the rule in lithotrity. Polished metallic surfaces carefully manipulated can hardly do such damage as the other agencies here mentioned.

Gentleness, dexterity, and experience are especially to be valued in lithotrity. If the bladder is pinched, the patient may die. A false passage or a lacerated inner meatus is a serious complication. It has been well said that no novice should undertake this operation. Civiale, with an almost unparalleled experience, introduced a small lithotrite with much less pressure than its own weight, and with uniform and great slowness; and yet in a healthy urethra it is only at the triangular ligament and beyond it that such extreme care is called for. The same author, who had no means of evacuating fragments in the bladder, restricted the length of his operation to two or three or perhaps five minutes. The like solicitude seems to have led Sir Henry Thompson, in his admirable and standard work upon this subject, to assign two minutes as the proper average duration of a sitting, — a period which his exceptional skill has often in his own practice enabled him materially to reduce. I have been gratified to find, however, that since he has availed himself of the advantage of etherization he recognizes the benefit to be derived from somewhat more prolonged manipulation. My own conviction is that it is better to protract the operation indefinitely in point of time, if thus the whole stone can be removed without serious injury to the bladder. I believe that in any case as favorable to lithotrity as the average, in these days when stones are detected early, this can be effected, — and that if the bladder be completely emptied of detritus, we have as little to apprehend from the fatigue of the organ consequent upon such manipulation as from the alternative of residual fragments and further operations. The duration of the longest sitting among the cases reported at the end of this paper was three hours and three quarters. The same result can be now accomplished in a very much shorter time. In a majority of cases the bladder can be completely and at once evacuated.

But has not this result been already attained by evacuating

instruments variously devised and modified? The following quotations from the latest authorities sufficiently answer this question in the negative: —

"We may here say, without fear of being accused of exaggeration, that evacuating injections practised after sittings of lithotrity have no apology for their use. *The whole surgical arsenal invented for their performance is absolutely useless. . . . It should be well understood that the best of evacuating catheters is worthless.*" [1]

"*The practice of injecting the bladder to wash out detritus is obsolete. . . . This apparatus of Mr. Clover should not be employed if it is possible to dispense with it,* as its use is quite as irritating as lithotrity itself." [2]

"Having used it [Clover's apparatus] very frequently, I would add that it is necessary to use all such apparatus with extreme gentleness, and *I prefer to do without it if possible.*" [3]

"*All these evacuating catheters are little employed.* They require frequent and long manœuvres, which are not exempt from dangers; besides, *they give passage, as a rule, only to dust, or to little fragments of stone, which would have escaped of themselves without inconvenience to the urethra.*" [4]

M. Voillemier here states the precise difficulty. The "evacuating apparatus" and the evacuating method hitherto employed do not evacuate. This fact is beyond question.

Such apparatus is not of recent contrivance. From the earlier days of lithotrity, the operation of breaking the stone has been followed by the obvious expedient of introducing a large and special catheter, through which water was injected and allowed to escape, bringing away a little sand, with a

[1] Article Lithotritie, by Demarquay et Cousin, in the Nouveau Dictionnaire de Médecine et de Chirurgie Pratique, pp. 693, 694. Paris, 1875.

[2] S. D. Gross: Diseases, etc., of the Urinary Organs, p. 232. Philadelphia, 1876.

[3] Sir H. Thompson: Practical Lithotrity and Lithotomy, p. 215. 1871.

[4] Article Lithotritie, by M. Voillemier, Dictionnaire Encyclopédique des Sciences Médicales, p. 733. 1869.

small fragment or two. This attempt at evacuation was aided by suction. With this object, and before the year 1846, Sir Philip Crampton employed an exhausted glass globe.[1] For the same purpose a rubber enema-syringe has been used, or a hydrocele bottle, with which fluid could also be injected and the bladder washed. By entering the catheter well within the bottle, or syringe, fragments were dropped inside the neck, where, lying below the current, they remained when the bottle was again compressed. When this neck was made of glass by Clover, the fragments became visible, as in Crampton's globe; and to this neat arrangement the accomplished lithotritist, Sir Henry Thompson, refers as Clover's bottle. But neither the previous practice nor the efficiency of evacuation by suction through a tube had been materially advanced. In the mean time the syringe was modified in France by a rack and pinion attached to the piston, so that water could be injected and withdrawn with great force, — a procedure not only useless, but detrimental to the bladder, if inflamed and thickened.

Before describing my own instruments, it may be well to say a word in regard to the introduction of large instruments

[1] The apparatus here alluded to was intended more particularly "for clearing the bladder of detritus, in cases in which the expulsive power of that organ has been, as so frequently happens in old persons, impaired or destroyed." In Sir Philip's own words: "The apparatus consists of a strong glass vessel of an oval form and six or eight inches in length by three in diameter, and capable of holding about a pint and a half of water; to this vessel is attached a tube of about half an inch bore, furnished with a stop-cock. The air being exhausted by means of an exhausting syringe, and one of Heurteloup's wide-eyed steel evacuating catheters being introduced into the bladder, it is next attached to the exhausted vessel; the stop-cock is then turned, and a communication being thus established between the bladder and the glass, the pressure of the atmosphere is by this means brought to bear on the bladder, and supplies an expulsive power, which may be increased to any required amount." — *The Dublin Quarterly Journal of Medical Science*, vol. i. p. 22. 1846.

into the bladder. The successful introduction of the large straight tube is so important that it deserves especial mention. It throws light upon the successful passage of the lithotrite, and also of the large-sized curved tubes.

Urethra to be measured.—In order to ascertain the maximum calibre of the urethra before introducing a tube, it should be measured by an instrument which will enter more readily than the tube. Such instruments we have in Van Buren's Sounds, which are slightly curved at the end and a little conical. Being made of solid metal and nickel-plated, they traverse the urethra with singular facility. Both Otis's Sounds and the conical probe-pointed elastic bougie also answer admirably for this purpose.

How to pass a straight instrument into the bladder. — A syringe facilitates the copious use of oil both in the urethra and within the tube. Into the normal urethra a straight instrument can be introduced with more accuracy than a curved one. Either may be passed rapidly as far as the triangular ligament, unless the instrument is very large, in which case great care is required not to rupture the mucous membrane. Having reached this point, which implies that there should be no premature endeavor to turn the instrument, but that it should be passed as far as it will go in the general direction of the anus before its direction is changed, the extremity of the instrument depresses the floor of the urethra in front of the ligament.

How to pass the triangular ligament.— Traction upon the penis next effaces this depression, and adds firmness to the urethral walls; so that if the instrument be withdrawn a little, and again advanced after lowering the handle until it is almost horizontal, it can be coaxed without difficulty through the ligament in question, — a natural obstruction which physicians often mistake for a stricture. The straight tube may be advantageously rotated through the aperture like a corkscrew. This obstruction passed, the rest of the canal is short, and corresponds to the axis of the body, to the line of which the instrument is now depressed.

Presence of an enlarged prostate.—Even the enlarged prostate can often be traversed with facility by a straight instrument. In fact, the metallic prostatic catheter, before it was superseded by the modern rubber one, consisted essentially of an inch or two of straighter tube added to the extremity of a common catheter, to reach through the unyielding prostate before the hand was depressed and the beak turned up.

Obstruction by fissure in the prostate.—An occasional difficulty in passing the enlarged prostate deserves mention here; namely, that resulting from a series of cracks or fissures, having their apex at the verumontanum, and radiating toward the bladder. I have a specimen of large prostate where these fissures readily engage a medium-sized catheter.

In such a case a large instrument may pass more readily than a small one. The finger in the rectum is here also of especial service. The handle of the tube may be also lowered to tilt up the tip in passing the inner meatus.

Obstruction at the inner meatus. — In passing either a sound, catheter, or lithotrite, the extremity of a straight instrument, and curiously enough the convexity of a curved one, is sometimes arrested just at the entrance of the bladder by the firm lower edge of the inner meatus. The fact that water now dribbles through the inner meatus thus dilated, or that a stone is felt with the tip of the curved instrument which has really entered the bladder, may lead the operator into the mistake of supposing that the instrument is fairly within; and I have known its further entrance, after sliding over this obstacle, to be erroneously explained by assuming the existence of a second or hour-glass cavity in the bladder itself.

How to overcome it. — To obviate this difficulty, and so soon as the triangular ligament is passed, a catheter, if curved, should be pressed fairly through the indurated neck, or prostate, in the direction of the axis of the body, by the hand on the perinæum, — a most efficient manœuvre when the prostate is large. If there be further difficulty, the tip should of course be sought and guided in the rectum (see p. 206). After introduction, a straight tube, or the shaft of a curved one, often returns to an angle of about 45° with the recumbent body; and if the patient is not etherized, a feeling of tension may then be relieved by depressing, with the hand upon the pubes, the suspensory ligament of the penis, — an expedient also useful during the passage of the instrument.

Anæsthesia in lithotrity. — My own practice has always been to etherize for lithotrity.

Position of the operator. — Each operator prefers the position to which he is accustomed; and when the urethra is healthy, this is of very little importance. But if there be obstruction, a position at the patient's left side enables the operator to introduce a catheter or lithotrite to advantage with the right hand, leaving the left hand free to act in the perinæum. After the instrument is introduced and both hands are required above the pubes, they are most available if the surgeon changes his position and stands upon the patient's right. I also introduce the straight tube on the right side.

Passage of a lithotrite. — The lithotrite is to be passed as a straight instrument, and not as a curved catheter. When it reaches the triangular ligament, the tip is insinuated into its aperture, and then the handle previously perpendicular, or nearly so, is depressed to an angle of about 45°. In this position it should remain, with but little further depression, while the blades are gently urged forward through the prostate. The convexity of the heel thus depresses the lower wall of the canal as it moves along and makes room. It moves as a boat, rising neither at prow nor stern (see Fig. 19, p. 313).

Water to be injected before crushing.—In injecting water before using the lithotrite, the capacity of the bladder may be estimated by the tension of the urethra behind the point of constriction. By attention to this indication we prevent over-distention. In the etherized subject a short pipe or nozzle suffices for introducing water. I have usually employed a common Davidson's syringe. An unetherized patient may for a moment resist this injection through a short tube, by contracting the sphincter of the bladder; but this readily yields. A distention by five or six ounces suffices. The smaller the injection of water the more readily, indeed, do crushed fragments fall into the blades of the instrument; but unfortunately so also does the mucous membrane. In fact, with too little fluid in the bladder the use of a lithotrite in unpractised hands is attended with danger; and in a long sitting an injection which will separate the walls is the only really safe way of keeping the bladder from between the blades. A careful examination of the action of a lithotrite through an opening in the summit of the bladder has confirmed me in this opinion, which was that of the older writers on this subject. From time to time the diameter of the collapsing bladder should be estimated by slowly opening the blades of the lithotrite. Water may be introduced as often as necessary; but care should be taken to guard against the serious injury to a contracted bladder which might result from suddenly injecting the contents of the syringe or aspirating bottle when it is already distended. On the other hand, distention of the bladder is a common symptom of retention. When extreme, it is often followed by inflammation and atony. But in a common case we do not anticipate such serious results, even when micturition has been frequent, and the bladder by inference small. It has occurred to me whether a moderate forced distention might not be of service in certain cases of contracted bladder, as it is in a permanently contracted anus.

Water retained by an elastic band.—A tape or an elastic band wound lightly once or twice around the penis near the scrotum retards the escape of injected water, and yet allows the movements of the tube or lithotrite.

The successful evacuation of the bladder depends upon several conditions both in the apparatus and in its use, which for distinctness may be enumerated separately.

1. A large calibre of the evacuating tube.

2. The shape of its receiving extremity.

3. Manipulation of the bulb.

4. Capacity of the bladder.

5. Evacuation of the fragments.

6. Immediate recognition and removal of any obstruction in the tube.

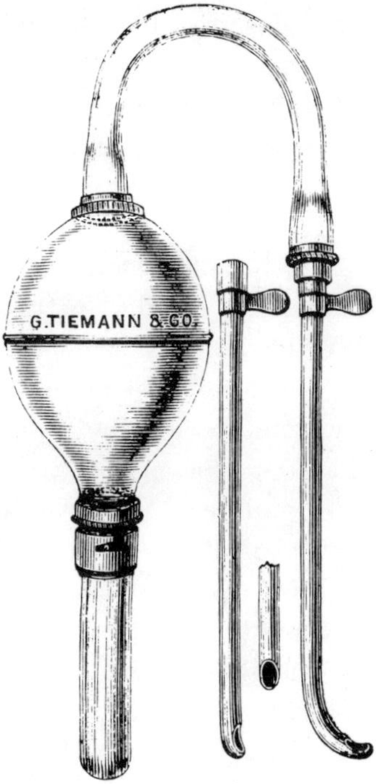

FIG. 1.[1]

1. *A large calibre of the evacuating tube.*—Whether or not we adopt the view of Otis that the average calibre of the normal urethra is about 33 of Charrière, there can be no question that it will admit a much larger tube than that commonly attached to either Clover's or the French apparatus. The efficiency of the process of evacuation depends much upon using the largest tube the urethra will admit. This fact has been stated by Sir Henry Thompson,

[1] Evacuating Apparatus. 1. Elastic bulb. 2. Curved rubber tube. 3. Curved evacuating tube of silver. 4. Straight evacuating tube, which is preferable to the curved one. 5. Front view of same. 6. Glass receptacle, with bayonet joint for débris. (Tiemann and Co., New York.)

but with a different significance. He recommends for the glass cylinder or trap which is to admit this tube a "perforation at the end the size of only a No. 14 catheter," = 25 Charrière.[1] This perforation is too small; and the tube which is designed to enter it is further reduced by its collar to the diameter of only 12, = 21 Charrière. In fact, this is the calibre of the evacuating catheters now attached to Clover's instrument, and is of itself fatal to their efficiency. An effective tube has a calibre of 28 to 31 or even 32 Charrière, and the meatus, which is the narrowest part, may if necessary be slit to admit it, if the urethra is otherwise capacious. Again, in the instrument as sometimes constructed by Weiss a joint is made by inserting an upper tube into a lower one, thus obstructing the calibre by a shoulder. The joints should become larger as the tube approaches the bottle, so that the tube may deliver without difficulty fragments of its own calibre. Whatever be the size of the catheter, the rubber tube with its metal attachments should have a calibre of at least seven sixteenths of an inch, = 31 Charrière, and there should be nowhere any approach to a shoulder inside.

My evacuating tubes are of thin nickel-plated metal of sizes 27, 28, 29, 30 and 31 *filière* Charrière, respectively. These are the sizes, including also perhaps 26 and 32, which I have designated as "large" in distinction to the calibre 21 of previous apparatus.

2. *The shape of its receiving extremity.* — The receiving extremity should depress the bladder when required to do so, and thus invite the fragments, while its orifice remains unobstructed by the mucous membrane. Upon the floor of the bladder when not indented a fragment of stone lying at the distance of half or even quarter of an inch from the tube extremity may not be attracted by the usual exhaust of the expanding bottle, which requires that the fragment should

[1] Diseases of the Prostate, p. 337. Fourth edition, 1873.

lie almost in contact with the tube. A very slight obstacle impedes the entrance of a fragment; and this fact renders inefficient all tubes like catheters with orifices along the side or upper wall. The orifice of a tube cut square is at once occluded by drawing in the vesical wall, while the spoon-shaped beak of the French instrument, made like the female blade of a lithotrite, allows fragments to lie too far from the opening in the tube.

The best orifice is at the extremity, and is made by bending the tube at a sharp right angle, carefully rounding the elbow, and then cutting off the bent branch close to the straight tube (Fig. 2*a*). The tube is then practically straight, while the orifice, which is slightly oval, delivers its stream laterally. The edge should be thickened and rounded to slide smoothly through the urethra; any rim inside the orifice should be masked by a false floor, but the calibre should be nowhere contracted. If the side walls of this orifice be removed a little, it gives an unguiform extremity to the tube, which is advantageous; and in introducing such a straight tube, this tip should be insinuated through

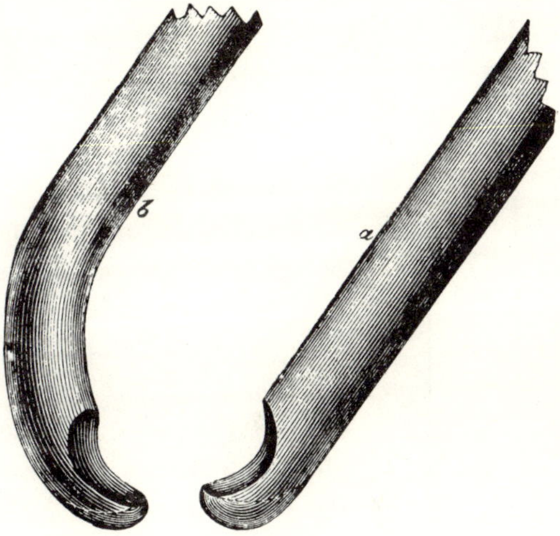

FIG. 2.[1]

[1] Evacuating tubes, with unguiform extremity. *a.* Straight tube. *b.* Curved tube. The dotted lines show the false floor of the extremity. The tubes are here of a diameter 31 Charrière. The straight tube is preferable.

the triangular ligament by rotation. If a couple of inches of the end of such a tube be bent, it may be inverted after introduction, and will bury itself in the floor of the bladder, which it depresses, while the orifice looks forward and is unobstructed (Fig. 2 *b*); or it may be used as introduced. An effective instrument may be made of a straight tube cut square at the end, if a disk convex outwardly, to repel the bladder, be attached to it at the distance of a diameter from the orifice. This was the original of the straight tube already described. When such an instrument is introduced, the interval can be filled by a rod. Indeed, the orifice of a tube should be contrived with a view to its introduction. Too large an orifice impairs the suction and admits fragments that become wedged higher up. Whatever be added to the extremity of the tube, in order to facilitate its introduction or to repel the bladder, should not prevent the orifice from lying, if required, in the floor of the bladder at the apex of an inverted tunnel.

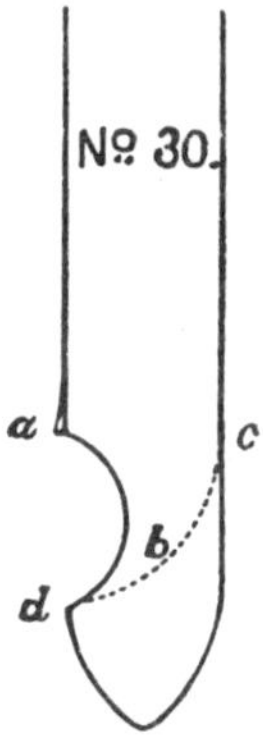

FIG. 3.[1]

3. *Manipulation of the bulb.* — The bulb, together with its tubes, contains about ten ounces. If compressed with one hand until the sides meet, only about five ounces are displaced. If half compressed and then worked with a shorter movement, about two ounces are moved back and forth; so that, provided the tube itself be handled carefully and skilfully, the bladder is not greatly disturbed. The

[1] The outline here given of the orifice and extremity of the tubes I use is more correct than that of Fig. 2. If the straight tube be closed by an extremity symmetrically round or ovoid, to facilitate its introduction, the orifice *a d* should have a length but little greater than the diameter *a c* of the tube. The curve of the inside floor *b* is a quarter circle described upon *a* as a centre. The tube is then proved by a close-fitting ball rolled through it from above. At *a* the edge is a little thickened on the outside, and at *d* rounded to protect the urethra.

object of more water is to prolong suction when fragments are passing freely; also occasionally to stir up the débris, and especially to relieve obstruction in the tube when it occurs. The best position for the surgeon is at the right hand of the patient, resting his left wrist on the pubes to steady the tube, while the bulb is supported in a stand on the table between the thighs (Fig. 4).

4. *Capacity of the bladder.*—It is desirable, in each case, to form an idea of the habitual capacity of the bladder. The previous frequency of micturition throws some light upon it. Better than this, the tension of the urethra behind the elastic band is a valuable indication of the fluid pressure in the bladder during evacuation. If the patient strains for a moment, the bladder may become very tense, and I think it then important to let the water escape through the hose (see p. 278). The bladder can be immediately replenished. Without a hose this manœuvre is impossible.

PROCESS OF EVACUATION.

Quantity of water needed during evacuation.—Unless the amount of débris is very abundant, there should be just enough water in the bladder to prevent the *thud*, or *fish-bite*, hereafter described (p. 217). While more than this needlessly scatters the fragments, a smaller amount allows the bladder to be constantly drawn into the catheter, giving rise to the quivering sensation above alluded to as the *fish-bite*. Nothing so facilitates evacuation as the power exactly to regulate the amount of water in the bladder and apparatus; and no contrivance so well accomplishes this desideratum as the hose.

5. *Evacuation of the fragments.* — Evacuation of the fragments is quite an entertaining art, requiring as much skill to accomplish the desired result in the shortest time as does the act of crushing. Dexterity in the process will hardly be

acquired without practice outside the bladder.[1] No jerk is required in pumping. The compression and expansion of the bulb equally divide a second or two of time. While the tube is held just above the débris, the fragments should fall

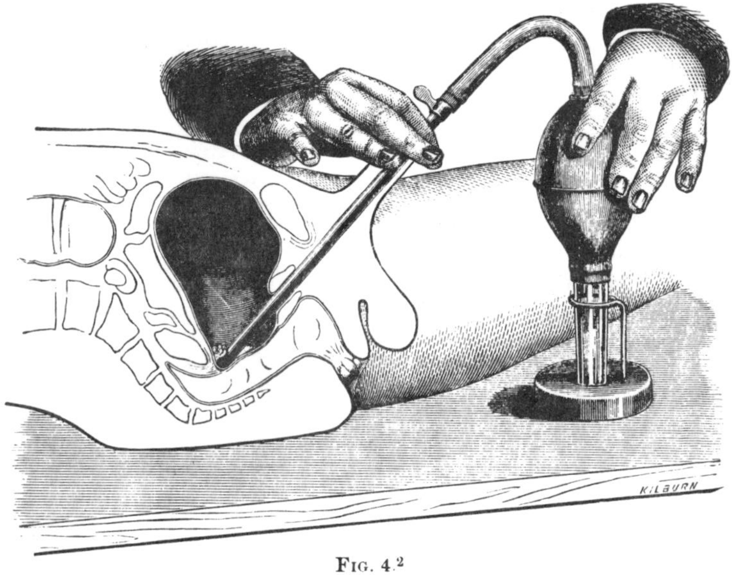

FIG. 4.[2]

[1] The bladder may be imitated by the lower two-thirds of an ox-bladder (carbolized for cleanliness) suspended inside a vessel having a mouth of four or five inches diameter, to which it is tied. The vessel should be previously nearly filled with water. To show the efficient action of circular currents in the closed bladder, the ox-bladder may be tied to the evacuating tube, and held before a bright light. With a tin funnel secured to the summit of a human bladder (*in situ*) to aid in replacing the fragments, the process of evacuation can be rapidly repeated. Such practice is very instructive. Calculi may be imitated by coal of varying hardness, or by a bit of old grindstone; a lighter and tough material for crushing, and liable to impact, is the cheap compressed meerschaum.

[2] The trap is here placed in a stand upon the table. The remaining fragments are few, and the capacious bladder is depressed to assemble them. The operator stands on the patient's left, and supports his right hand firmly upon the pubes. This position is, on the whole, the most advantageous.

in a shower into the trap. The operation may be divided into a first and a last half. During the first half, while the fragments are numerous, the secret is to separate and float them by the injection, so that they may enter the tube as

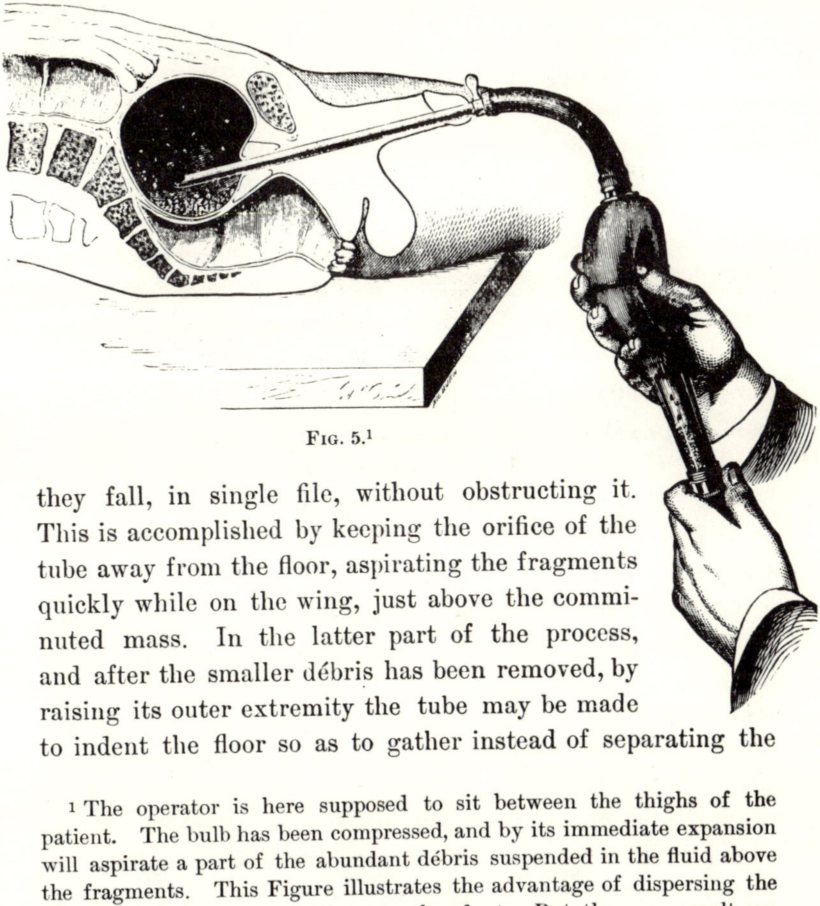

Fig. 5.[1]

they fall, in single file, without obstructing it. This is accomplished by keeping the orifice of the tube away from the floor, aspirating the fragments quickly while on the wing, just above the comminuted mass. In the latter part of the process, and after the smaller débris has been removed, by raising its outer extremity the tube may be made to indent the floor so as to gather instead of separating the

[1] The operator is here supposed to sit between the thighs of the patient. The bulb has been compressed, and by its immediate expansion will aspirate a part of the abundant débris suspended in the fluid above the fragments. This Figure illustrates the advantage of dispersing the fragments for aspiration, when too abundant. But the same result can be better accomplished by withdrawing the tube a little from the floor, with the hand supported on the pubes as in Fig. 4. (From a photograph of a frozen section, in which the rectum and the bladder were previously distended with plaster.)

fragments. Some of the chips are apt to collect about the tube orifice; but the tube thus raised is carried behind them. It is important occasionally to turn the orifice forward to wash the fragments from beneath the shoulder of a high prostate. A very slight movement of the tube sometimes makes much difference in the rapidity of the evacuation; so that when it is on the floor of the bladder or quite near it, and steadied by the hand upon the pubes or the thigh, if any one expansion of the bulb proves more successful than another, the precise position then occupied by the tube should be carefully maintained. On the other hand, when the tube is choked at each expansion, if it be withdrawn, or tilted up a quarter or even an eighth of an inch, it may happen that a shower of débris at once appears in the trap. Higher in the cavity, while the débris is abundant, the orifice may be turned downward or partly sideways, so as to project horizontal currents around the bladder, the fragments being aspirated as they whirl. At the different stages of the process there is opportunity for a little tact in placing the tube, just as there is in discovering fragments with a lithotrite.

6. *Immediate recognition and removal of obstruction in the tube.*—If a short interval elapses without the fall of débris, it may be presumed that there is obstruction. This happens not only when the bulb will not expand, when its dimple disappears reluctantly, and when compression is difficult, but also when the current passes so freely that an impediment would hardly be suspected. Obstruction occurs in several ways:—

(1) In the elastic tube, which may be accidentally bent at an angle or compressed. This should be looked at first. A bit lodged in the elastic can be displaced by pinching it.

(2) In the bladder, the most common obstruction is at the orifice of the evacuating tube. A little practice will enable the operator to distinguish the encouraging rattle of débris

passing this tube to appear at once in the trap (if held upright) from the valvular click of fragments too large to enter it. This click is quite constant at the end of the process, after the smaller chips have been aspirated off. If the orifice be choked, an effort should be made to expel the fragments in the ordinary way,—first raising the tube into clear water above the débris, and then compressing the bulb with a short and forcible squeeze. A half-dozen such efforts rarely fail; but the rod may be introduced, if necessary.

(3) It sometimes happens that nothing appears in the trap, although the current passes quite freely and the click of the abundant débris is still felt. A scale is then wedged higher in the evacuating tube, which admits water but excludes fragments. This is worth remembering. The rod removes it.

(4) A source of obstruction, and the most common one, is the wall of the bladder when drawn against the tube orifice with a dull thud, or a rapid succession of jerks not unlike the bite of a fish. It naturally interferes with the process, and if the patient has not been etherized is painful. The tube orifice may be moved to another part of the bladder where aspiration is more free. Perhaps the orifice has been accidentally turned sideways; it then readily engages the floor. But the usual explanation is that the walls of the bladder are slack, and more water is needed to distend them. This will be further noticed.

After a dozen or more aspirations it may be found that all the fragments which can pass the tube have done so, and that many of them have its full diameter. The passage of débris has ceased, and the larger bits are clicking against the catheter. The lithotrite should now again be introduced. When no click has been heard for several minutes the bladder may be considered as practically cleared, and the patient should be remanded for subsequent examination.

Lithotrite (Fig. 8). — It would be plainly desirable, if it were easy, to crush the whole stone before attempting to evacuate it; but this is rarely possible. The lithotrite becomes so choked with impacted débris that the convex surface of the mass prevents the engagement of other fragments between its blades. The character of this impaction varies. The powder of some varieties of soft stone, compressed in this way with mucus, is singularly hard, being scarcely indented with a sharp probe. A clean lithotrite always works to best advantage; and the operator frequently withdraws the loaded instrument to evacuate it, sometimes with fatal injury to the neck of the bladder. It would be obviously better if the instrument could be emptied at will within the bladder, especially if we distinctly recognize that what can be withdrawn in a lithotrite would come better through a tube, and that *the province of the lithotrite should be to pulverize, or indeed merely to comminute, and not to evacuate.* Fergusson's operation consisted largely in bringing away the finer débris, a pinch at a time, between the blades of the lithotrite. I cannot understand why, when a tube is to be introduced into the urethra to distend and protect it, and to deliver the débris at once, such a practice should still find advocates.

Although all lithotrites are made a little loose for the purpose of working out the débris, and although I have had one constructed with an especial device for this motion, I do not find it easy to clear the female blade by a lateral movement of the male blade, chiefly because the impaction is so firm that the dense mass, instead of yielding, twists the female blade from side to side. Nor does an instrument like that of Reliquet fulfil the indications. It is like the old fenestrated *brise-pierre;* but, as in the *brise-pierre*, its high sides are an obstacle to the approach of fragments. The male blade also of Reliquet's instrument is that of the lithoclast, and we need only close the blades between the thumb and finger to be satisfied of their scissor-like action upon the bladder. Lastly, it does impact badly.

The instrument about to be described keeps its blades

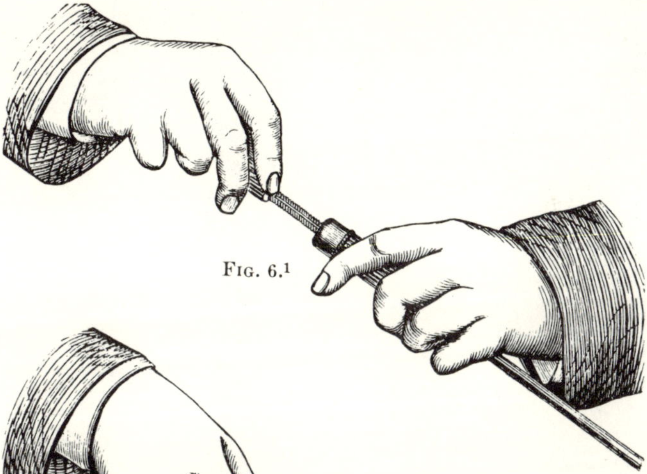

FIG. 6.[1]

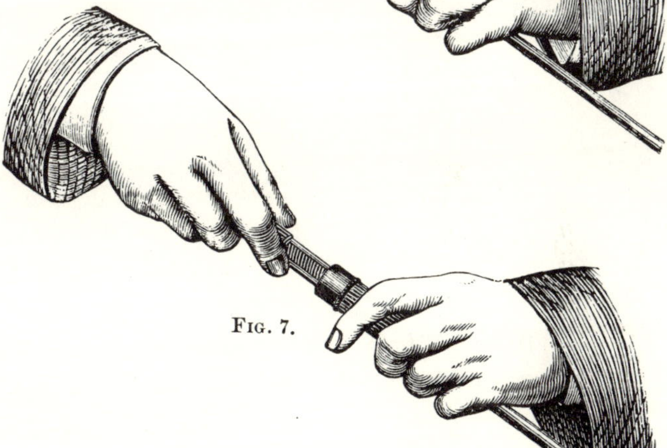

FIG. 7.

clear, and secures certain other desirable ends pertaining to the lock, handle, etc.

Lock. — The general acceptance of the wheel-shaped handle of Thompson's instrument testifies to its convenience as a

[1] Figs. 6 and 7, — position of the hands in holding and locking this lithotrite. Fig. 6, lithotrite unlocked; Fig. 7, lithotrite locked by a quarter rotation of the right wrist.

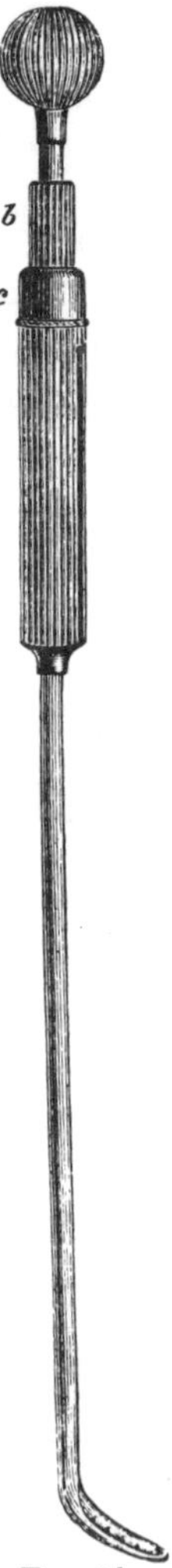

FIG. 8.[1]

hold for the left hand. But it is always a little awkward to disengage the thumb of this hand, or indeed of either hand, in order to close the lock of a lithotrite at the critical moment of grasping the stone. This objection I have obviated in closing the lock by rotation of the right wrist, without relaxing the grasp or displacing the fingers of either hand (Figs. 6 and 7).

Wheel. — In a protracted sitting the wheel is an inconvenient handle, its chief merit being that it affords so insecure a grasp that the operator is supposed to be unable, with its prescribed radius, to break the blades. But in a larger instrument these blades are stronger, and a ball may be substituted for the wheel (Fig. 8 *a*).

Injecting Tube. — If the sitting be protracted, as proposed, the water dribbles away, and the collapsing bladder, especially if trabeculated, is liable to serious damage from the lithotrite. To meet this difficulty, the injection of water, by means of a short, flat tube introduced into the urethra from time to time by the side of the lithotrite, is a valuable resource in a long operation.

Blades. — The blades of this lithotrite consist of a shoe, or female blade, the sides of which are so low that a fragment readily falls or slides upon it; while the male blade, or stamp, offers

[1] Lithotrite by Collin et Cie., from a working model. *a*, Ball which turns the screw. *b*, Revolving cylinder-handle attached to the screw-guard, which also revolves. This guard consists of two rods, which slide through notches in the cap of the lock. By their revolution the cylinder-handle turns the cap and operates upon the lock. *c*, Cap of the lock, which by its revolution wedges up the screws.

a series of alternate triangular notches by whose inclined planes the detritus escapes laterally, after being crushed against the floor and rim of the shoe. At the heel of the shoe, where most of the stone is usually comminuted, and where the impact is therefore greatest, the floor is high and discharges itself laterally, while its customary slot (Fig. 9 *f*) is made to work effectively. It may be unnecessary to say that the female blade of the common lithotrite, when drawn from a thin, flat plate as in the French instrument, has a disadvantageous cavity at the heel, where the greatest impaction occurs by gravitation.

One of the dangers of lithotrity, which has been already emphasized, is the liability of the bladder to be nipped in the instrument. The common lithotrites, even the best, have thin extremities which seize the bladder like forceps. I have known a strip of mucous membrane brought away in the instrument from the floor of the bladder without serious harm; but my belief is that if the face-wall of the bladder be included in the firmly closed jaws the patient will die. It cannot be too carefully provided against, not only by skill in the operator, but also in the construction of the instrument itself, and especially during a protracted operation, while water is escaping and the bladder collapsing. With this object, the shoe is here wider and longer than is usual, to repel the vesical walls (Fig. 9).

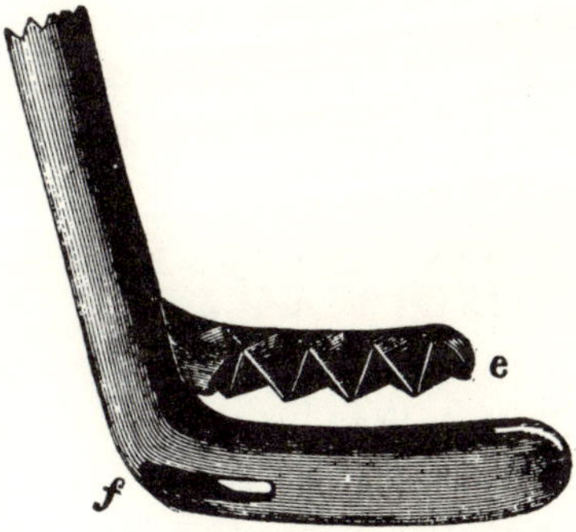

FIG. 9.[1]

[1] *e*, Male blade, presenting on alternate sides triangular notches. The small portion of débris not discharged laterally by these notches is driven through the slot in the female blade. *f*, Slot in the female blade.

It can hardly be doubted that in practice dexterous operators secure most stones and fragments as they gravitate into the female blade while it depresses the floor of the bladder, perhaps a little to one side or the other, where the stone is felt. A simple and efficient manœuvre, especially for a small fragment, is that of opening the blades of the lithotrite widely in the vertical position, then slowly turning them to one side and closing them along the floor of the bladder. If in attempting this the instrument be opened after it is turned, the male blade displaces the fragment without securing it; and it is of course understood that in opening the lithotrite the blade in contact with the bladder, commonly the female blade, is stationary. The inverted lithotrite works efficiently in a depression, if the bladder be kept out of harm's way by a special device; but with the common lithotrite it is essential to turn the blades up before crushing, and move them, in order to be sure they are free. Indeed, whatever be the position of the lithotrite, it is important always to give it a little rotation before screwing down, to see if it is free from the mucous membrane. This habit also keeps the operator informed whether he has room, or needs more water in the bladder. In the exceptional case of a stone behind the prostate, it may be necessary to invert the lithotrite and seek it. Fragments, however, are readily washed from this region within reach of the evacuating tube by occasionally turning the orifice and directing the stream from the tube upon them.

While, many years ago, I had not infrequently prolonged lithotrity to ten or fifteen minutes, and longer, it is only within two years that I have aimed at the evacuation of a considerable stone during a single sitting; and although experience will perhaps be necessary to determine precisely what cases are unfavorable to such an operation, there can now be no question that it is practicable to remove at once a far greater quantity of débris than has hitherto been considered possible. The conditions most favorable to lithotrity are obviously most favorable to this modification of it, — a stone neither very large nor hard, and especially a large urethra, promising its best results. But if the preceding views are correct, the future of lithotrity lies in the direction of a fast-working lithotrite, which while it effectually protects the bladder is more powerful than the usual instrument, and better proportioned to the work it is to do, — a rapid comminution of the stone. This is necessary in order to secure its immediate and complete evacuation by means of a large tube with an efficient orifice. *It will be no longer essential to pulverize the stone, but only to comminute it;* and if in so doing the lithotrite can be kept free from impaction, the process will be more rapid and efficient.

During the last year I removed by lithotomy two soft stones, weighing 1272 and 1230 grains, from two male adults, aged forty and twenty-four respectively, who recovered after various risks. I cannot but think that with a tolerably sound bladder, a urethra of good size, a large lithotrite, and a large tube, the operation might have been performed with less risk by the method of lithotrity now described.

We get a useful view of the interior of the bladder by examining it in position through an opening in its summit. This part of the organ with the free and thin posterior wall is mainly concerned in distention. The floor of the bladder is comparatively firm and flat, and if the subject be in good condition adheres to a thick mass of cellular tissue in and near the ischio-rectal fossæ upon which it rests. This mass is traversed by the rectum variously distended; and this canal in a thin subject may be advantageously filled with air during an operation to facilitate its indentation by an instrument, — reversing for the operation of lithotrity one of the precepts of lithotomy.

NOTE.—Figs. 10 to 14 show plaster casts of bladders variously distended, and holding instruments to show the effect of a slight pressure in indenting the floor of the bladder in order to facilitate the approach of fragments. The dotted line near the summit of each represents the level of an air cavity, which makes it possible to place the cast in the exact position it occupied in a horizontal subject.

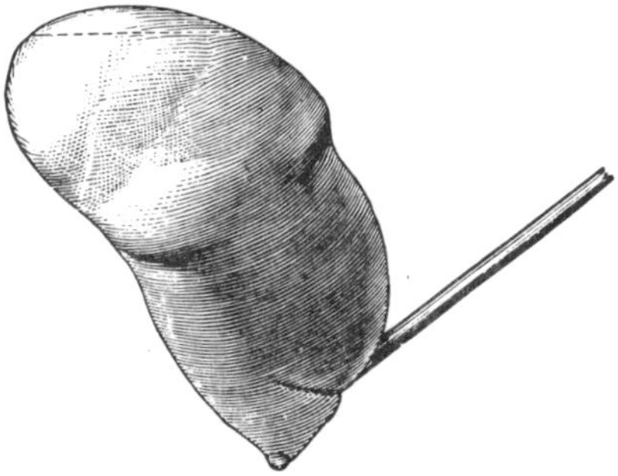

FIG. 10.[1]

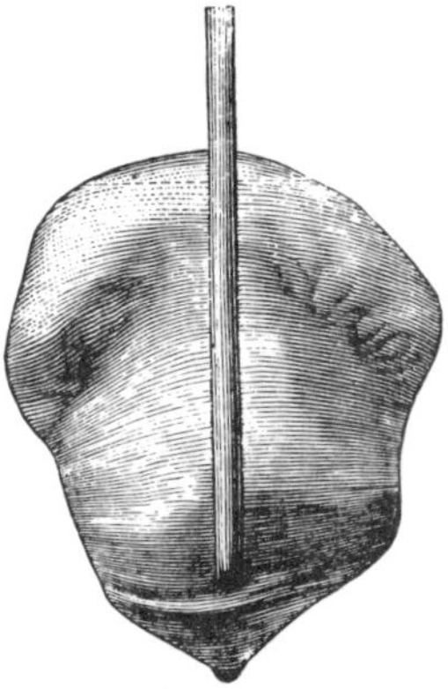

FIG. 10 *a*.

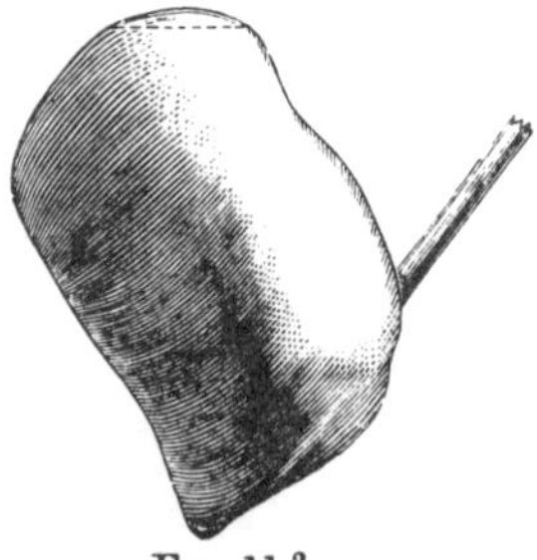

FIG. 11.[2]

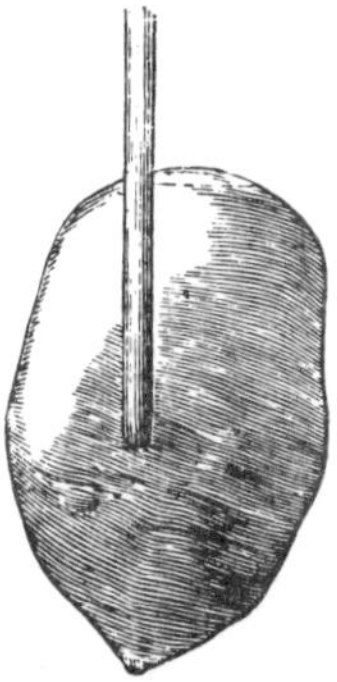

FIG. 11 *a*.

[1] Figs. 10 and 10 *a* present side and front views of a distended bladder of singular symmetry. The original suggests in profile the torso of a Silenus, the pectoral pouches overhanging the pubes, the abdomen beneath the symphysis, while the hollow loins were cushioned on the sigmoid flexure which indented them. The extremity of a curved tube is seen below, at the apex of an inverted tunnel, and just above it is a trace of the vesical valve. These figures are one fifth larger than the others

[2] Figs. 11 and 11 *a* show a less distended bladder, containing a straight tube which indents the posterior wall.

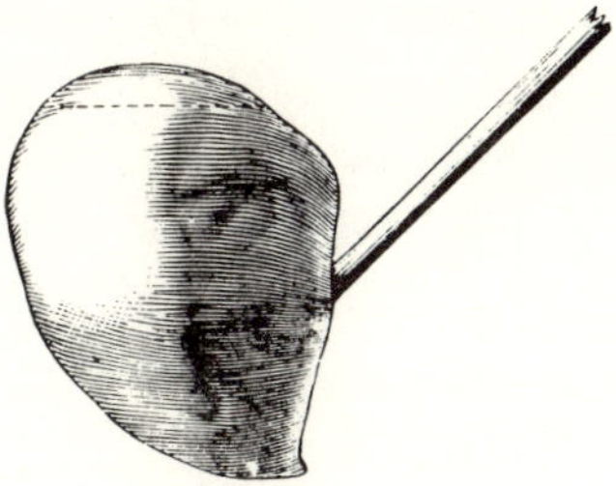

FIG. 12.[1]

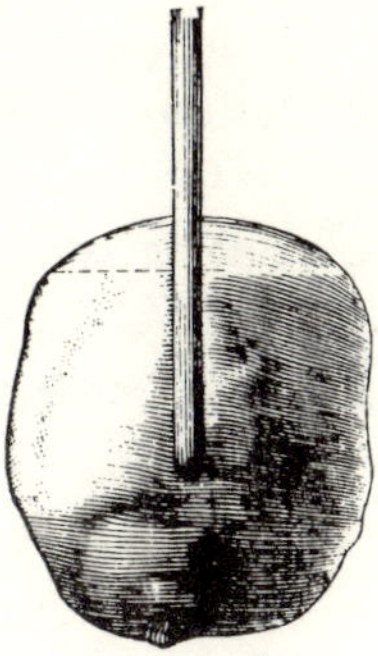

FIG. 12 *a*.

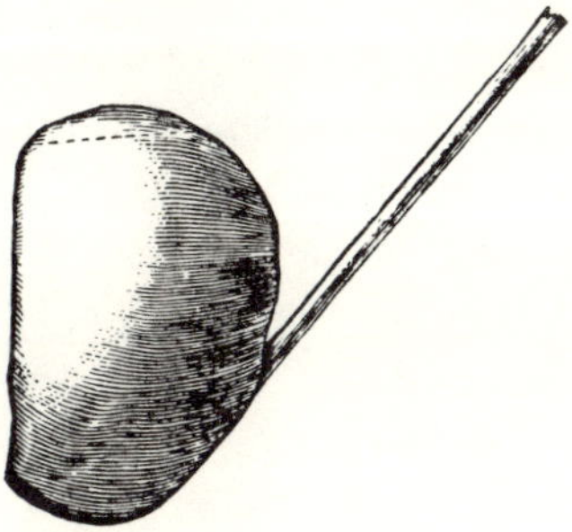

FIG. 13.[2]

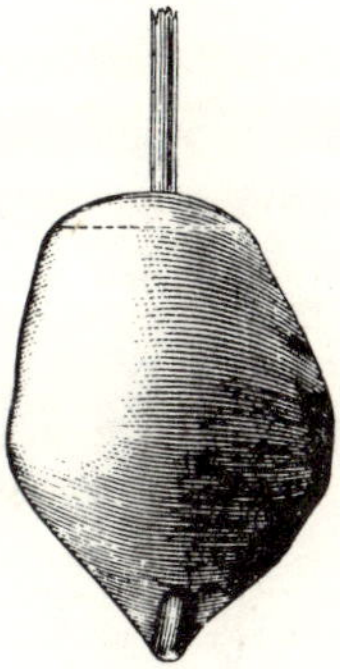

FIG. 13 *a*.

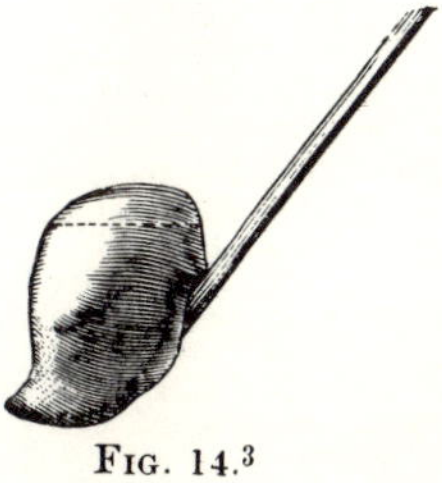

FIG. 14.[3]

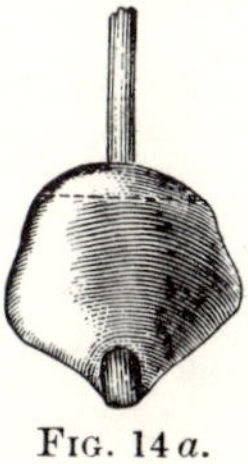

FIG. 14 *a*.

[1] Figs. 12 and 12 *a*, — a bladder with a curved tube brought forward behind the prostate, slightly indenting the floor.

[2] Figs. 13 and 13 *a*, — a bladder containing a large lithotrite, which has so depressed the floor that the posterior wall rises perpendicularly.

[3] Figs. 14 and 14 *a*, — a bladder with a very small injection, imprisoning a lithotrite.

The sigmoid flexure is largely concerned in compressing the bladder behind. The posterior wall of this viscus may be so crowded by the intestines as to become flat or even concave. A horizontal section of the bladder is then transversely oval, flattened between the intestines behind and the pubes in front, each of these indenting it. A well-filled or tense abdomen tends so to shorten the antero-posterior diameter of the bladder, that, while a large stone may gravitate backward into that part of the bladder which is compressed by the intestines, carrying the thin wall with it, it is not so with a small fragment, which unless the floor be artificially depressed may lie on one side or the other of the vesical orifice more readily than at a considerable distance behind it. So, in sounding with a curved sound, it may sometimes be a little difficult to move the instrument back and forth in the urethra, although its extremity may be readily turned down upon the floor of the bladder on either side. It is seen also (Figs. 11, 13, 14), as a result of this conformation, that a lithotrite, or straight tube, standing at an angle of forty-five degrees with the recumbent body, abruptly buries its extremity in the floor of the bladder near the foot of the posterior wall, which then becomes more upright, and that it does not lie upon the centre of an extended concave surface as sometimes represented. The deep pit at the extremity of the straight tube and the similar depression made farther forward by the curved and inverted tube (Figs. 10 and 12) show how readily fragments can be made to gravitate to the lithotrite, or to the tube orifice, provided the latter be not plugged by the mucous membrane. The curved tube when inverted rests on the adherent floor; but a straight tube bearing upon the free and thin posterior wall (Fig. 11) should not be urged too forcibly against it. In either case, the nearer the instrument approaches a vertical position the deeper will be the indentation. A pit of this sort formed in the elastic floor by an almost insensible pressure of the instrument explains the observation of Thompson, that when a fragment is caught by the lithotrite many more are likely to be caught, like fish in a pool, in the same place. A central indentation of the floor also explains how in certain cases of large stone a lithotrite or sound may be passed back and forth beneath it without touching it, unless the beak is tilted up. The stone may then seem to adhere to the upper wall of the bladder, and to be suspended from it. During an operation of lithotomy, I have myself been deceived in this way up to the moment of introducing the finger into the bladder. I am not aware that this common source of error in diagnosis has been before pointed out. An adherent stone is rare.

Case I. — December 14, 1875. Age, sixty-four. Date of symptoms, six years. Two or three stones measuring from half an inch to more than three quarters. Three sittings. First sitting: no fragments were removed through a tube. Second sitting: interval, seven days; duration, forty-five minutes under ether; quantity removed, "a large mass of fragments;" size of tube, twenty-seven. Third sitting: interval, twelve days; quantity removed, "a few fragments." Result: the patient was discharged well one week after.

Case II. — May 15, 1876. Age, sixty. Date of symptoms, twenty years. Two stones of one and one quarter inches and three quarters of an inch diameter respectively. One sitting: duration, one hour and a half under ether; lithotrite introduced three times; quantity removed, one hundred and sixty-seven grains; size of tube, twenty-nine; there was afterward a slight cystitis; no fragments were passed; in two weeks the patient was again sounded, and no fragments were found. Result: discharged well.

Case III. — August 6, 1876. Age, sixty-two. Date of symptoms, eighteen months. Several stones, none larger than three quarters of an inch. The patient was confined to the house in great pain, drawing his water every half-hour or less. The prostate was unusually large. One sitting: duration, about one hour and three quarters under ether; size of tube, twenty-nine. He afterward passed a few grains of sand only. Result: no unfavorable symptoms; almost entire relief from pain; later, no difficulty in retaining water, but continues to pass a catheter; gained flesh and former health, and resumed avocation.

CASE IV.—December 14, 1876. Age, sixty-six. Date of symptoms, two years. Single stone. One sitting: duration, about an hour under ether; quantity removed, one hundred and eleven grains; size of tube, twenty-eight. Result: the patient did well for two days; then there was a chill with higher temperature, pain in the back, and pain referred to the left hip; a gradually failing pulse; moderate meteorism, with but little tenderness; death on the sixth day. An autopsy was not permitted.

CASE V.—January 8, 1877. Age, fifty-five. Date of symptoms, one year. Single stone. "A severe chill followed the primary examination." Seven days after, the meatus was incised and enlarged from twenty-eight to thirty-one. One sitting: diameters of stone, ten to twenty millimetres; duration, one hour under ether; size of tube, thirty-one. Result: no sand or fragments were afterward passed; nor were there any subsequent symptoms.

CASE VI.—April 21, 1877. Age, forty-three. Single stone with nucleus of dead bone. Five years ago the pelvis of this patient was crushed. Sinuses discharging dead bone opened on both hips. Six months after the injury symptoms of stone existed. One sitting: duration, one hour and a half under ether; meatus incised; size of tube, thirty; quantity removed, sixty-six grains, and also three small pieces of bone, doubtless nuclei, one of which was incrusted; an indurated spot was detected by the tube where the bladder seemed to adhere to the pelvis. Four days after, under ether, the lithotrite brought away with difficulty through the urethra a square scale of bone too elastic to be broken, measuring five eighths of an inch by seven sixteenths, but no sand or fragments. Result: there were no unpleasant symptoms at any time; and after another careful examination for bone the patient was discharged well.

CASE VII.—(Dr. T. B. Curtis's case.) March 6, 1877. Age, fifty-four. Date of symptoms, two years. Single stone. One sitting: diameter of stone, one inch and a quarter; duration, one hour and twenty-five minutes under ether; lithotrite introduced three times; size of tube, thirty-one; quantity removed, when dry, two hundred and fifty-seven grains; the six largest fragments weighed together twenty-four grains; the strained urine yielded during the next week two and one half grains. Result: rapid recovery, with no subsequent symptoms.

CASE VIII.—(Dr. C. B. Porter's case.) August 19, 1877. Age, sixty-one. A large, flabby man, with a feeble pulse. Date of symptoms, twenty-six years. Two stones: one so large that it was barely possible to lock the lithotrite. Passes water every fifteen or twenty minutes. Three sittings. First sitting: duration, one hour and a half under ether; size of tube, twenty-eight; quantity removed, two hundred and twenty-eight grains; passed afterward one hundred and eight grains. Second sitting: interval, four days; duration, three hours under ether; size of tube, thirty; quantity removed, seven hundred and forty-four grains; passed afterward sixteen grains; no after symptoms of importance. Third sitting: interval, five days; duration, three and three quarter hours under ether; size of tube, thirty-one; quantity removed, seven hundred and six grains; no pain or discomfort afterward; total number of grains after drying, one thousand eight hundred and two. Result: discharged well two weeks from the date of the first operation; after a few weeks the patient could retain his water from three to four hours.

The details of the earlier of these operations are expressed with less exactness than I might now desire, but were dictated by myself at the time, and are within the fact as to the duration of each operation and the size of the stones. The cases, all of soft stones,—that is, not oxalate of lime,—are the only ones by which the method that is the subject of this paper has been tested. As statistics, they are not so numerous as to have importance. But they abundantly illustrate what this operation is able to accomplish in removing at once a large quantity of stone by the urethra. The fatal case without an autopsy, the absence of which is greatly to be regretted, must pass for what it is worth. The other cases demonstrate a tolerance by the bladder of protracted manipulation which has not hitherto been recognized.

Since the above was published, six cases have been successfully treated by the new method, — making fourteen cases in all, with one death, which is about the proportion of fatality in Sir Henry Thompson's list of four hundred and twenty-two cases, with sittings of three minutes' duration. Among the later cases, two of the three which occurred in my own practice offered exceptional interest. In the first case, a calculus lodged deep in the urethra was removed. A contracted urethra was then enlarged by divulsion with Voillemier's instrument, a No. 31 tube was introduced, and a considerable quantity of thick mucus was immediately evacuated. This was found to contain twenty-five grains of phosphatic fragments, the whole mass being so voluminous that it could not probably have been otherwise as well withdrawn. In the second case, the extremity and wings of a red rubber catheter had been lost in the bladder. After the stone of which these formed the nucleus was broken, the fragments of catheter came through the tube at once. The following are the cases: —

Case IX. — Patient aged fifty. Twenty-five grains of phosphatic deposit evacuated; time, four minutes. 1861, the urethra was opened to remove impacted gravel. 1863, he was cut for stone, and has occasionally passed gravel since. 1876, he was operated on for stricture, and has passed a No. 12 sound until within two weeks; one week ago he voided a stone "as large as the end of his little finger." Now he has frequent micturition, and an impacted stone is felt in the urethra just behind the scrotum. This stone was broken, and ten grains were removed with long forceps. The rigid and cicatricial urethra was next divulsed. The bladder was evacuated through a twenty-nine tube, yielding about one and a half ounces of mucus and gravel, the latter weighing when dry twenty-five grains. The walls of the urethra were now scraped with the female blade of a small urethral lithotrite, to remove an abundant and closely adherent calculous deposit. During the succeeding five days the temperature and pulse remained nearly normal, frequent micturition being somewhat relieved by opiates. For a dull pain in the urethra after urinating, water was injected to wash the passage after each micturition,—an expedient I have long employed in the treatment of gonorrhœa, and also, in imitation of the usual practice after strong applications to the eye, to terminate abruptly the action of strong gonorrhœal injections in the urethra. The patient did well. At the end of three weeks, a single phosphatic concretion as large as a small pea was discovered and removed through a twenty-six tube.

Case X.—Patient's age fifty. Eighty-two grains of stone with a rubber catheter nucleus were evacuated; whole time, twenty-five minutes. Eighteen weeks ago, during the treatment of a traumatic laceration of the urethra, a winged rubber catheter was kept in the bladder. A portion of this was broken off and remained there, causing in a few days frequent micturition and cloudy urine. Five weeks ago a stone was discovered. Now there is frequent micturition, and abrupt stoppage followed by pain in the glans penis. The bladder was filled and emptied,—the fluid measuring half a pint, which quantity was again injected. By the lithotrite the stone measured nearly an inch and a quarter, being doubtless caught lengthwise. A certain elasticity of the closed blades led to their withdrawal with a small fragment of brittle rubber. This withdrawal was twice repeated with bits of rubber, including the two wings and also twenty-seven grains of stone. The whole operation had now lasted nine minutes. A straight evacuating tube, No. 31, was next introduced, and the bladder pumped during four minutes, after which it yielded no more foreign material. Almost all the stone thus evacuated (fifty-five grains), together with three bits of rubber catheter measuring respectively three fourths, seven eighths, and one fourth of an inch in length, and No. 23 Charrière in diameter, came through the tube within the first minute. The lithotrite was now again introduced, but nothing more discovered; after which the bladder was again washed out. The entire operation lasted twenty-five minutes, much of which was occupied in determining the fact that the bladder had been evacuated. The next night the patient had no pain, and micturated but twice instead of six times as habitually before. Two days after, the temperature suddenly rose to 102° Fahrenheit, but as quickly subsided without other sign or symptom, the patient being entirely relieved.

CASE XI. — Patient's age, sixty-two. Date of symptoms, three years. Two stones, lithic; largest diameter, thirty millimetres. One sitting: duration, one hour and twenty minutes; size of tubes, twenty-nine and thirty; quantity removed, three hundred and nineteen grains; urethra somewhat contracted in front of scrotum. In evacuating these stones the time was found to have been occupied as follows: crushing, twenty-nine minutes; evacuating, twenty-four minutes; the rest of the time being consumed in passing and withdrawing the instruments, renewing the water, etc. As usual, most of the fragments passed the tube early in the operation, and readily, much of the time occupied by the evacuation being consumed in making sure that no fragments were left behind. Micturition before the operation once every hour and a half; after the operation about once an hour, and obstructed by purulent mucus. The patient had a large though yielding prostate. The water was drawn during eight days; at the end of which he was generally able to relieve himself, the purulent mucus having diminished in quantity. The testicles were somewhat swollen. Though still under treatment, the patient is fairly convalescent.

A discussion of the relative values of lithotrity and lithotomy, at a recent meeting of the Royal Medical and Chirurgical Society,[1] has interest in this connection, because it exposes the current English views upon this subject, while it gives prominence, by contrast, to the advantages of the new method of lithotrity over the old one. It is evident that the large tubes offer a ready means for preventing the recurrence of stone by either nuclei or fragments, which is "by no means uncommon" after lithotrity, as Mr. Cadge remarked, and "one of its serious defects;" also, for removing the phosphatic deposits which, in the words of Sir Henry Thompson on that occasion, are "not unfrequently left after lithotrity," "being due to the injury done to the mucous membrane by sharp fragments of stone, and by continued instrumentation." Sir Henry looked upon them as "unavoidable, and as a price

[1] March 12, 1878. See "The Lancet," March 16, 1878.

paid for the greater security to life which lithotrity affords." Again, Sir James Paget said "he must confess to a general feeling in favor of lithotomy over lithotrity," unless "the calculus can be got rid of in two or three sittings." Sir Henry Thompson on this subject said, "Three, or at most four sittings, at which point he should distinctly prefer to cut."

The obvious question then is whether in adult patients, when the stone requires more than three or four sittings of a few minutes each, by the old method, it is safer to cut, or to employ the new and rapid lithotrity, with evacuation. The latter must be preferred to lithotomy, in cases now rejected by the lithotritist, unless it can be shown that its mortality amounts to one in three, — this being the death-rate of lithotomy in such cases, as stated during the discussion. So great a mortality from the new operation is improbable.

There can be no doubt of the importance of the complete evacuation of final fragments, renal nuclei, phosphatic masses, and foreign bodies.

In the matter of crushing, stress was justly laid upon the difficulty of withdrawing the impacted lithotrite from the bladder, — both Sir Henry Thompson and Mr. Coulson speaking of fragments actually "preventing the withdrawal of the instrument," and "requiring in one case incision in the perinæum." This difficulty is obviated by the new notched lithotrite, which effectually clears itself. It also permits more expeditious work. The larger size, as made by Collin, is much more powerful than the usual lithotrite, while it can readily be introduced into a bladder that will admit a No. 27 tube.

As the female urethra is so easily dilated, the new lithotrity will doubtless prove to be the easiest way to dispose of calculi in the female, the tubes being made shorter and larger than for the male urethra.

I may again say, in conclusion, that since its first announcement this method of evacuation has been, by repeated experiment, so modified and reduced to a system, as to have become much more rapid and efficient. The time then consumed by the operation, although it showed a surprising tolerance of the bladder, is no criterion of the time now required for accomplishing the same result. The improvements relate chiefly to the systematic dispersion or collection of fragments in the bladder, to the position of the tube, and to the recognition and immediate removal of obstruction. A considerable part of the time is still consumed in ascertaining whether the stone is wholly evacuated, — a large part of it being usually removed at the beginning of the operation.

The following are the chief points connected with the modification in lithotrity which I have described: —

1. The calculus, although not necessarily pulverized, is crushed as rapidly and completely as is practicable. The dust and fragments are immediately evacuated, and a serious source of irritation is thus removed.

2. This can be generally effected in a single operation.

3. The operation (performed of course under ether) may be, if necessary, of one or two hours' duration, or even longer.

4. The method applies to larger stones than have been hitherto considered to lie within the province of the lithotritist. It also applies to small stones, nuclei, phosphatic deposits, and foreign substances.

5. Evacuation is best accomplished by a large tube, preferably straight, — with a distal orifice, the extremity of which is shaped to facilitate its introduction and (during suction) to repel the bladder wall, — and by an elastic exhausting bulb which acts partly as a siphon. Below the latter is a glass receptacle for débris.

6. The best size for the tube is the largest the urethra will admit.

7. Such a tube is usually introduced with facility, if passed vertically as far as it will go toward the anus before changing its direction, and afterward directed almost horizontally, and passed by rotation through the triangular ligament. The first part of this rule applies also to the introduction of a lithotrite, and even a curved catheter. A free injection of oil is important.

8. A small meatus should be enlarged, or a stricture divulsed, to allow the passage of a large tube.

9. If the bladder be not small, a large and powerful lithotrite is always better than a small one.

10. That this may have room for action, the escaping water should be replaced occasionally through a tube inserted a few inches into the urethra by the side of the lithotrite. But the bladder should not be over-distended.

11. To save time, and also to prevent undue dilation of the vesical neck, a non-impacting lithotrite is desirable. The jaws of a non-fenestrated instrument will not impact if the male blade is furnished with alternate triangular notches by which the débris is discharged laterally, and also with a long thin spur at the heel fitted to a corresponding slot in the female blade, — provided the floor of the female blade, especially at the heel, be made nearly on a level with its rim. To repel the bladder, the female blade should be longer and a little wider than is usual. It should have also low sides easily accessible to fragments, — relying for strength less upon these than upon a central ridge below the heel. In the male blade of such a lithotrite, the apices of the triangles should be a little blunted. Lastly, a non-fenestrated female blade protects the floor of the bladder during a long sitting. A fenestrated instrument directs sharp splinters against it. The latter also delays the process of disintegration by

delivering through its opening the same fragments many times.

12. In locking and unlocking a lithotrite repeatedly in a long operation, it takes less time and is easier to turn the right wrist, as in my instrument, than to displace the thumb of either hand in search of a button or a lever, as in previous instruments.

The efficiency of evacuation has recently been further illustrated by the removal through the urethra, under ether, without crushing, of thirty-five small calculi, during a single sitting of half an hour, in which the bladder was completely emptied. The patient was sixty-five years of age, the prostate large. The stones were lithic, nearly spherical, and almost destitute of facets. The two largest had a diameter = 34 of Charrière. Of these stones thirteen were drawn through a tube of the calibre 31 Charrière. Twenty-two were arrested in the tube, — the smaller being detained by other larger stones simultaneously engaged in its extremity, into which they closely fitted. Thus obstructed, the tube was withdrawn ten times, always with one or more calculi. The stones, when dry, weighed two hundred and forty grains. I used in this instance a tube having a long oval orifice with a thick edge, passing the latter through the meatus, and especially the prostatic portion of the canal, with facility, by rotating the tube.

Such an operation can hardly be called lithotrity. I have therefore proposed for the new method the name Litholap′-axy, — λίθος, and λάπαξις (*evacuation*).

RAPID LITHOTRITY, WITH EVACUATION.[1]

To the Editor:

An article by Dr. Keyes in your last issue (May 18) gives me occasion to refer to one or two misapprehensions which pervade his allusions to "Modern Lithotrity," as he terms the new operation for stone.

In this article, which is devoted mainly to a description of the jaws of a lithotrite, the writer states that my lithotrite "must sometimes clog," because "it is made on the principle of Reliquet's." He is mistaken. In the first place, Reliquet's instrument is fenestrated; mine is solid. In the second place, as an ascertained fact, my lithotrite does not impact. The male blade is furnished with lateral notches forming inclined planes by which the detritus is extruded right and left, except where a small portion at the heel is driven through a slot by an effective spur. Reliquet's non-impacting lithotrite is identical with the obsolete fenestrated *brisepierre*, with teeth in the opening below to insure pulverization. Dr. Keyes proposes to remove these added teeth, and return to the *brisepierre à mors fenêtré* (*porte à faux*) of Charrière.[2] In fact, he goes back to the flattened jaws of the "slightly indented and fenestrated or open female blade" figured by Costello,[3] with a male blade as small as in the common lithotrite, to avoid pinching the mucous membrane,[4] — in short, to a common lithotrite with the floor removed.

1 New York Medical Record, June 8, 1878.

2 Nouveau Dictionnaire de Médecine et de Chirurgie, tom. xx. p. 667. Paris, 1875.

3 Cyclopædia of Practical Surgery, vol. iii. pp. 21, 50. London, 1861.

4 The mucous membrane would be more secure if care were taken always to blunt, or round a little, the edge of the sole of the male blade.

I am gratified to find that the writer of the article indorses my statement (which is an important corollary of the new system) that "*in future it will be no longer essential to pulverize the fragments, but only to comminute them.*" This may be accomplished by either a fenestrated or a solid instrument. Any fenestrated lithotrite that sufficiently reduces the size of fragments driven through it, enables them to pass the evacuating tubes, the use of which characterizes the new method. But although instruments of this class will doubtless do well enough with small stones, as does indeed a common lithotrite, my objections to a fenestrated instrument, of which I considered and rejected several (including that proposed in your journal), are these: —

1. Sharp fragments, while firmly engaged in the opening, or driven through it, are likely to injure the floor of the bladder. During a long operation, such as I propose, it is hardly possible to prevent the frequent contact of the floor of the bladder with the extremity of the instrument; in which case the latter does not present to the mucous membrane a rounded and polished surface, but irritates it with protruding splinters of calculus, continually coming in contact with the same limited region of the floor.

2. The sides separately are not as strong as when united by a floor of metal, and if they are made low enough to be readily accessible to fragments (which is important) are consequently liable to break, especially should the strain come on one alone. The strength of a fenestrated blade lies in the height of its sides, and is but partially compensated by their breadth, unless the latter is extreme. Moreover, the male blade must be disadvantageously narrow. When it is wide, the corresponding opening not only impairs the strength, but delivers large fragments.

3. Now, although fragments, if small enough, pass the tube readily, dust and small débris pass more readily, and first.

Therefore when a fragment has been fortunately seized, the operator loses an opportunity if he fails to crush it, — as happens when he drives it through a fenestrated blade to be again seized. Although by the new method pulverization is no longer essential as before, our aim is still to accomplish a maximum disintegration at each closure of the jaws; and this is better done with a solid upper and lower jaw than when either of them is fenestrated. A non-impacting instrument is very desirable, but not at the sacrifice of efficient and rapid crushing, or with danger to the mucous membrane.

I may add that, to prevent impaction, when the blades are closed it is quite unnecessary that the male blade should project below the female blade, — an arrangement Dr. Keyes has devised and emphasized for this purpose, and a description of which, indeed, occupies a considerable portion of his paper. It is sufficient that the blades of a fenestrated instrument occupy the same level at the outlet.

Again, the heel of the instrument figured in your journal has the form of the segment of a circle. Such curved blades admit fragments, and crush them at great disadvantage.

Blades should be as straight, set at as nearly a right angle with the shaft, and as little rounded at the heel as is compatible with their introduction.

In my non-fenestrated lithotrite the blades are nearly straight, and the triangular notches deliver on alternate sides. This lateral action not only clears the jaws, but makes their hold very tenacious. It also secures to the blades the incidental advantage of grinding while they crush.

Your contributor finds my instrument too large (or, as he says, "clumsy"). It is made large with a distinct object; namely, to break larger and harder stones than have been hitherto considered within the province of the lithotrite. It comminutes, with safety to the bladder and without impaction, as no lithotrite hitherto devised has done. The new method of treatment is grounded in the fact that the normal urethra admits larger instruments, and is an easier road to the bladder, than the lithotritist has hitherto recognized. The operator soon becomes not only accustomed to the use of a large lithotrite, but reluctantly foregoes the power it gives him, even when the stone is small. Collin has, however, made a second size.

While the power possessed by this lithotrite and the fact that it does not impact are its more important features, and especially adapt it to the requirements of the method now proposed, almost as useful is the change in its lock. I believe that this will ultimately be adopted by those not already educated to the old system, because it is based upon the readiest movements of the hand and wrist.

But a modification of the jaws and lock of the lithotrite is an inconsiderable feature of the proposed new method. Rapid work is indeed thereby facilitated; and an empty instrument can safely be withdrawn as often as the operator pleases, to relieve the bladder of what will come through the tubes, and so clear the way for more rapid crushing.

A far more important point to the lithotritist is *the comparative harmlessness of long sittings*, which I think was unsuspected until the publication of my paper. In the first trials, what was wanted was not so much an improvement of the existing crushing apparatus, as *an efficient means of evacuation*, capable of removing all the débris at one sitting. For this purpose, the large tubes criticised in your journal are absolutely indispensable. Their use is precisely what makes the new operation practicable, and together with their manipulation is perhaps its chief innovation. The set of tubes described in my paper ranges from 27 to 31 Charrière; but they can be procured of any smaller size, and should of course be adapted to the previously ascertained calibre of the urethra.

It will, however, be found that the efficiency of the tubes diminishes very rapidly with their size, and that a canal narrowed by stricture, or by a small meatus, will require to be enlarged so that the introduction of a large tube may be made possible. In such a case as that reported, where the urethra admitted only a No. 20 instrument (French), and in which the operator of course found my largest tubes too large, I should prefer to increase the size of the passage rather than attempt to extract the fragments of a calculus through the small calibres formerly in use, even though the tube were otherwise modified as I have recommended. With a normal urethra I do not believe that the tubes supplied by Tiemann will be found any too large.

The change proposed in the new procedure, and the consequent advantages, will appear in a clearer light if we consider the limitations of the usual dilatory method explicitly acknowledged, quite recently, by both Sir Henry Thompson and Sir James Paget. These distinguished authorities gave their opinion that lithotrity should be restricted to stones requiring only two or three or at most four sittings of two or three minutes each. For larger stones, in their judgment, lithotomy does better, though resulting, in adults, in a mortality of one in three. It should be added that when lithotrity was thus pronounced unsuccessful in such cases, all attempts at the immediate evacuation of débris had resulted in practical failure.

The new method not only crushes calculi exceeding in size the limits hitherto affixed to crushing alone, but at the same sitting evacuates by the urethra the fragments and débris. This is done under ether, in a sitting of one or two hours' duration, or even longer. So far, its results have been better than could have been anticipated, — being sixteen or seventeen cases of complete evacuation with but one death, against one in thirteen by the usual method. Several of these patients would have been, by accepted rules, subjected to lithotomy, and consequently to a risk equal to one death in three cases. I cannot but think that with due care in its application the method now proposed will be found to yield results at least as favorable as those before obtained.

HENRY J. BIGELOW.

BOSTON, May 25, 1878.

LITHOLAPAXY.[1]

The object of this operation is to remove at once, by the urethra, the débris created by the lithotrite. It is based on the belief of a tolerance by the bladder of protracted manipulation, which has not been hitherto recognized. It is also based on a theory that a brief manipulation, in the bladder, of polished and blunted instruments is less irritating to that organ than is the protracted presence of fragments, especially in view of the fact that the bladder hugs the latter more or less sharply at each micturition. When lithotrity is properly done, the process of crushing is easy and safe. The real question relates to the subsequent disposal of the fragments. If the purpose of the surgeon is to get rid of them, and if their evacuation has hitherto been, for the want of proper appliances, slow and injurious to the bladder, it is fair to consider whether this object cannot be attained with the aid of an instrument devised to evacuate the bladder more quickly through the urethra, while its walls are held apart at their full normal dimensions, — such, for example, as this canal attains when the meatus is compressed during the passage of urine.

It is quite safe to leave this question to be settled by such further experiments as shall be deemed wholly satisfactory. In the mean time, in order that the operation of evacuation may be accomplished in the readiest and safest way, it may be well to offer a few explanatory suggestions in respect to it.

One difficulty at the outset may be illustrated by a simple experiment. If a small catheter, surmounted by a funnel, be

1 The Lancet, Nov. 2, 1878.

tied in an ox's bladder and held vertically, water introduced by the funnel will distend the bladder very forcibly. Similarly, the hydrostatic pressure of a column of water but a few inches higher than the pubes will distend the human bladder beyond its safe capacity. So that it may be assumed that any catheter surmounted by a bulb is more liable to injure the bladder by over-distending it than when the bulb is lowered to the level of the bladder or below it. The weight of a full bulb in the former position also prevents accurate manipulation of the catheter. It is more easily handled in a stand.

The instrument now employed is a siphon, at one of whose extremities is a large metal tube that takes advantage of the full normal capacity of the urethra, while the other terminates in an elastic bulb and glass receptacle. The tube extremity is shaped to facilitate its introduction, and also so that its orifice may be placed, if necessary, at the lowest point in the bladder, at the apex of an inverted funnel, among the fragments, without being occluded by the usual valve-like action of the bladder-wall. A straight tube has advantages over a curved one: the surgeon can more readily direct it and regulate its pressure; it is less liable to obstruction, and better cleared by a rod. Again, a straight instrument, when of the size 29, 30, or 31 of Charrière, is more easy to introduce than a curved one. In order to carry it into the bladder with least resistance, it should be passed as far as possible in a nearly vertical direction toward the anus, before the handle is depressed; its extremity then lies not only in front of the aperture in the triangular ligament, but, what is of more importance, below it, and is afterward tilted up to this orifice by depressing the handle of the instrument to the axis of the body. The tube should next be rotated through this aperture like a corkscrew; and during this process its point, which is made a little eccentric for this purpose, revolves in a small circle until it discovers the orifice. A common difficulty in introducing a catheter or lithotrite results from depressing the handle prematurely, by which the beak is arrested above the aperture in the ligament instead of below it. This error should be carefully avoided in introducing the large straight tube, which so fills the urethra that it needs every advantage in traversing its less yielding parts. Indeed, it is not superfluous to say that even a free use of oil injected with a syringe both into the urethra and into the tube may sometimes determine the question of the passage of the larger sizes. And yet, with these precautions, the whole manœuvre is a very easy one. Before introducing the tube, the calibre of the urethra is ascertained by a common olive-pointed elastic bougie, or a sound. I have not found much advantage in trying to dilate it, unless at the moment of the operation, by incising the meatus, which is the narrowest part, or by "divulsing" a stricture when it exists. Such preliminary enlargement of the contracted canal, unless especially contra-indicated, suggests itself.

But there is another important measure that does not suggest itself, and yet deserves careful attention. In order to protect the bladder from over-distention, the first movement of the aspirator should be to withdraw water from it, and not to inject water into it. This cannot be too strongly emphasized. As a preliminary to this precaution, the surgeon ascertains exactly the capacity of the bladder. For this purpose it should be emptied by a catheter, and tepid water slowly injected, until the fluid is forcibly expelled between the catheter and the loosely grasped urethral walls. This reaction of the organ, which anæsthesia does not prevent, may be relied on to furnish a sufficiently accurate indication of the size of its cavity. If the fluid be now drawn off and measured, the same amount may be safely reinjected through the large tube, which is next to be introduced, the injected fluid being retained in the bladder by a tape tied round the penis, with the thumb or a cork at the extremity of the tube. Here is, I think, a critical moment of the operation; because if the contents of the bulb are added to those of the already distended bladder, the organ may be over-stretched. It should not be forgotten, therefore, that the elastic bulb, before it is attached to the tube, should be compressed until the sides meet, *in order that its first action may be to withdraw from the bladder, by its expansion, such an amount of fluid as can be reinjected with safety.* The present instrument holds ten ounces; by compression it loses five ounces. This amount would then be aspirated from the bladder by its first expansion, after which the usual pumping action displaces only about two ounces of fluid at each stroke, and can hardly injure the bladder. In order to direct attention to the importance of compressing the elastic bulb, a clamp is provided with the instrument to compress the bulb before it is attached to the tube. Other details, relating especially to the signs and avoidance of obstruction, may be found elsewhere. Briefly, when fragments are still felt, and yet cease to fall into the trap, there is either obstruction, — which usually occurs in the tube, and should be removed by compressing the bulb or introducing the rod, — or the fragments are too large to pass the tube, and need further crushing. In respect to the time occupied by the whole operation, I would suggest that if the surgeon will crush the stone as usual and then remove the fragments, he will probably find his patient to be still in so good a condition that he will be tempted again to introduce the lithotrite, followed by the tube. At the end of half an hour or more he will have repeated this several times, and will then find that the stone, if of average dimensions, has been evacuated. He will also find, in a common case, that the patient is no worse for the operation.

As these remarks apply chiefly to the mechanical part of

lithotrity, — an operation which, indeed, depends more than any other for its success upon a careful and economical adaptation of its instruments to their employment, — a few observations may be here added respecting the lithotrite.[1]

It is very desirable, during a long operation, to prevent the impaction of the lithotrite, which interferes with crushing, and sometimes injures the neck of the bladder. This may be effected by raising the floor of the female blade, and by adding lateral notches to the male blade, which should be also provided with a central septum at the heel. The lateral grooves for the male blade should also extend through the heel of the female blade. I am persuaded that the simplest movement for locking a lithotrite is a quarter rotation of the right wrist, without displacing the fingers of either hand. Further, it seems not to be always remembered by surgeons that the " rapidity " of a lithotrite depends upon the inclination of its screw thread; and that while the slowest screw gives most power and requires the strongest blades, " rapidity" sacrifices power. In the longer and more rapid operation now contemplated, larger and stronger blades than have been commonly employed, and which also better protect the bladder than do the latter, seem to me desirable.

I have elsewhere said that the blades of a lithotrite should be as nearly at right angles with the shaft, and their floor as straight, as is compatible with their convenient introduction into the bladder. Many instruments are made with oblique blades, which are also so rounded at the heel as to curve their floor. This is a mistake. A cubical stone, for instance, would exactly fit a right-angled lithotrite. But when the same blades are made oblique, at an angle for example of forty-five degrees with the shaft, then in order to grasp the same stone they must not only be opened wider, but they will

1 The aspirating siphon and the lithotrite have been made by Weiss and Son, with great mechanical perfection.

not reach so far out upon the stone. In other words, the size of their grasp rapidly diminishes with their obliquity. They must be opened wider, and they seize less of the stone. Their power also diminishes, because if they are made longer with the view of preserving their grasp, their increasing leverage increases friction in the slide. This is readily seen by increasing the obliquity until they reach the line of the stem of the instrument. The shaft and blades are then in a continuous straight line, and they merely roll the fragment between them. The latter acts only as a wedge to separate them, while the friction of the slide is at its maximum. In other words, right-angled blades crush best and wedge least. Oblique blades, on the contrary, wedge more and crush less, and the depth of their grasp is also less. And what is here true of the whole blade is true of any part of it, — the heel, for example, which should not be oblique nor much rounded, but as nearly at right angles with the shaft and with as straight a floor as is compatible with its convenient introduction. It is only the difficulty of introducing right-angled blades that compels us to make them a little oblique and curved. But the slanting and hooked blades, sometimes still made, act at great disadvantage. It may be added that the tip of the female blade should be bevelled, so that (if we compare it to a bent finger) it may impinge against the upper wall of the prostate, while passing it, rather with its pulp than with its nail.

In conclusion, it may be said that a small stone does not usually entail a serious operation of any kind. On the other hand, a large stone does. It may be better to resort to lithotomy in the case of a large stone, with a diseased bladder or kidney, however fatal the former operation may be in such cases. But there has hardly been any material change of late years in the operation of lithotomy, unless it be in a greater attention to cleanliness and in the general treatment of the patient. It is certain that no *bona fide* Lister dressing can be applied to the wound. The danger also of hæmorrhage remains the same as heretofore. So that I think any very great increase in the percentage of recoveries from lithotomy would, perhaps, result chiefly from a resort to the operation in more favorable cases than formerly, — by which I mean in certain cases of stone which have been of late relegated to lithotrity, and which might as well be subjects for experiment with the operation now proposed, as for lithotomy.

The question then presents itself thus: —

1. Whether, when any stone, large or small, has been crushed, it is not better to distend the urethra to its natural limits, and remove the detritus at once by a few strokes of the siphon, than to leave it to be expelled through the contracted urethra by the unaided and comparatively ineffectual efforts of the bladder.

2. Whether, by thus assisting the bladder, we may not so increase the amount evacuated, and so diminish the time of the operation, that it may be possible by the method now proposed to treat with success larger stones than heretofore by lithotrity.

LITHOLAPAXY.[1]

To the Editor:

The Lancet of February 1 contains a paper by Sir Henry Thompson, entitled "A Lecture on Lithotrity at one or more Sittings." In another communication, February 15, he promises to give his views more completely "in the fifth edition" of his Clinical Lectures "now going through the press." The publication of this volume will be looked for with the more interest because the Lecture on Lithotrity fails to give a clear exposition of the author's existing views. It mixes new and old ideas, its tendency being to obliterate rather than define the line between what has been done by lithotrity hitherto and what can be accomplished now, leaving the reader uncertain how far Sir Henry discriminates between the new and old method.

The new operation enlarges the range of lithotrity, and encroaches upon that which has hitherto been regarded as belonging exclusively to lithotomy. This is all I claim for it. Cases can be relieved by litholapaxy which would not have been treated by the old lithotrity; as, for instance, one case where eighteen hundred and two grains of soft stone were removed at three sittings, — one of nearly four hours' duration, the patient travelling home four days afterward. Such a result, till now wholly unprecedented, would have been before regarded as bordering on the impossible. Experience alone can decide the limits of the new operation.[2] I am surprised

[1] The Lancet, May 17, 1879.

[2] So early as 1846 Sir Philip Crampton said: "It appears, then, that cystotomy and lithotrity are not to be considered as rivals, and that the question as to which of these operations should be the rule and which the exception should never be brought into discussion; each operation

that Sir Henry should attribute to me a disposition "to make the rule absolute to remove at one sitting an entire stone, no matter how large it may be, or what may be the condition of the patient." He adds: "Invariable conformity to such a rule, I do not hesitate at the outset to say, will lead to results which though often successful will not seldom be disastrous." This is obvious.

In attempting to identify the old operation with the new, Sir Henry relies mainly upon his having used Clover's form of Crampton's instrument, with which Sir Philip, before 1846, drew "upwards of two drachms of pulverized calculus at once from the bladder."[1] He dwells much on what he calls "that useful instrument, the aspirator of Clover." It is figured in his former works with half-a-dozen differently curved catheters attached to it. He now figures it (see Lancet) with "a slight modification," as he says, based upon what he calls a "hint" from my "aspirator." It is quite extraordinary that Sir Henry should claim such efficiency for Clover's apparatus. Except in cases where the prostate is so enlarged that the bladder retains even sand, his is the only voice, so far as I know, that has spoken in its favor.[2]

has its special province, the boundaries of which (if, indeed, they admit of being fixed at all) can be determined only by a comparison of a vast collection of facts carefully noted, and above all faithfully reported and properly authenticated." (Dublin Quarterly Journal of Medical Science, 1846, vol. i. p. 25.)

[1] Dublin Quarterly Journal of Medical Science, 1846, vol. i. p. 22.

[2] For the information of those who have not seen my paper, I here cite the latest authorities on this point: —

We may here say, without fear of being accused of exaggeration, that evacuating injections practised after sittings of lithotrity have no apology for their use. *The whole surgical arsenal invented for their performance is absolutely useless. . . . It should be well understood that the best of evacuating catheters is worthless.* — DEMARQUAY ET COUSIN: *Nouveau Dictionnaire de Médecine et de Chirurgie Pratique*, pp. 693, 694. (Paris, 1875).

Having used it [Clover's apparatus] very frequently, I would add that it is necessary to use all such apparatus with extreme gentleness, and *I*

Clover's instrument is a very good bladder-washer. But as an evacuator of anything but sand and minute fragments that can also pass the urethra without it, it is unequivocally worthless. It cannot be otherwise. Its size, with its collar, is only No. 21 French calibre, through which nothing of importance can escape from the bladder. In fact, to adapt it to the new system, Sir Henry has been compelled to enlarge its calibre from 21 to 26. Again, the bulb of Clover is so weak that in a vertical position it cannot expand to its own full dimensions; much less can it aspirate effectively. For this slender bag Sir Henry has now substituted a bulb, "stiff," as he describes it, like mine. The short curve which I had selected from the arsenal of old catheters and sounds for the end of my

prefer to do without it, if possible. — SIR HENRY THOMPSON: *Practical Lithotrity and Lithotomy*, p. 215 (1871).

All these evacuating catheters are little employed. They require frequent and long manœuvres, which are not exempt from dangers; besides *they give passage as a rule only to dust, or to small fragments of stone, which would have escaped of themselves without inconvenience to the urethra.* — M. VOILLEMIER: *Dictionnaire Encyclopédique des Sciences Médicales*, p. 733 (1869).

In short, the "evacuating apparatus" and the evacuating method, hitherto employed do not evacuate. This fact is beyond question. BIGELOW: *Litholapaxy, etc.*, pp. 6, 7 (London, 1878).

Sir Henry Thompson also testifies to the inefficiency of Clover's instrument by admitting that when, in the old lithotrity, he wanted to evacuate the fragments as rapidily as possible, he employed several sittings. "It is desirable," he says (Lancet, January 8, 1876, p. 38), "to treat any cystitis that may occur during the course of the sittings, especially if it is severe, by freely crushing the stone without delay. . . . Under these circumstances, I place the patient under the influence of ether, crush freely all the large and sharp pieces, and wash out the débris with Mr. Clover's aspirator."

But as Clover's instrument evacuates inefficiently, Sir Henry is compelled to add: "If some large pieces still remain after the fresh crushing, the former symptoms of cystitis re-appear in two or three days, and may be again relieved by another sitting,—this time altogether or nearly so, as a succeeding crushing will no doubt dispose of the principal part of the stone, and leave at all events no considerable fragments."

curved tube he now discovers to be the "more generally useful form."[1] He has also adopted my terminal trap below the bulb. With these modifications, he gives what he entitles "an admirable illustration of the existing method." This flattering adoption of the essential features of my plan, which Sir Henry calls "taking a hint," is rather like taking the apparatus. If not, let Sir Henry endeavor to evacuate a stone of moderate size with "Clover's original instrument" as now "slightly modified" by him, omitting only the "stiff" bulb and enlarged tube.[2]

Although my pump acts perfectly, the operator will doubtless modify it a little to suit himself, adopting the necessary conditions of an adequate exhaust of some sort, an adequate evacuating tube, and an efficient trap. I find also that an elastic tube interposed between the bulb and the bladder, to avoid the jar of pumping, is desirable.

But what I insist upon, as characterizing the new lithotrity, is —

1. A practical recognition of the tolerance of the bladder, which is far less sensitive to instruments than to fragments,

[1] Hitherto Sir Henry has designated as the most useful form a squarely cut extremity. "In most cases," he says, "the best kind is that which is cut transversely at the distal end" (The Diseases of the Prostate, etc., p. 337, fourth edition, Philadelphia, 1873). Such an extremity is really the worst, because it is at once closed by the bladder.

[2] Sir Henry does not seem to appreciate the full use of a large tube. This is shown by his figure of the "modified" instrument (See Lancet, February 1), where, although the calibre of the evacuating tube is 26, its hole for the admission of fragments is but little more than half its diameter. Where lies the utility of so large a tube, if only small fragments can get into it? This hole is a relic of the Clover instrument.

As regards the size of the tube, the operator can fairly take advantage of the full size of the urethra. The larger the tube, the larger will be the fragments released. I have employed, without any objectionable result, a 30 French calibre, often 31; and I prefer a straight tube. Although these largest sizes are not essential to the operation, they admit many fragments that would otherwise have to be crushed.

with the obvious corollary that when the operator crushes a stone it is better to remove the fragments by protracting the operation than to leave them, — as has been hitherto the usual practice of distinguished operators, including Sir Henry Thompson; and —

2. The use of a tube large enough to afford an easy passage from the bladder, not (as with Clover's instrument) for sand, which does not need it, but for detritus, which, owing to its size or quantity, would not pass the urethra without it, — this being an application of Otis's discovery of the previously unrecognized capacity of the urethra, of which the meatus is the narrowest part.

This is not in accordance with the former teaching of lithotritists. At the late litrotrity meeting of the Medico-Chirurgical Society there was no question about the traditional few minutes,[1] as the limit of time beyond which it is not usually safe for the lithotritist to try the endurance of an average bladder. The error is a natural one. Surgeons have hitherto attributed to instruments of polished metal the damage really due to the roughness of fragments. With Sir Henry Thompson, they believed that "the mere sojourn of the instrument in the bladder is a source of irritation precisely corresponding to the time, within certain limits, it continues there. Anything, therefore, that will diminish the time of the operation, and the amount of movement and concussion, will necessarily give a greater prospect of success."[2] This mistake prevailed for half a century, because the real cause of the injury could not be ascertained. There was absolutely no way to extract fragments large or abundant enough to

[1] A sojourn, say of two minutes, in the bladder, which I will allow you, although you know I do not occupy so much time myself. — Sir Henry Thompson: *Clinical Lectures on Diseases of the Urinary Organs etc.*, p. 188 (Fourth edition. London, 1876).

[2] Clinical Lectures, etc., p. 172.

make trouble, and to show what would be the behavior of the bladder when thus relieved. The new instrument first accomplished the evacuation of bulky débris, and by removing this source of inflammation disclosed the comparative harmlessness of the lithotrite and the pump. The discovery of the tolerance of the bladder could have been made in no other way. What Sir Henry Thompson would call a little modification of method involved an important difference in result, making it easy to accomplish what was before impracticable, — a trite occurrence in the history of inventions.

There can be no doubt about Sir Henry Thompson's teaching. So lately as 1876 he writes: —

"You heard me say in the theatre the other day . . . that you should not encourage the early passing of the fragments. They rest at the bottom of the bladder. I usually keep the patient in bed, and pretty much on his back, for thirty-six hours or so, afterwards. He should at all events, for that period of time, pass urine in that position, so that the sharp angular fragments are left at the bottom of the bladder and are not forced into the urethra."[1]

With unparalleled opportunities for observation, Sir Henry seems to have been well satisfied with the old lithotrity and its instruments. In the lecture to which he refers for an exposition of his latest views, he says: —

"I do not mean to say that any striking novelties in the instruments, or in the system of operating, have recently been achieved. The mechanical procedure has probably long been too nearly perfect to permit us to expect results of that kind."[2]

When this conservative view was again expressed at the lithotrity meeting of the Medico-Chirurgical Society in 1878,[3] it elicited nothing from Sir Henry concerning the tolerance of the bladder to instruments, the advantage of removing

[1] Clinical Lectures, etc., p. 188.
[2] Clinical Lecture, Lancet, January 8, 1876.
[3] The Lancet, March 16, 1878, p. 385.

all fragments, or any other essential feature of the new operation.

I may here allude to a small matter. Sir Henry insists upon the importance of making the movements of the bulb keep time with the respiration of the patient. I think this will be found both unnecessary and impracticable. The first part of any long aspiration, whether it is or is not synchronous with the breathing, suffices to clog the orifice of the tube with débris ; the last part of the aspiration is then useless. Nor does a "stiff" bulb need to be aided by the diaphragm of the patient. Nor need danger be apprehended from any expulsive effort to which the bladder is accustomed, like respiration, cough, or even vomiting. In fact, this last is not unusual with an anæsthetic. I let the water off while it continues.

Although a long stroke is occasionally useful, I commonly pump at the rate of about twice in three seconds, moving only about two ounces of water back and forth. The main difficulty is to find for the extremity of the tube the best place for gathering fragments, and to prevent its obstruction, whether by fragments or by the bladder. This somewhat nice adjustment is experimental, and, I think, is easiest when the left hand, holding the evacuating tube, rests on the pubes. The manipulation is provided for in my instrument by the intervention, between the evacuating tube and the bulb, of an elastic tube eight inches long. If the operator prefers, it may be shorter; my first one was only two inches long. The facility and delicacy of the manipulation, it is needless to say, are greatly impaired if the bulb be rigidly attached to the evacuating tube, as in Clover's apparatus and Sir Henry Thompson's figure, — especially if, as there, it is placed above the tube.

In my present method of evacuating the débris, the bulb full of water is coupled with the evacuating tube introduced into the empty bladder; and when the pump is in action, water is added to distend the bladder, if its walls prove to be slack enough to fall into the eye of the tube and obstruct it. The earlier cases naturally occupied more time than is now necessary; but I still find, as at first, that the most time is spent in searching for and removing the last fragment, and in incidental delays, — not in evacuating the mass of débris, which is drawn out with surprising rapidity. With ether, rapid surgery has become less essential; and lithotrity is now, perhaps, less than any other surgical operation, to be performed against time. I doubt whether the hurried operation mentioned by Sir Henry Thompson would bear frequent repetition even by himself. There would seem to be need rather of deliberation than of haste. A remaining fragment may be easily overlooked; and in less skilled hands haste might be mischievous. Removing a stone of one hundred and twenty grains, with two lithotrites and an assistant to clear them, is mainly the operation of Fergusson, who relied for evacuation on repeated withdrawals of the loaded instrument.

Litholapaxy is now no novelty in America; and its success here will, I think, recommend it elsewhere. Allow me to add a few recent examples.

An operation which I performed January 26, in the case of a medical gentleman aged sixty-seven years, lasted fifty minutes, and consisted of two crushings, occupying fifteen minutes; three evacuations of fragments, nine minutes; changes, and other delay, twenty-six minutes. Two hundred and sixty grains of phosphatic stone were thus removed. The patient had no trouble from the operation, and on the thirteenth day went home to the country, well. There were no fragments left in the bladder.

In another case, February 10, that of a man aged fifty years, one diameter of the stone measured $1\frac{5}{8}$ inches. The operation continued one hour and twenty-one minutes. The crushings occupied twenty minutes; the evacuation of fragments, thirty; while the changes, etc., were recorded at thirty-one minutes. Three hundred and two grains of hard oxalate calculus were crushed and drawn out, — with some delay in the operation, due to fragments lodged behind a high prostate. I was unable to break the stone with Charrière's, or rather Collin's, instrument. The patient had no unfavorable symptoms, hardly a trace of blood, and no fragments were left.

This case, which involves, so far as I know, the largest hard stone yet evacuated at one sitting, is an example of what can be done by the new process. In evacuating such stones, it need only be said that the smaller the tube the more minutely must the fragments be broken, and the greater will be the liability to obstruction. Small stones, common in these later days of lithotrity, especially soft ones, are not infrequently crushed at one sitting, by any lithotrite, without ether, and, if reduced to sand, may really need no tube to evacuate them.

The following case is as good a test of the new operation as I could wish.

The patient, aged thirty-three, entered the hospital October 31, about four months and a half ago. His condition was so bad that it was thought unadvisable to attempt any operation, even lithotomy. The urine was ammoniacal and fetid, always containing a large quantity of blood, — also pus and mucus to the amount sometimes of nearly one half, by measurement. Micturition was very frequent, occurring at intervals of from ten minutes to half an hour, day and night, during much of this time. The straining was excessive, ineffectual, and productive of great suffering. Three unsuccessful attempts having been made on previous days, a sound was first introduced into the bladder, under ether, November 10. The next day the temperature rose to 103°, and remained thereabout till the fourth day, when another complication presented itself. The left knee became suddenly inflamed and swollen. It has remained so ever since. During the next two months the temperature ranged from 100° to 102° daily, — afterward slowly receding, though the other symptoms did not abate.

I saw the case, for the first time, March 7. With so diseased and irritable a bladder, it was evident that litholapaxy could be considered only as an experiment. It was a last resort, being perhaps better than lithotomy. Should it succeed, it would testify strongly in favor of the new method; should it fail, it could hardly be counted against it.

On the 9th of March I operated. In the neighborhood of the triangular ligament an obstruction prevented the passage of sounds larger than a No. 15 French calibre. After snipping the meatus, this obstruction was divulsed by Voillemier's instrument, and it then admitted a full-sized lithotrite, and a straight tube, 29 French, for which, later in the operation, 30 was substituted. Two hundred and forty grains of stone were now slowly and carefully removed in sixty-eight minutes. An abundance of flocculent and fibrinous material concealed the fragments when lying in a basin, and testified to the inflammation.

At 4 P. M., four hours after the operation, the temperature had fallen from 99° to 96°. In eight hours more, at midnight, it had risen to 103° with a pulse of 130, where it remained through the second day, the tongue being red, smooth, and dry. A general pain in the region of the bladder and urethra required opiates. Yet, on the third day, the tongue became moist, with a light coat, the temperature had fallen to 99°, and the pulse to 84. This improvement still continues. The patient has had no such comfort for many months. During the first week after the operation he passed his water six times in twenty-four hours almost without pain, and there has been no tenderness over the bladder. The urine contains very little sediment, and apart from the knee, which remains as it was, the patient is rapidly convalescing.

I have only to add a few words regarding the new lithotrite. Sir Henry does not seem so heartily satisfied with mine as I could wish, nor, in fact, with anything connected with the new operation, unless possibly its results. This lithotrite, he says, is "surely some resuscitated relic of the early history of lithotrity, . . . reminding him very forcibly of the terrible engines used by Heurteloup."[1] The present tendency of London lithotrites is to small size, because it has been believed that the smaller the instrument the less the danger. With long operations, large stones, and the general use of ether, they will again be larger. With size we gain power. There is no more reason for employing small lithotrites to empty, under ether, an average bladder, than small catheters to draw the water. In fact, the surgeon who becomes accustomed to the efficient action of a large lithotrite does not willingly relinquish it; a little more care is necessary in introducing it, but if non-impacting it need not be withdrawn, loaded with sharp fragments, through the neck of the bladder, at short intervals, to be cleaned by an assistant.

My new lithotrite proves to be very efficient, and I am recently indebted to London makers (Weiss and Son) for an instrument that works perfectly. It is a good size for general use; a smaller one, if preferred, may be used in special cases. This instrument is non-impacting, and keeps clean in the bladder for an indefinite time. Its rounded tip protects the bladder in a protracted operation, — as it also does the prostate during introduction. For the old wheel, which hurts the hand in long crushing, the ball is a welcome substitute;

[1] Of Heurteloup's operation Crampton says: "Nothing could exceed the dexterity and skill, unless it be the gentleness, with which it was performed." (Dublin Quarterly Journal of Medical Science, vol. i., p. 17.)

and unless the human hand undergoes some modification of what are now its easiest movements, the system of *a right-hand lock*, here first employed, must, as I believe, whatever be the size of the lithotrite, supersede in time any previous method of locking.

Your obedient servant,

HENRY J. BIGELOW.

BOSTON, March 25, 1879.

LITHOLAPAXY.[1]

To the Editor:

An editorial paragraph in the "Record" of May 31 mentions that the letter from Sir Henry Thompson to Professor Van Buren, which appeared in the previous issue, was written for publication.

Sir Henry's reiterated criticisms of lithotrites should not be allowed to obscure the main facts, be their value more or less, of rapid lithotrity, — which means long sittings for the immediate and complete evacuation of the fragments by large tubes, and depends upon the newly discovered tolerance of the bladder to the smooth surfaces of instruments; while the old lithotrity meant repeated short sittings and sharp fragments left in the bladder.

The size of a lithotrite has little to do with litholapaxy. Stones are so frequently soft and small that a small lithotrite of any kind may be large enough. Of course the operator will be careful not to break such a lithotrite upon a large or hard stone. Like other lithotrites, mine is made in various sizes. It is not, however, the large lithotrite that I have desired to bring to the attention of surgeons, but the new lock, and the protective and non-impacting blades, designed to promote safe and rapid work at a moment when the hand or the attention of the operator is fatigued by a long operation. I prefer a large lithotrite if it possesses these qualities, even in dealing with common calculi. Sir Henry prefers a smaller one, whether it clogs or not, and frequently withdraws it to clean it. His prejudice against a large instrument is connected with a life-long and erroneous theory that the dangers of lithotrity result mainly from the instruments used in the

[1] The Boston Medical and Surgical Journal, June 19, 1879.

operation. This was the general mistake of the day. It was not known that the irritation was really occasioned by the fragments which it was the custom to leave in the bladder. When these fragments were drawn out by my apparatus, and that source of danger to the bladder was removed, it was found that the instruments themselves did but little harm. Sir Henry, perhaps, might long ago have discovered this fact of the tolerance of the bladder to instrumentation if he had possessed any means of evacuating it thoroughly. But he had only Clover's instrument, the tube of which was so small (21 French) that it drew out only sand and left the fragments. Hence his error and failure to discover the new facts of what is now known as rapid lithotrity.

Sir Henry devotes the last half of his letter to the expression of creditable sentiments in relation to his attitude toward surgical progress. A little explanation may be here desirable.

A year after the publication of my paper, he published a lecture in the "Lancet" (Feb. 1, 1879), in which he says: "My own system has for a long time past been gradually inclining to the practice of crushing more calculus at a sitting, and removing more débris by the aspirator than I formerly did," — which might very well be true, his former sittings having been limited to two minutes or less; but the hindrance to his "removing more débris" was the small size of Clover's tube. The editor of the "Lancet" replied (February 15): "We cannot close our eyes to the fact that the views advanced in his lecture of the 1st inst. do involve an abandonment of his old position. Lithotrity as hitherto practised by him and lithotrity as recommended and performed by Professor Bigelow are different operations, and based on opposite and contradictory principles." This "editorial observation" in the "Lancet" Sir Henry, curiously enough, chooses to regard, in his letter published in the "Record," as "adverse criticism of himself personally, not of his mode of operating."

Sir Henry's position will now be understood. It is in this connection that he expresses the opinion that the terms "abandonment of position" and the like, "adapted as they are to military men," do not accord with the aims of men who "'live and learn.' . . . It is an error," he says, "to look for a life-long consistency in matters of opinion from men who think for themselves." The world will not question the right of Sir Henry to "live and learn," nor to "think for himself," but only the propriety of his claiming to have originated by "thinking for himself" ideas he has learned from others.

A friend has to-day sent me the fifth edition, just published, of Sir Henry's "Diseases of the Urinary Organs." I find that in this edition Sir Henry both honors rapid lithotrity with his indorsement and appropriates as his own its essential details. He adopts large tubes, increasing the ineffectual catheter of Clover from 21 to 29, which latter calibre I often employ, my smallest tube being 27, my usual size 30, and the largest 31. "You are first to introduce," he says (page 173), "an evacuating silver catheter fitted with a flexible stylet, — in size, say, from No. 14 to No. 16, English scale," calibres equivalent to 24 and 29 French.[1] Here being the essential feature of the operation, Sir Henry at this point definitively abandons

[1] Handerson's comparative scale, from which these equivalent numbers are taken, is made by Reynders & Co., New York. It is accurate, and very convenient in having instead of holes a long triangular slit like a wire gauge. "In England," says Sir Henry Thompson, "we cannot be said to have a uniform scale; all our measurements are very arbitrary. One maker has one scale, and another another." (Diseases of the Urinary Organs, 1879, p. 47.) On page 48, however, he gives a scale, of which the largest size 14 is the equivalent of 24; and this corresponds to Handerson's scale (New York Medical Record, 1877, p. 638). The French numbers increase more rapidly than the English. Larger calibres have hitherto been but little known either in France or England. The main point is the necessity of enlarging Clover's tube.

"consistency" and the 21 tube of his previous editions in favor of "large evacuating catheters and a good aspirator" (page 177). Neither of these he used before I described them. This gives him the whole key to rapid lithotrity, and he is able to accomplish thorough evacuation at once by prolonging the sitting till evacuation is complete, demonstrating at the same time that the bladder tolerates instrumentation if the fragments are removed, — which is the new principle that underlies litholapaxy. The large tube once appropriated, what remains is easy. The aspiration of his new edition means effectual aspiration with large tubes, and his lithotrity becomes rapid lithotrity.

A comparison of this, Sir Henry's present practice, with his recent opposite teaching of frequent repeated crushings — each confined to a few minutes, lest the polished instrument injure the bladder, but leaving the bladder nevertheless to struggle in the intervals with sharp, broken pieces of stone, which he had no means of extracting — will show the significance of the criticism by the editor of the "Lancet."[1]

In conclusion, I may venture to hope that the valuable example set by Sir Henry in accepting large tubes will aid in doing away with whatever apprehension still exists of danger from their use.

HENRY J. BIGELOW.

[1] The Lancet of May 17 contains a letter on this subject.

LITHOLAPAXY.[1]

To the Editor:

Dear Sir, — Will you allow me to correct an erroneous statement contained in one of your recent editorial articles upon the new lithotrity (vol. xvi., Nos. 7 and 8)? It relates to the lithotrite devised by me. This particular instrument is not indispensable for the performance of litholapaxy, since almost any lithotrite can be made to crush the stone, — the novel and essential characteristic of the new method being the complete evacuation of the calculus by a long sitting and a large catheter. But although the error referred to is unimportant, it should, I think, be corrected in deference to surgeons who use my non-impacting instrument.

The writer says, referring to the lock of this lithotrite, "The liability to break is a serious objection. . . . Thompson's catch cannot be broken in this manner." Now, this is a mistake. My instrument, although employed by myself and others upon stones both large and hard, has never been, as your writer states, "broken." Nor do the parts he alludes to (the old screw-blocks of Charrière and their boxes) differ in strength from those of all other lithotrites, inasmuch as they are identical in all of them. If one breaks, others must be liable to the same accident.

This writer has misapprehended a trivial occurrence, incidentally mentioned many months ago, in connection with the then novel method. This was what happened. Tiemann and Co. borrowed from me, for examination, a lithotrite just arrived, one of the first of my instruments made in Paris, and lent it for use. The French workman, to whom the lock

[1] The New York Medical Record, Sept. 27, 1879.

was new, had miscalculated the width in this combination of the Charrière screw-blocks, so that when the instrument was locked and screwed up these blocks had little or no bearing. They were at once lifted out of their boxes, just as they are purposely lifted out by thumb and finger when they need cleaning. That was the whole of it. The skilful French maker, annoyed at the carelessness of his workman, made the lithotrite perfect in a few hours; and the surgeon, in whose hands the defective adjustment revealed itself, ordered one of my lithotrites from Weiss.

The error here corrected does not impair the general excellence of the other criticism, it being quite possible that the writer should be a skilful surgeon without being perfectly familiar with the locks of lithotrites, — just as a skilful navigator may not have investigated the construction of the chronometer he uses.

Several of the critical remarks of your able editorial writer are well founded. He rightly says that the evacuating process, though not more efficient, is drier and neater if all the water is kept inside the aspirator and all the air outside of it; which implies that there should be good joints and no leakage, with stopcocks at all the orifices, one of them being at the highest point to let air out easily. I would add, however, that it is important not to lose sight of convenience in other respects.

The progress of the new lithotrity was most liberally encouraged, at an early period, by New York surgeons. The attention now directed to some of the minor details connected with the instruments is rapidly contributing to their perfection.

Almost the only objection I have known made to the new method, either here or abroad, has been directed to the size of the instruments I generally use, which at first impressed persons accustomed to the use of Clover's aspirator and the

English lithotrite as "clumsy" or "unwieldy." Large-sized catheters are absolutely indispensable, and are now so recog nized. With regard to the size of the lithotrite, it is to a certain extent a matter of taste. My own instrument, with a wrist-lock, ball-handle, and non-impacting blades, is not necessarily larger than others. It can be had from Tiemann and Co. of any size the operator may prefer. I think, however, that large and hard stones will be found to require a more powerful instrument than those hitherto in use. In fact, it is very possible that a calculus should break a lithotrite. This accident happened from time to time in the practice of the old lithotrity, and we are now dealing with larger and harder stones. That is one reason for avoiding a slender construction, especially of the blades; but my chief reason for using a large lithotrite is the convenient command it gives of the stone. Having learned how easy, as well as safe, with proper care and skill, is the introduction of large instruments, I prefer to use a powerful lithotrite to crush even a moderate-sized calculus, provided the blades are so constructed as not to become impacted. With a small stone or fragment the choice of a lithotrite is wholly unimportant; while a bladder or urethra, if exceptional in any way, may require an exceptional instrument. But I do not see why some operators still enjoin the use in all cases of the smallest or lightest lithotrite that can possibly be made to crush the calculus.

HENRY J. BIGELOW.

BOSTON, Mass.

LITHOLAPAXY.[1]

In a paper upon litholapaxy published last year, I reported twelve cases with one death. Below is a record of nine cases upon which I have since operated successfully, under ether as before: —

Case XIII. — March 9, 1878. Age, thirty-three. Stone weighing two hundred and forty grains. Time, sixty-eight minutes. Rapid recovery. The patient, for many months very ill, was at once relieved.

Case XIV. — Dec. 20, 1878. Age, sixty-nine. Stone measuring eleven centimetres by fifteen. Time, forty-five minutes. Usual recovery.

Case XV. — Jan. 24, 1879. Age, sixty-seven. Stone weighing two hundred and sixty grains. Time, forty-six minutes. Usual recovery.

Case XVI. — Feb. 10, 1879. Age, fifty. Three hundred and two grains of hard oxalate stone. Time, one hour and twenty-one minutes. Usual recovery. This was the largest hard stone yet treated by immediate evacuation.

Case XVII. — April 7, 1879. Age, fifty-four. One hundred and eight grains of hard oxalate stone. Time, thirty-five minutes. Usual recovery.

Case XVIII. — April 26, 1879. Age, forty. Stone of the size of a marble. Time, twenty-seven minutes. Usual recovery. Only worthy of record as immediately relieved from great irritation of four years' duration.

Case XIX. — June 4, 1879. Age, sixty-five. Stone weighing two hundred and forty-two grains, mixed lithic and phosphatic. Time, forty-six minutes. Usual recovery.

Case XX. — Small stone. Usual recovery. The only case where I was unable to pass a straight tube, from obstruction at the internal meatus.

[1] The Boston Medical and Surgical Journal, Oct. 16, 1879.

Case XXI.—July 21, 1879. Age, twenty-one. A large stone of seven hundred and twenty grains. Measurement, two and one fourth inches. Time, one hour and seventeen minutes. Usual recovery.

It is unnecessary to say that these operations were done deliberately,—neither the anæsthesia, the crushing, nor the evacuation requiring haste. I have hitherto reported the time of my operations to illustrate and impress this fact, which was a new one. Surgeons familiar with the use of ether do not hesitate to continue anæsthesia almost indefinitely if there is anything to be gained by it. Nor is the bladder itself affected unfavorably by a protracted operation. Indeed, "rapid lithotrity"—a name intended to designate a long sitting for the purpose of removing the whole stone through a large tube—calls for greater deliberation and care than the old dilatory lithotrity by repeated two-minute sittings, with an interval of days between them. It is rapid only as a whole, and when compared with the old operation.

The details of a case may further illustrate this,—for example, the last here recorded, where seven hundred and twenty grains were removed in one hour and seventeen minutes, the stone being the largest but one as yet subjected to operation by the new method. Here four crushings occupied twelve, six, six, and four minutes; and five washings, six, four, twelve, and seven minutes, respectively, with intervals added. But a very large part of this stone was removed in ten minutes by the first two short washings; the remainder of the time was for the most part devoted to a leisurely and careful search for residuary fragments. As performed here now, the operation consists of litholapaxy, followed by thorough sounding with a tube. It may be made shorter by not completing it,—by postponing the final exploration. In other words, surgeons may prefer to leave the last fragments for a second operation. This has been proposed by one of the strongest advocates of haste, which is a habit connected with the two-minute sitting, insisted on when it was erroneously supposed that damage to the bladder was in proportion to the time occupied by instrumentation. The tradition has so strong a hold on surgeons that cases of rapid lithotrity are still reported, in which the operator seems to have been under pressure of some sort to finish the sitting quickly, at all hazards, as if it were essential to do so; and yet the performance of lithotrity against time will probably be soon as obsolete as is now haste in other operations under ether anæsthesia.

LITHOLAPAXY;

OR,

LITHOTRITY WITH IMMEDIATE EVACUATION.[1]

THE communication I have the honor to make relates to a modification of the operation of Lithotrity. It is a proposition to supersede frequent sittings, as nearly as may be, by a single sitting of sufficient length to enable the surgeon to crush the calculus completely and remove all the fragments.

In the opposite practice, which has hitherto prevailed, the calculus, unless it were very small, was broken, a little at a time, at intervals of a few days, and the pieces were left in the bladder. For this course there was a plausible reason. The inflammation that sometimes followed the operation was naturally attributed to the instrument used in crushing the stone; and the shorter the operation the less, it was supposed, would the irritation probably be. Under this impression, skilful operators, ever since Civiale, have reduced the length of the sitting to a few minutes, — hesitating to continue manipulation even with instruments of polished metal. They had no hesitation, however, in leaving the mucous membrane exposed for weeks to sharp, ragged edges of broken stone, — the fragments in the bladder remaining where they were, because there was no instrument for removing them.

The removal of mere sand and minute fragments by suction through the urethra is old, and dates from Crampton, who records two drachms of sand drawn out at once, — of which, I believe, no larger quantity has since been so removed at one sitting. This sort of detritus also escapes of itself, by the urethra, without inconvenience. But fragments large or

[1] Transactions of the Clinical Society of London, vol. xii., 1879. Read Oct. 25, 1878.

abundant enough to be important factors in producing irritation have never till now been got rid of. One insuperable obstacle has always been the small size of the evacuating catheter. The aspirator of Clover, for example, is inefficient, partly because the catheter, having the small calibre of 21 French, allows the passage only of sand and a few minute fragments.

So long as the two sources of injury, the crushing and the fragments left by it, were thus inseparable, their effects could not be distinguished, and there was a strong feeling against any protracted manipulation of the stone. To withdraw the offending fragments was the only possible way to discover what was the effect of the crushing itself, and how far it might be prolonged.

It has happened that I have always etherized patients for lithotrity; and as there was no pain in the operation, I not infrequently protracted the sittings to ten or fifteen minutes. The need I felt was not of more crushing, — for I was already doing as much of this as seemed advantageous, — but rather of some way to get rid of what was already crushed. The singular insensibility sometimes shown by the bladder not merely to the presence of calculi to which it had become accustomed, but also to lithotrity, and by the urethra to divulsion, was too striking to be overlooked, and made it probable that the mucous membrane would tolerate a good deal of interference if it were decisively terminated, and irritation were not kept up by the unwonted presence of sharp fragments left in the bladder. When Otis announced the great capacity of the urethra, now familiar through Van Buren's steel sounds, it became obvious that large fragments of stone might be removed. I therefore had some tubes of corresponding size made, and soon after adopted the evacuating catheters and the aspirator I now use, by which the bladder can be rapidly emptied of any common amount of débris. I experimented with caution, in view of the overwhelming weight of traditional and current testimony. A gentleman, then lately from abroad, who had had unusual opportunities for observation of lithotrity, told me, after seeing one of my earlier operations, that the mechanical procedure might be good, but that the patient would die. Yet he recovered. This and other similar cases, then first treated by the aid of large evacuating catheters and an efficient aspirator, showed a tolerance on the part of the bladder to the use of instruments, which had till then been unsuspected.

These considerations involve this new principle in lithotrity, that it is better to remove all the fragments immediately, because the bladder does tolerate a good deal of mechanical disturbance with the lithotrite and aspirator, if only that be all, — with the obvious rule that we may substitute, for the traditional few minutes of a sitting, time enough to remove the whole stone.

Experience has confirmed both the principle and the rule; and although it is impossible now to prescribe the limits of the operation, I have frequently continued it for an hour with successful results, and have known eighteen hundred grains to be removed in three sittings, of about three hours each, under ether, — the result being almost immediate relief.

The long sittings of the new method suggest other precautions besides those usual in common lithotrity. Instead of withdrawing the lithotrite frequently to clean it, I have devised blades that cannot become impacted with detritus. The old fenestrated instruments do not clog, — and in that respect work well, especially as the coarse gravel that passes the fenestra of the female blade will also pass through the large catheters. Dr. Van Buren and Dr. Keyes have used the fenestrated lithotrite successfully in the new operation. But this allows sharp fragments to be pressed through the instrument against the floor of the bladder; and I doubt if this is harmless. The sides also of a fenestrated blade are weakened, if made low enough to receive fragments readily. Therefore, while this mode of construction may be serviceable for small stones or fragments, I usually prefer a solid female blade to protect the floor of the bladder, relying on a self-cleaning male blade to prevent impaction. I like also a large lithotrite to crush common stones as well as large ones; but if the operator prefers, he can use different lithotrites for different stones.

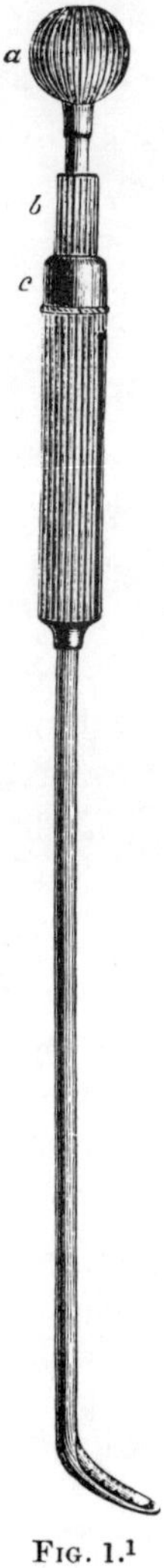

FIG. 1.[1]

In a long operation, when the attention gets wearied, the lithotrite is liable to catch the wall of the bladder. When the operation exceeds a few minutes, the average surgeon cannot be relied on always to turn up the instrument in the centre of the bladder before crushing; and the forceps-like blades of the best common lithotrites are well arranged to do injury. I find great advantage, and no disadvantage, in a long and blunted, as well as wide, female blade. This keeps the walls of the bladder back while the male blade is securing the fragments, either when they fall into a depression made in the floor by the female blade, or when the lithotrite, previously opened, is turned to one side and closed along the floor.

In crushing, the easiest movement, and the one that recurs most frequently, is the rotation of the right wrist in screwing down the male blade. The lock of my lithotrite is shut and opened by

[1] Author's lithotrite. *a*, Spherical handle substituted for a wheel; *b*, cylinder which operates upon the lock *c*.

this same movement, and can be applied to any lithotrite. The same movement that locks it begins the crushing, and the reverse movement unlocks it, — the requisite force being applied by a ball, in preference to the wheel commonly used.[1]

The Aspirating-Siphon is an elastic tube, having at one end an evacuating catheter, at the other an elastic oval-shaped bottle, terminated below by a glass receptacle and supported on a stand. The bottle itself is strong, and when compressed dilates with force. Fragments enter at the top and fall to the bottom, into the glass receiver, where they remain. They cannot return from the bottle to the bladder, as happens when, to reach the trap, they must pass the mouth of the evacuating tube. But if they could, no harm would ensue, — evacuation with large catheters being so rapid that a fragment or two returned to the bladder is very soon brought back again. When the fragments once enter the catheter, they pass so quickly to the bottle as to make it possible, without retarding them, to interpose between the catheter and bottle several inches of elastic tube to relieve the bladder from the vibration of the aspirator, and to make the catheter independent of any motion of the other part of the apparatus. If the surgeon guides the catheter with his left hand supported on the patient's thigh, the elastic tube allows a delicacy of manipulation which is hardly possible when the bottle is rigidly attached to the catheter, especially if it surmounts it.

[1] After careful experiment as to the easiest movement of the hand and arm in crushing, which is undoubtedly the rotation here spoken of, I adapted the lock to it. It requires no displacement of the fingers. If any easier movement be discovered, there will be an advantage in adapting a lock to that. I have heard, in apology for the traditional wheel as a handle, that the awkward hold it gives the hand prevents the application of sufficient force to break the blades; but the blades, without being too large to pass easily through the urethra, can be made strong enough to resist the better grasp allowed by a ball.

The calibre of an evacuating catheter determines the size of the fragments that pass it. Beginning with 27 French, I

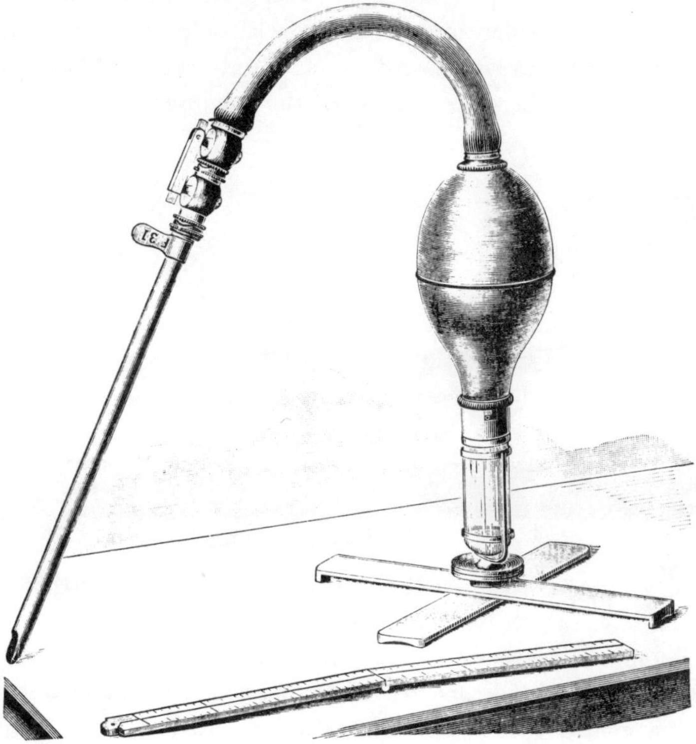

FIG. 2.[1]

gradually increased the size to 31,—employing, as a rule, a calibre of 30. Smaller tubes transmit smaller and fewer fragments; I therefore prefer at least 30, when it can be used. If

1 Aspirating-Siphon in a stand which has a ball and socket joint to allow the bottle to stand in an easy position. The glass trap is surmounted by an oval bottle and curved tube of rubber, terminated by a stop-cock. When the latter is coupled with the stop-cock upon the evacuating catheter, the two are kept open by a hinged clip, seen in the drawing.

the surgeon prefers 28 or 29, he can further crush the fragments that will not pass through these. The catheter should have its lower orifice of full calibre, with a prolonged blunt extremity or lip to facilitate its passage into the bladder, and to keep the vesical walls away from the opening.

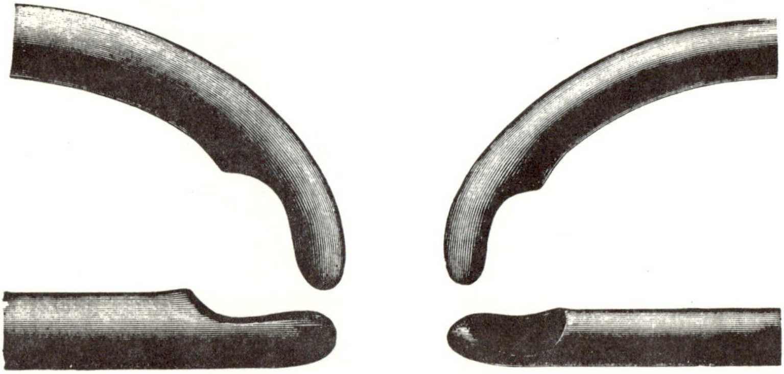

FIG. 3.[1]

I use a straight tube. It is introduced more readily than a curved one, and shows better how it lies in the bladder. The fragments, under aspiration, are so constantly moving that a curved instrument is not needed to find them, as in sounding; on the contrary, they find the catheter. If, however, a bent tube be preferred, the curve should be short, the hole close to the end, and of full dimensions.

To introduce a large tube, the urethra is copiously oiled with a syringe, and its calibre ascertained with a steel sound. The meatus, the narrowest part, may be snipped with scissors, if necessary, or a stricture be enlarged by divulsion; but a calibre of 30 will usually enter the normal passage. Whether straight or curved, the evacuating catheter is passed perpendicularly as far as the rectum. The straight catheter is then laid horizontally, — a movement that tilts up the end to the

1 Extremities of straight and curved tubes, of the sizes 27 and 31.

orifice in the triangular ligament. This entered, the instrument is, by a screw-like motion in the axis of the body, passed through the prostate, the eccentric extremity readily finding its way. In one form of enlarged prostate a further elevation of the point of the catheter may be required to find the aperture in the triangular ligament. But the common difficulty of passing an instrument of any sort results from a premature depression of the handle, which raises the other end above the orifice. This observation is not new, but requires to be emphasized in connection with large-sized instruments. It is also useful to press the bent part of a curved instrument in the direction of the axis of the body, with the left hand on the perinæum. It need not be said that all the movements are gentle and deliberate. Rapid lithotrity should be done slowly.

The stone is crushed as usual, except that a non-impacting lithotrite may be kept in the bladder to advantage until the fragments are lost in the detritus. When the latter is removed, the crushing is repeated. Detritus is withdrawn better by a catheter than by an impacted lithotrite, and a few alternate operations of crushing and aspiration suffice to evacuate a stone of considerable size.

As preliminary to aspiration, the evacuating catheter is introduced and the bladder emptied, leakage being prevented by a band tied round the penis. The bottle is filled by letting it dilate while the elastic tube is immersed in water; and, the stop-cock being then closed, it is placed in its stand. To expel the air from the evacuating catheter, this may be also filled by means of a syringe, and its stop-cock also closed. It remains to couple the full bottle with the catheter in the empty bladder. The apparatus is now ready.

An aspiration that withdraws two or three ounces of water about twice in three seconds brings a continuous shower of detritus into the glass cylinder. If the bottle expands reluctantly, a fragment is lodged in the catheter, and a sharp compression of the bottle will probably eject it; but if not, it may be pushed back with a rod. Several successive jerks, similar to the bite of a fish, signify a valve-like stoppage of the opening in the catheter by the elastic walls of the bladder. The latter is then too flaccid, and needs a few ounces more of water from the bottle to distend it; after which the stop-cocks are shut, and the bottle is replenished. This common sign is generally a valuable one, because it indicates a good-sized bladder; but it sometimes happens when the opening of the catheter is turned sideways, and does not occur with a curved catheter.

The operator sits on the patient's right. Evacuation is very rapid when the catheter is held properly; and the best place for the end of the instrument is ascertained by trying. It is a little curious that a continued shower of detritus is sometimes brought into the trap by changing the direction or elevation of the catheter only a quarter of an inch. Any good position should be maintained accurately. A good place for aspiration is just off the floor of the bladder; higher, when the first fragments are crowding into the tube and need to be received in single file; and lower, in a depression of the floor, when the débris require to be assembled. The last fragment, if small enough, is sure to enter the catheter after a while. By a few minutes' aspiration in a tumbler covered with a napkin, I can always isolate, from a mass of broken coal, the only bits too large to enter the catheter. As the sand is cleared away, fragments announce their presence by clicking against the tube; a long, full-sized one may be arrested half-a-dozen times before its final withdrawal and appearance in the trap. When the clicking has ceased for a minute or two, the bladder is practically clear; and there remains only a final exploration with a tube or lithotrite at a convenient time.

A little air, mostly from the evacuating catheter, may get into the bladder during the operation, — but does no harm, if it does not over-distend a small bladder. The air is readily discharged with the urine; but it is well from time to time to open the evacuating catheter and expel it, by compressing the bladder above the pubes.

The pulse and temperature, usually higher the day after the operation, soon subside, the general treatment of symptoms being much the same as after lithotrity.

By this method, which I have called Litholapaxy, its peculiar feature being evacuation, tenacious mucus with phosphatic deposit, as well as nuclei and certain foreign bodies, can be better removed than in any other way.

LITHOLAPAXY.

AN IMPROVED EVACUATOR.[1]

THE operation for the complete removal of a stone at one sitting has been as successful as its most sanguine advocates could have hoped. Several years may still be needed to determine precisely its relative value; but in the mean time it has been abundantly proved that the bladder tolerates long operations, — provided the fragments of the stone, which are the principal cause of inflammation, be removed, — and that fragments need no longer be a source of inflammation. Although several cases of litholapaxy have terminated fatally, the cause of death was not the usual one after such operations; it was not an inflammation of obscure origin, connected with previous disease of the bladder or of the kidneys. The few deaths that have occurred were due to mechanical injury, which with greater experience in operations of this kind will doubtless in the future be avoided.

It has been remarked by more than one writer that the new lithotrity requires even more care than was necessary in the old method by short sittings. This is true. Each repeated act of crushing or of evacuation is obviously liable to its own casualties; and we must add to this liability any that may arise from the gradual abatement of the operator's vigilance. It was once an object, in persuading surgeons to forego their traditional prejudices, to show that the new operation was safer than they supposed; but this being now generally conceded, it is at present important to insist that it should be attempted only by practised lithotritists, or by a beginner only after familiar practice upon the cadaver. I know no other

[1] Boston Medical and Surgical Journal, Jan. 8, 1880.

surgical operation in which a little want of skill or of care is so insidiously liable to fatal accident. The skill here is of a particular kind; and though a surgeon may use a knife well, it does not follow that he also uses a lithotrite well. Before considering this instrument, however, let us examine the evacuator, or "rubber bulb."

It was an alteration of the evacuator that made litholapaxy possible, and led to the discovery of the tolerance of the bladder. This was the enlargement of its tubes from the size of the common catheter to the largest the urethra will admit without injury. In evacuating a small stone the smaller of the new large tubes (26 or 27 French) works well enough; but in order to evacuate a considerable stone with comfort either to the surgeon or to the patient, we need a tube of from 28 to 31; and for its introduction it is often well to enlarge the meatus, which is the narrowest part of the urethra. I cannot but think that the preference of some operators for the curved tube I at first employed is connected with their previous familiarity with curved catheters; and yet when a curved evacuating tube is in position its entire curve is in the bladder, and in the manipulation of the instrument there exists the disadvantage of not knowing, as readily as with a straight tube, where its point lies. The orifice in either case is on the side of the extremity, and there is a quarter of an inch, more or less, of tapering solid metal beyond it, necessary to make its introduction easy and to keep the bladder from obstructing it.

The large evacuating-tube being the essential instrument in the new operation, a vacuum produced by almost any apparatus will draw fragments through it. Certain principles, however, observed in their construction will make them more convenient and efficient.

An apparatus I early employed consisted of a stiff bulb and Clover's trap, attached to the large catheter by a short elastic tube. The combination was a good one; for the elastic tube allowed the bulb, when in use, to be bent down to the level of the bladder. The bulb could thus be laid on its side, and by further depression reversed; which brought the catheter tube to the top. It then remained only to construct a glass trap at its lowest point, so that the fragments should be left where they fell. This arrangement, placed in a stand, is practically the evacuator I still use.

A strong rubber bulb is an indispensable substitute for the former slender one.

In the glass trap at the bottom of the instrument the fragments are kept out of the current at a point distant from the catheter. After entering at the top of the bulb, they settle at once to the bottom and remain there undisturbed.

If fragments are drawn through the tube with the force and rapidity that are given to the current by a strong rubber bulb, a few inches added to the length of the route are of no consequence. A short and curved elastic tube five inches long, — but which I have varied from two inches to two feet, — between the bulb and the evacuating tube, makes it possible to move one without the other. It relieves the surgeon and protects the patient. The surgeon can explore the bladder in search of fragments without having to move the bulb, which weighs a pound or two; while the jar of pumping does not reach the bladder. The discomfort to the unetherized patient resulting from this jar is a serious objection to the rigid attachment of the bulb of water to the tube. The bulb should have a support of its own, placed upon the table or bed between the patient's legs, which may be separated a little as in the case of the introduction of a catheter or a lithotrite. The surgeon's hand, instead of supporting the evacuator, is then supported by it.

The bulb, when thus near the level of the bladder, acts as a siphon. This is desirable. By experiment it will be found

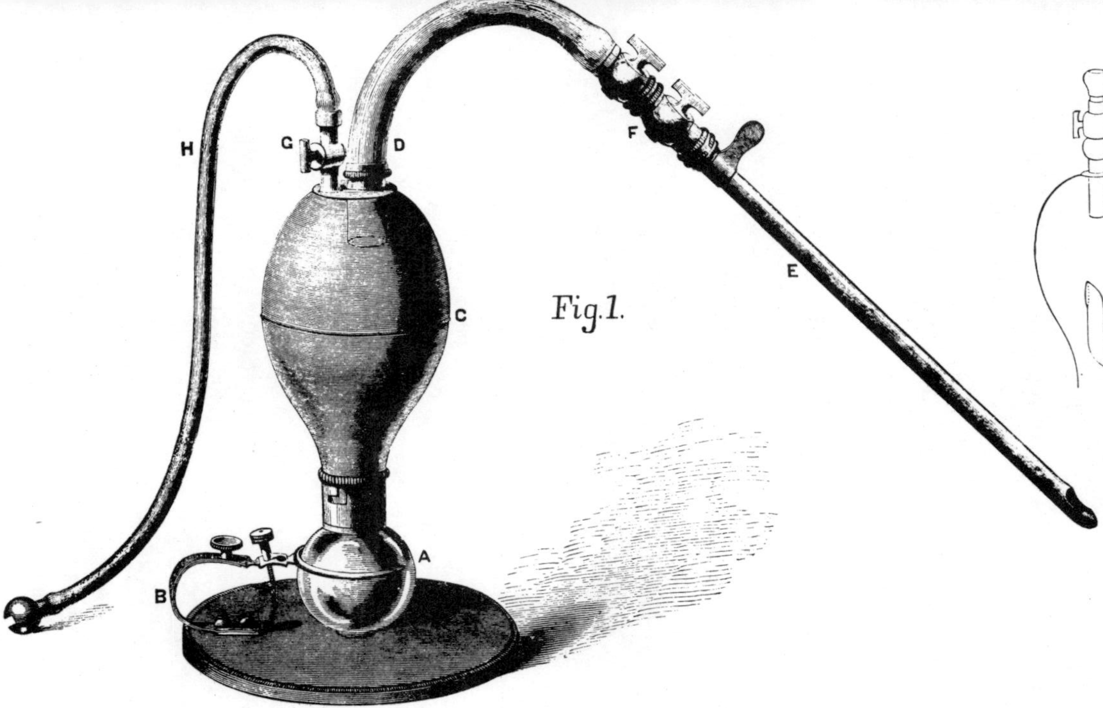

Fig.1.

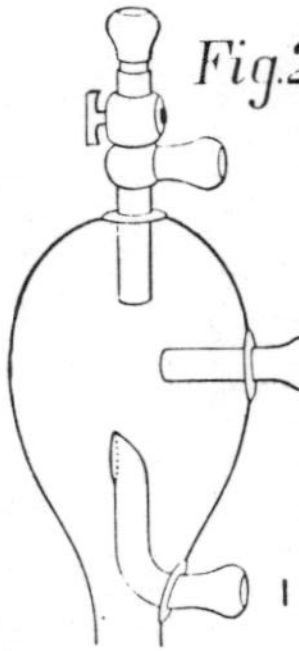

Fig.2.

FIG. 1. A, Glass trap, forming with the screw-catch B, which supports it, a ball-and-socket joint. C, Elastic bulb. D, Elastic tube, five inches long; one end attached to E, the evacuating catheter, the other continued into the bulb to form a chamber above its orifice. F, Coupling between the evacuating catheter and the elastic tube. G, H, Hose for air and water, with a movable attachment at G.

FIG. 2. Diagram of a bulb used for experiment.

that the difficulty of suction increases as the bulb is held higher than the evacuating-tube; it is very marked in Clover's instrument. There is great advantage in keeping the bulb low, near the level of the bladder.

The evacuator thus described works very well. I have used it in most of the operations I have performed. Its imperfections are that if by accident a little air gets inside, the bulb has to be uncoupled to get rid of it, and a few drops of water may escape and wet the bed. By a simple expedient I have remedied these inconveniences. In the instrument I here show (Fig. 1) the air can be removed, or water withdrawn from the bulb, or added to it, without a drop being spilled. Indeed, the operation would be absolutely dry did not a sensitive bladder occasionally contract and squeeze out a little water by the side of the lithotrite or catheter, in spite of the elastic band I usually tie around the penis to prevent it. When this happens, it is perhaps best not to try to stop it.

In this instrument the large evacuating tube at the top of the bulb extends an inch or more downward into its cavity. A space is thus formed where any accidental air collects, but cannot pass to the bladder. This space is emptied at will through an elastic tube or hose, a little more than a quarter of an inch in diameter, placed by the side of the first. The arrangement is a very simple one. Through this small hose, which can be attached and detached in a moment, the turbid contents of the bulb may be replaced by clear water without unfastening it from the catheter; or the contents of a tumblerful of water can be transferred to the bladder and back again, absolutely without loss, and with the elimination of all the air. With one end of the apparatus in the bladder and the other in a tumbler of water, the operator, even while he is evacuating the fragments, can vary the volume of water at will and put it where he pleases. The catheter and the elastic tubes, large and small, are each provided with a stop-cock.

If before using the lithotrite the surgeon desires to add or withdraw water from the bladder, this may be done through a common-sized catheter coupled with the bulb, — thus obviating the necessity for a syringe, and rendering this part of the operation as dry as the rest.

Instead of the metal ball-and-socket joint in the stand of my former instrument, I have substituted another, of which a strong glass trap forms the ball. This is supported in a metal socket, which allows all necessary motion or, if it is desirable, fixes the trap upon the flat disk.

The operation is as follows. The urine is drawn through a small catheter, and replaced by water from the bulb. The lithotrite is then introduced, and the stone is crushed. A large tube is next passed into the bladder to evacuate the fragments. Before the tube is introduced, its stop-cock must be closed. If during the pumping the bladder indicates, by repeatedly stopping the tube, that its parietes are hanging loose and acting as a valve, it should be distended by a little water injected from the bulb. This water is retained in the bladder by closing the cock of the evacuating-tube; while the bulb is replenished through the small hose.

When the empty evacuating tube is first introduced, a few bubbles often rise from it, and are caught in the bulb by elevating it; but when the current is established, air takes care of itself, and goes to the air space in the top of the bulb. In fact, there is none unless by accident. By opening the cocks and compressing the abdomen, it is easy to drive all air out of the bladder through the bulb.

In pumping, only a couple of ounces of water need be moved between the bladder and the bulb, backward and forward gently, without a jerk, once in a second or two. The tube is advantageously held just off the floor of the bladder, — a little higher at first, when the débris clogs it, and lower when only a few fragments remain.

As regards the amount of time necessary for an operation under ether, take as much as is necessary, precisely as in an amputation or excision. I usually add to the evacuation a thorough sounding. This requires more time. Some operators leave a few fragments in the bladder, to make the sitting shorter; but I doubt the expediency of doing so. Great care is essential, — also practice. How to pass instruments, large and small, curved and straight, with absolute facility, should be learned upon the dead body before practising upon the living. Notwithstanding an occasional assertion to the contrary, I am sure that if a common tin sound bent successively into a variety of different irregular curves can be introduced with ease into the bladder of a dead subject,—not empirically, but with a reason for each movement (and a few hours' intelligent practice, based upon anatomical considerations, will enable this to be done), — a catheter can be adroitly passed in any difficult case upon the living subject, and the accidents avoided that sometimes follow the introduction of common instruments, such as laceration of the mucous membrane and false passage. Obstructions from strictures or the irregular walls of an enlarged prostate will also be skilfully dealt with.[1]

1 The evacuator of Thompson illustrates the objections mentioned in the text. Latterly (Gazette Hebdomadaire, Oct. 31, 1879), Thompson has arranged a single stop-cock to do the duty of two in closing its lower orifices to keep the bed dry; but the instrument is virtually the same. (1) The bulb, or bottle, like Clover's, is above the catheter, so that the water has to be drawn up into it; and if the cocks happen to be simultaneously opened for a moment, it will all run into the bladder and distend it. (2) Its weight must be supported by the operator, or rest upon the catheter. (3) Being rigidly fixed to the catheter, it communicates the jar of pumping to the bladder, — this old "short connection" thus retained between catheter and bulb, upon which Thompson insists, yielding, so far as I can discover, no equivalent advantage. (4) Lastly, the mouth of the catheter enters *low down, into the narrowest part* of the bulb. Consequently fragments, after rising into the bulb with the current, must, on their way to the glass trap, again crowd in front of the catheter; and thus débris is needlessly returned to the bladder. It

would be better, if it be desired to connect the catheter low down, to prolong it a couple of inches inside the bulb, and to let the fragments escape at a higher point, where the cavity is wider, as is represented in the lowest tube of the annexed diagram (Fig. 2). With such an instrument I experimented some time ago. This arrangement also keeps the contents of the trap quiet, and there is no return of fragments.

But even an imperfect or inconvenient apparatus may suffice to empty the bladder. The only feature of an evacuator absolutely essential to rapid lithotrity is the large evacuating tube I have elsewhere described, which Thompson has adopted without change. It is this that enables his instrument to evacuate. The want of this large catheter (in combination with good suction and a trap) was fatal to the success of previous instruments, and to all attempts at the immediate evacuation of any considerable amount of débris. With such a catheter Clover's instrument could have evacuated the bladder slowly, and might have led, in the face of traditional prejudice, to the discovery of the tolerance of that organ, and of lithotrity at a single sitting. But the catheter of Clover's instrument was too small, being only 21 French (12 English), beyond which the English scale did not go. Its eye was also defective. The new method was impossible to those who were using this small catheter. They could not empty the bladder of all its fragments, and therefore knew nothing of its great recuperative powers after the complete removal of this source of irritation. Authorities agreed that evacuating instruments were worthless. When Otis directed the attention of surgeons to the fact (see a paper by R. F. Weir in the New York Medical Journal, April, 1876) that the capacity of the average urethra was very nearly 33, rapid lithotrity was made easy. Sittings were lengthened from a few minutes to an hour or two.

LITHOLAPAXY.

FROM A CLINICAL LECTURE.[1]

GENTLEMEN, — Within ten days we have had two cases of litholapaxy, one of which you saw. After both, the temperature rose from 98° to above 100° F. On the third day it fell to 99° F., and now, three days later, it is normal. This reaction is like that from the effect of a bougie, and the temperature like that of urethral fever. A patient readily recovers from the operation of litholapaxy if we remove from the bladder all the fragments of the stone. In fact, the new method has succeeded beyond expectation.

Small stones are easily ground up, especially if soft, and then come away of themselves. Serious consequences may follow if fragments are left in the bladder. In former times cases that did not admit of lithotrity had to be cut; likewise those in which, from any reason, lithotrity was hazardous. A recent number of the London "Lancet" reports a case in which Mr. Smith, of St. Bartholomew, removed four ounces of stone from the bladder of an elderly man, who left the hospital in a week. This is the largest quantity of débris ever removed by litholapaxy.

The operation, of course, is purely mechanical, and any reference to it is chiefly to its mechanics. The principles of litholapaxy and of complete evacuation are pretty well settled and accepted. It is now mainly a question of certain minor details of convenience in the apparatus. I am satisfied that one point which contributes as much as, if not more than, any other to rapid and complete evacuation is the power of regulating and of frequently varying the quantity of water in the

[1] The Boston Medical and Surgical Journal, March 4, 1880.

bladder. You require just enough water to prevent the *thud* of the slack walls when they are drawn into the eye of the catheter. When you feel that, the bladder must have a little more water to distend it. Too little water crowds the fragments together. When there is too much, you may have to chase a single fragment a long time.

The arrangement of hose I show you here is the only one that allows the operator to diminish the quantity of water in the bladder without disturbing the apparatus. If one end of this hose, which is not much larger than a pipe-stem, be kept in a tumbler of water it does not in the least interfere with the convenience of the operator; but on the other hand it does enable him, by turning the cocks, to vary from one minute to another, if he please, the amount of water in the bladder. There can be no doubt of the advantage of being able to do so.

Another point relates to the size of the tubes. The smallest tube used in litholapaxy is larger than the largest tube that was used for evacuation in previous operations. But you will find that the largest tubes I use are sometimes not preferred by other surgeons. They are in the habit of using a No. 28 or 29 tube, and these often serve the purpose. The fact is this: a stone after evacuation is found to have been mostly reduced to powder and minute fragments; large fragments are rather the exception. Now, the fine débris may be evacuated through a 28 or 29 tube, though perhaps not quite so rapidly as if the tube had a calibre of 30 or 31. It then remains only to crush the larger fragments and repeat the process. I prefer a larger tube, when there is no objection to its introduction, because it not only evacuates the dust more rapidly, but at the same time allows me to remove the large fragments without having to crush them again.

I am sure that in the end operators will all use a stand to support the weight of the bulb, because it is very inconvenient to hold it through a long operation. But there should be a device (as in the stand I show you here) for supporting the bulb at different heights, which can be varied during the progress of evacuation.

I also think surgeons will connect the bulb with the evacuating catheter by means of an elastic tube, so that one can be moved without the other. This to me is a *sine qua non*.

DE LA LITHOLAPAXIE;

OU, LITHOTRITIE AVEC ÉVACUATION IMMÉDIATE EN UNE SEULE SÉANCE.[1]

Il s'agit ici d'une modification de la lithotritie, ayant pour effet de renverser les traditions qui avaient, jusque dans ces derniers temps, réglé cette opération, et de la rendre applicable à des calculs plus volumineux que ceux qu'on avait eu l'habitude d'opérer par la méthode du broiement. Ce mémoire a pour but d'exposer brièvement l'historique de la découverte du procédé nouveau, et de décrire l'appareil instrumental au moyen duquel il a pu être mis à exécution. Certains perfectionnements portés à cet appareil se trouvent décrits ici pour la première fois.

La méthode nouvelle qui se trouve exposée dans ce mémoire est basée sur un fait nouveau : à savoir, la tolérance inattendue qu'offre la vessie pour les manœuvres instrumentales prolongées de la lithotritie avec évacuation. Au moyen du nouvel appareil qui se trouvera décrit plus loin, et qui est le seul qui ait permis d'atteindre de pareils résultats, on peut maintenant évacuer complètement, en une seule séance, les débris d'un calcul de volume considérable.

En présentant une méthode opératoire nouvelle, dont les principaux détails sont cependant déjà connus du monde médical depuis près de trois ans, l'auteur a cru qu'il serait superflu de soumettre à l'Académie de Médecine un travail complet et circonstancié où tous les détails ayant trait à son procédé se trouveraient exposés. Il a pensé qu'il se conformerait mieux aux désirs de l'Académie en se contentant de

[1] Mémoire soumise au Comité de l'Académie de Médecine de France, pour le prix d'Argenteuil de l'année 1881.

présenter une description sommaire de sa méthode et de son appareil instrumental.

Civiale, après plusieurs essais, parvint à améliorer ses instruments de telle sorte qu'il put atteindre un résultat qu'à tort il avait cru avantageux, consistant à restreindre la séance de lithotritie à une durée de quelques minutes. Chose singulière, depuis cette époque-là jusque vers l'année 1878, les chirurgiens se sont fourvoyés en cherchant à dépasser les résultats ainsi atteints par Civiale et en abrégeant encore davantage la durée de la séance. On s'est imaginé que les séances de très courte durée témoignaient de l'adresse du chirurgien, tout en rendant l'opération moins dangereuse pour le malade. Ainsi, Sir Henry Thompson recommandait à ses élèves de ne pas dépasser pour chaque séance une durée de trois minutes, tout en leur faisant remarquer que, grâce à une habileté manuelle particulière, il avait lui-même pour habitude d'accomplir la besogne d'une séance de broiement en un espace de temps moitié moindre. Il était alors convenu que la durée d'une séance ne devait pas dépasser un nombre de minutes très limité. Maintenant, cependant, des opérations ayant une durée d'une demie heure sont communes, et, dans un cas exceptionnel à cet égard, l'opération, suivie d'ailleurs d'un heureux résultat, a eu une durée de plus de trois heures.

Cette innovation si frappante s'explique de la manière suivante. La vessie est moins sujette à être lésée par le contact d'instruments métalliques arrondis et lisses, convenablement maniés, que par la présence des fragments anguleux qu'on avait autrefois l'habitude de laisser séjourner dans sa cavité pendant toute la durée du traitement par la lithotritie. La vessie tolère de bonne grâce une opération prolongée pourvu qu'elle ait pour résultat l'ablation complète des fragments. Pendant une cinquantaine d'années, il n'existait aucun appareil qui permît d'opérer l'extraction des fragments à travers les voies naturelles. Il était, par conséquent, impossible de déterminer, d'une manière quelque peu précise, jusqu'à quel point la vessie pourrait tolérer les manœuvres chirurgicales. Pendant un demi-siècle, il n'éxistait à ce sujet que des notions tout-à-fait erronées.

Le procédé nouveau, grâce auquel l'auteur de ce mémoire, il y a près de quatre ans, fit la découverte du degré de tolérance offerte par la vessie pour les manœuvres prolongées, fut l'emploi d'une grosse sonde évacuatrice ayant le calibre de l'urèthre normal, c'est-à-dire, entre les numéros 25 et 31 de la filière Charrière, au lieu d'un calibre ne dépassant pas le numéro 21, comme celui de la sonde qui fait partie de l'appareil à aspiration de Clover. Il fallait, en outre, un moyen efficace quelconque pour retenir les fragments qui auraient été entraînés à travers la sonde et pour empêcher leur retour dans la vessie.

Une forte sonde de calibre suffisant, d'une part, et un appareil destiné à empêcher le retour des fragments dans la vessie, d'autre part, constituent donc les parties absolument indispensables de l'instrument évacuateur. Une poire élastique en caoutchouc constitue le meilleur moyen de propulsion pour communiquer à l'eau d'injection le mouvement réquis de va-et-vient; mais, à vrai dire, l'agencement réciproque des parties constituantes essentielles de l'appareil, — à savoir, forte sonde, réservoir, et poire élastique, — peut varier de toutes les façons, selon les préférences de chacun; du reste, les diverses manières de combiner ces éléments ont au fond peu d'importance.

Je me permettrai d'ajouter ici quelques détails relativement à chacune de ces parties constituantes principales d'un appareil évacuateur efficace et commode tel que je le conçois.

Il s'agira d'abord de la sonde, — dont le calibre pourra varier entre les numéros 25 et 31, — qui a été imaginée pour cette nouvelle méthode de lithotritie avec évacuation immédiate. Cet instrument peut être droit ou courbé, selon le goût ou les habitudes du chirurgien. Quoi qu'il en soit à cet égard, il doit être muni d'un œil arrondi, situé tout auprès de son extrémité, et ayant un calibre non moindre que la lumière intérieure de l'instrument. Le bec doit être un peu prolongé, en forme de lèvre arrondie, pour faciliter le cheminement de l'instrument à travers le canal. La sonde ainsi conformée a été adoptée partout sans modification aucune.

Tous les appareils évacuateurs qu'on avait déjà imaginés avaient l'inconvénient de réinjecter dans la vessie un certain nombre des fragments qui en avaient été extraits, défaut qui rendait l'opération plus longue et le succès définitif moins certain. J'ai complètement remédié à cette imperfection en ajoutant un petit réservoir avec soupape, s'adaptant au pavillon de la sonde, de telle sorte que les fragments, ayant parcouru toute la longueur de la sonde et franchi son orifice extra-vésical, ne peuvent plus rentrer dans la vessie.

Ce réservoir se compose d'un petit cylindre creux en verre, à l'intérieur duquel se meut, sans bruit, une boule en caoutchouc faisant soupape, en s'acculant, pendant la compression de la poire, contre un grillage en entonnoir qui laisse passer l'eau, tout en s'opposant au retour des fragments dans la vessie. Ce détail de l'appareil, qui n'avait pas encore été décrit, est pour moi presqu'aussi important que la grosse sonde évacuatrice.

La bouteille en caoutchouc doit avoir plus de résistance, plus de force élastique que celle de Clover. Elle s'adapte à la sonde par l'intermédiaire d'un court tube en caoutchouc, grâce auquel la sonde et la bouteille peuvent se mouvoir indépendamment l'une de l'autre. La poire peut reposer à la hauteur voulue sur un support quelconque, et grâce à celui-ci et de l'interposition du tube de caoutchouc, le chirurgien peut s'épargner la fatigue de supporter le poids considérable de l'appareil rempli d'eau pendant toute la durée de son emploi.

La bouteille a une forme sphérique, et la sonde s'adapte sur son équateur. Si par hasard il venait à pénétrer de l'air dans l'appareil, il irait de suite se loger au sommet de la poire, tandis que les fragments se trouveraient entraînés par leur poids vers le fond. L'air accumulé en volume suffisant pour gêner l'opérateur peut de suite être expulsé à travers un petit tube avec robinet qui surmonte la poire. Le chirurgien peut alors remplacer cet air par de l'eau qu'il aspire en sens inverse à travers ce même tube.

Les fragments, ayant franchi le trajet à travers la sonde et étant parvenus jusque dans l'intérieur de la poire, tombent dans le réservoir transparent qui se trouve placé sous celle-ci. Ce réservoir peut être facilement détaché lorsqu'on désire extraire son contenu.

Tout brise-pierre suffira, à la rigueur, à effectuer le broiement de la pierre, pourvu qu'il soit d'une force suffisante. Il ne s'agit pas ici de la manière dont il faut s'y prendre pour l'introduire dans la vessie. Je me contenterai de faire remarquer qu'un instrument d'un volume excessif ne peut pas être conduit à travers l'urèthre sans danger ; et que l'urèthre profond et le col vésical tolèrent encore moins que la vessie les lésions traumatiques qui pourraient être infligées pendant l'opération.

Puisque le chirurgien se propose à présent d'achever le broiement du calcul en une seule séance, afin de pratiquer l'extraction immédiate des débris, il est devenu fort avantageux de se trouver muni d'un brise-pierre pouvant fonctionner longtemps dans la vessie sans que les mors soient sujets à s'engorger. J'ai donc été conduit à imaginer une conformation particulière des mors qui rend leur engorgement impossible. A cet effet, le mors mâle de mon brise-pierre présente, sur la surface qui se porte à l'encontre du mors femelle, une série d'encoches latérales, à plans inclinés dirigés alternativement à droite et à gauche. J'ai également fait construire un instrument à mors fenêtré qui broie sans s'engouer. Il n'est pas avantageux de se servir du brise-pierre pour extraire les débris du calcul. Leur ablation s'opère d'une manière plus salutaire par l'aspiration à travers la sonde que par l'extraction au moyen du brise-pierre, dont les mors, lorsqu'ils sont chargés de débris et entr'ouverts, peuvent infliger aux parois uréthrales des lésions très graves, sinon fatales. Afin d'empêcher l'engouement, qui est surtout sujet à se produire à l'angle du mors femelle, j'ai fait pratiquer dans cet endroit une fenêtre assez large, destinée à être complètement traversée par l'angle de la branche mâle se prolongeant en forme de talon, et repoussant devant lui les débris du calcul. Pour augmenter la force de l'instrument, sans toutefois nuire à la facilité de son introduction, j'ai fait construire les mors avec un coude dépassant de bien peu de degrés l'angle droit ; et, finalement, pour rendre le bec de l'instrument aussi inoffensif que possible pour les parties à travers lesquelles il doit cheminer pendant son introduction, et surtout pour garantir la paroi supérieure de l'urèthre, j'ai fait légèrement allonger, infléchir en avant, et arrondir l'extrémité du mors femelle. Cette conformation nouvelle ne nuit aucunement à l'efficacité des prises opérées par le chirurgien.

J'ai encore modifié la poignée du brise-pierre d'une manière que je crois avantageuse, en y adaptant des armatures nouvelles de deux espèces, destinées à faciliter son maniement. Il s'agit toujours du brise-pierre usuel, à vis et à écrou brisé, avec poignée à barillet cylindrique. Dans l'un de mes brise-pierres le chirurgien fait fonctionner l'écrou brisé au moyen d'un anneau qui entoure le barillet, et auquel on communique avec les doigts de la main droite un mouvement de va-et-vient, en le faisant glisser dans les deux sens, longitudinalement. L'autre brise-pierre, dont le mécanisme diffère de tous ceux qu'on avait déjà imaginés, fonctionne par l'intermédiaire d'une armature à rotation dont le jeu alternatif dans les deux sens, dextrorsum et sinistrorsum, en quart de cercle, est effectué par les doigts de la main droite. L'ouverture et la fermeture de l'écrou brisé s'opère ainsi très facilement, sans effort et sans tâtonnements des doigts, au moyen de mouvements très naturels de pronation et de supination de la main droite, du même genre que ceux qui servent à faire marcher la vis du brise-pierre. J'aime à croire qui cette poignée finira par remplacer toutes celles qui ont été imaginées jusqu'à présent.

En faisant pénétrer un instrument quelque peu volumineux, le chirurgien doit veiller à ne pas violenter la partie profonde de l'urèthre. Le broiement peut continuer jusqu'à ce que les débris se soient accumulés en quantité suffisante pour gêner le jeu du brise-pierre. Pourvu que les forces du malade ne soient pas trop délabrées, il n'est point nécessaire, pas plus que dans tout autre genre d'opérations, d'imposer d'avance des limites précises à la durée totale de la séance.

Le broiement du calcul ayant été effectué, le brise-pierre est retiré, la sonde évacuatrice est introduite, et la bouteille en caoutchouc est adaptée à son extrémité extra-vésicale. Un lien élastique est alors fixé autour de la verge pour empêcher la vessie d'expulser son contenu liquide ; en tâtant la paroi inférieure de l'urèthre derrière cette ligature, le chirurgien peut, jusqu'à un certain point, apprécier le degré de la distension subie par la paroi vésicale. La quantité d'eau à employer varie naturellement selon la capacité de la vessie. Il suffit que la vessie soit suffisamment distendue d'eau pour empêcher l'aspiration de sa paroi trop flasque contre l'œil de la sonde ; lorsque ce phénomène vient à se produire, le chirurgien en est averti de suite par une série de petites secousses transmises à la sonde et même à la bouteille en caoutchouc au moment où l'aspiration s'exerce ; il suffit alors de distendre davantage la vessie en y ajoutant une certaine quantité d'eau, que l'on peut puiser dans un vase au moyen du petit tube situé au sommet de la bouteille.

L'évacuation a lieu d'une façon très simple et facile, au moyen de petits mouvements de va-et-vient communiqués au contenu de la vessie par l'intermédiaire de la sonde, et produits par la compression et par l'expansion de la poire élastique. Les fragments du calcul ne tardent pas à se faire voir et à s'accumuler dans le réservoir en verre. La sonde est tenue d'abord de manière à ce que l'œil soit un peu élevé au-dessus du bas-fond vésical ; plus tard, et au fur et à mesure que les fragments deviennent moins abondants dans la vessie, le bec doit être abaissé de plus en plus. Les fragments trop gros pour traverser la sonde viennent heurter contre les rebords de l'œil avec un cliquetis facile à percevoir, et exigent alors un nouveau broiement.

La recherche d'un dernier fragment de faible volume, ou d'un petit calcul, s'effectue mieux au moyen de cet appareil à aspiration qu'avec la sonde exploratrice qu'on a l'habitude d'employer pour reconnaître la présence de calculs ou de fragments dans la vessie. Grâce à l'emploi de l'aspiration le fragment vient à la rencontre de l'instrument explorateur. Celui-ci l'évacue de suite, ou bien fait savoir au chirurgien que le broiement sera de nouveau réquis pour venir à bout de ce fragment encore trop volumineux.

Telle est ma nouvelle méthode de lithotritie rapide en une seule séance. Je peux dire que cette opération a reçu un accueil favorable presqu'universel en Europe comme en Amérique. On n'entend presque plus aujourd'hui de voix dissidentes à ce sujet. Les calculs petits et moyens se laissent facilement broyer et évacuer en une seule opération. Des pierres plus volumineuses ont été traitées de la même façon, et la guérison des malades a été prompte et complète. Porter, Thomas Smith, Teevan, Green, et d'autres chirurgiens encore, ont rapporté des cas heureux où les quantités de débris évacués par ce procédé, en une ou deux séances, d'une à trois heures de durée, ont varié entre mille et près de deux mille grains (de 65 à 120 grammes environ). Ces faits si frappants témoignent de la révolution complète qui s'est opérée dans nos esprits relativement aux limites qui doivent maintenant être imposées à la lithotritie. Il n'est pas encore possible de prévoir jusqu'à quel point la méthode nouvelle, que je viens de décrire d'une façon très sommaire, pourra, chez l'adulte, remplacer la taille ; les données existantes ne suffisent pas encore pour que nous pouissions déterminer l'étendue du champ dans lequel elle pourra être employée avec profit.

J'ai proposé pour cette méthode de broiement avec évacuation d'emblée des fragments le nom de *litholapaxie*. Nous pourrions, cependant, nous passer de ce néologisme, peut-être quelque peu cacophone, si la vieille lithotritie de Civiale, en séances courtes et multipliées, venait à être abandonnée. La lithotritie, quelles que puissent être les modifications qu'elle subira, sera toujours la lithotritie, — mais dorénavant cette méthode, je crois, sera caractérisée par l'évacuation immédiate et complète des fragments tout autant que par le broiement de la pierre, qui autrefois constituait à lui seul toute l'opération.

Certaines complications préexistantes peuvent donner lieu à des indications particulières. Le méat uréthral, qui constitue généralement le point le plus étroit du canal, doit souvent être élargi au moyen d'une petite incision, pratiquée au moyen d'un bistouri boutonné, ou bien avec des ciseaux. C'est là une opération insignifiante.

D'autre part, il est parfois nécessaire, dans certains cas, de pouvoir écarter, séance tenante, l'obstacle constitué par un rétrécissement uréthral plus profondément situé. La divulsion s'est trouvée être un excellent moyen pour atteindre ce bout ; et, à cet effet, j'ai quelque peu modifié l'instrument qui était affecté à cette opération. Mon divulseur est ainsi constitué : la bougie filiforme conductrice s'attache comme d'ordinaire, par un pas de vis, à un mandrin métallique droit. Celui-ci sert de conducteur à une longue et forte olive métallique qui, ainsi que la tige en tube qui lui sert de manche et de moyen de propulsion, est perforée dans toute sa longueur d'un canal central, de manière à pouvoir cheminer par glissement le long du mandrin conducteur, en dilatant les points rétrécis du canal de l'urèthre. Pour pratiquer la divulsion, on introduit d'abord le mandrin droit central à la suite de la bougie filiforme. Ce mandrin conducteur est immobilisé pendant le cheminement d'avant en arrière de l'olive dilatrice à travers les points rétrécis, au moyen d'une sorte de pavillon en forme d'hémisphère creuse, qui coiffe le gland, en appuyant contre celui-ci, et fournit ainsi un point d'appui.

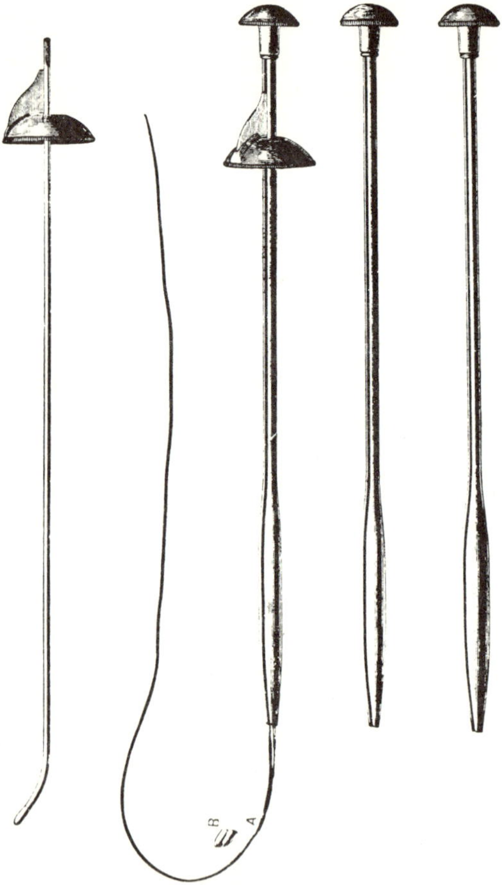

Fig. 1[1].

[1] Divulseur Bigelow.

L'opérateur, étreignant la verge de la main gauche, pousse l'olive le long du mandrin conducteur central de la main droite, pendant que la propulsion en avant de celui-ci est empêchée par le pavillon évasé qui coiffe le gland et s'y appuie. Il y a en outre certains détails qu'il serait inutile de décrire ici. Il suffit d'inspecter l'instrument pour comprendre de suite sa construction et la manière de s'en servir. Je me contenterai de dire que cet instrument à divulsion a l'avantage sur ceux qui existaient déjà, de n'exiger pour son maniement qu'une seule paire de mains, et qu'il remplit parfaitement le but pour lequel il a éte imaginé.

Tels sont l'appareil instrumental nouveau et la méthode opératoire nouvelle pour le traitement des calculs vésicaux que j'ai l'honneur de soumettre, très respectueusement, à l'appréciation du Comité de l'Académie de Médecine pour le prix d'Argenteuil de l'année 1881.

MODERN LITHOTRITY.[1]

My object in the present communication is to show in what the modern operation of lithotrity consists, and to explain the instruments which have made its performance possible; for the removal of a vesical calculus through the urethra is now mainly a question of apparatus, of which certain essential details are new. And as it is by no means necessary that the different parts of the apparatus should be put together exactly in any particular manner, it will be perhaps better to illustrate the principles of its construction than to insist on any special form of it. It will also be unnecessary for me to dwell on those parts of the subject which belong as well to the old lithotrity as to the new.

From the days of Civiale to the year 1878 there was little change in the operation. The duration of a sitting was as brief as the skill of the surgeon, stimulated by his fear of producing cystitis, could make it. Three minutes or less was the limit inculcated by standard books and teaching of specialists, and the use of anæsthesia was exceptional. At present anæsthetics are the rule. The instruments have been already modified in an important manner, while sittings often last half an hour, and have been successfully extended to three hours and more.

Had Clover (whose catheter had a calibre only 21 of the French standard, — about 12 English) or Mercier employed larger catheters (between 25 and 31 French, — 15 to 20 English), they might have evacuated the bladder completely. They would have found how little affected it was by a long operation if no fragments were left behind, and that polished

[1] Transactions of The International Congress of Physicians and Surgeons, Seventh Session; Vol. II., pp. 292–306. London, 1881.

instruments were not injurious to it, while sharp fragments were. They would have discovered a *tolerance on the part of the bladder* wholly at variance with the traditions of half a century. Upon this tolerance modern lithotrity is based.

The new and essential instrument of the operation is *the large catheter* (25 to 31), whether straight or curved (Fig. 1). This is indispensable. It has an orifice at the extreme end, one side of which is prolonged so as to make its introduction easy.

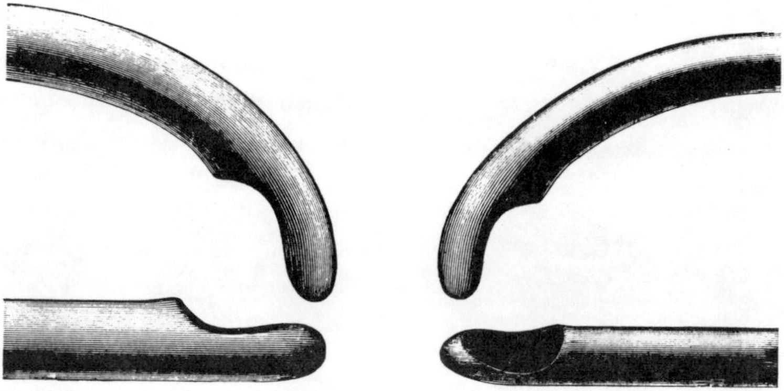

FIG. 1.[1]

It has been adopted with little or no change, so far as I know, everywhere. Although my first apparatus was provided with efficient means of suction and a detached trap, neither of which was used before, its distinctive feature was the large catheter. The small size of the previous evacuating catheter delayed surgical progress for half a century. All the fragments could not pass through it, and it was impossible for surgeons to ascertain how the bladder would behave when once completely emptied of all fragments.

Assuming all this to be admitted, let us examine the rest of the apparatus, and see how the operation is modified by it.

[1] Large and small evacuating catheters, straight and curved (Nos. 25 and 31 French).

As even a single minute fragment left in the bladder may be the nucleus of a future stone, it is important to get rid of it with certainty, and once for all. Now, although a fragment remaining in the catheter after the bulb has ceased to expand goes back to the bladder, yet if it has once passed beyond the catheter, its return to the bladder ought to be made impossible: the surgeon should be able to secure it. And yet no evacuator hitherto devised, whether with a long or a short connection between the bulb and the catheter, accomplishes this important end; they all inject fragments from the apparatus back into the bladder. I find by experiment that a few added inches of elastic tube make little difference; *it is from the bulb or bottle that fragments are chiefly returned before they settle into the receiver, and not from the tubes.*

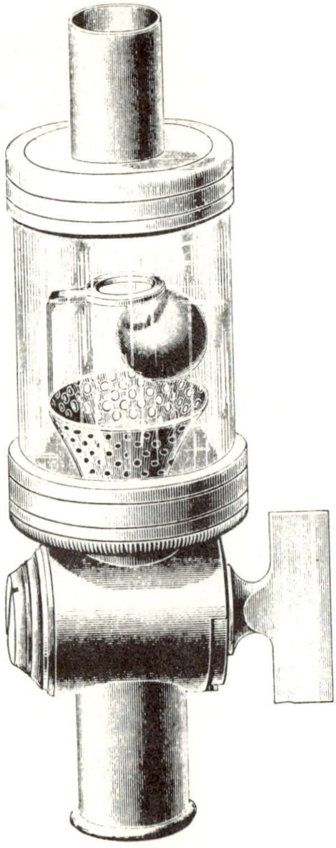

Fig. 2.[1]

To prevent this I have fixed a simple contrivance to the head of the catheter, which is absolutely effectual in securing every fragment as it comes through it (Fig 2). It consists of a small, light glass cylinder, containing a ball-valve of rubber acting noiselessly, the valve seat of which is perforated so as to strain the return current and to keep back any fragment that

[1] Catheter-valve, or strainer. A rubber ball, acting as a valve, has a seat of perforated metal, which strains the water. It prevents the fragments which pass it from returning.

has once passed it. Such a *catheter-valve, or strainer*, to which I alluded in my first paper (1878), is, I think, nearly as important as the large evacuating catheter itself, of which it may indeed be considered as a part.

Other parts of the apparatus admit of endless variations which are less important.

If to the essential large catheter and trap we merely attach a strong elastic bulb, we have an excellent and simple instrument for a short washing or for sounding for a last fragment. I have called this an evacuating sound (Fig. 3). No fragment drawn by it from the bladder can get back. This apparatus resembles Clover's, which was the first of the straight variety. It differs from it in having a large catheter, a valve or strainer, and a stiff bulb, all of which are either necessary or important to success.

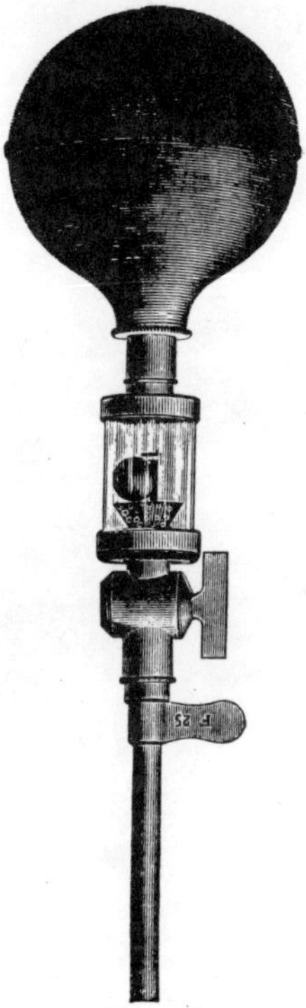

FIG. 3.[1]

One of the early additions to my own first instrument with which, in its original form, Thomas Smith successfully evacuated nearly two thousand grains of débris, was a hose. This contributes greatly to the convenience of the operation. When, for example, at each aspiration of the bulb the wall of the bladder is drawn with a painful jerk, or series of jerks, into the orifice of the catheter, evacuation is obstructed. More water is then needed to distend the walls. This is conveniently supplied by a small hose attached to the top of the bulb (Figs. 4, 6, 7).

[1] The evacuating sound. It consists of an evacuating catheter, a catheter-valve, and a rubber bulb.

Should the patient strain or vomit, and the bladder be forcibly distended in consequence, we have here a means whereby the superfluous water can be quickly removed from it. When air rises to the top of the apparatus from the empty catheter or a leaky joint, it can escape by this hose and be replaced by water. Valves in the hose itself, or in the vessel into which it delivers, allow the bloody water to be changed for fresh. By its means the amount of water can be regulated, and the operation becomes a dry one, while the apparatus is as simple as a common enema-syringe.

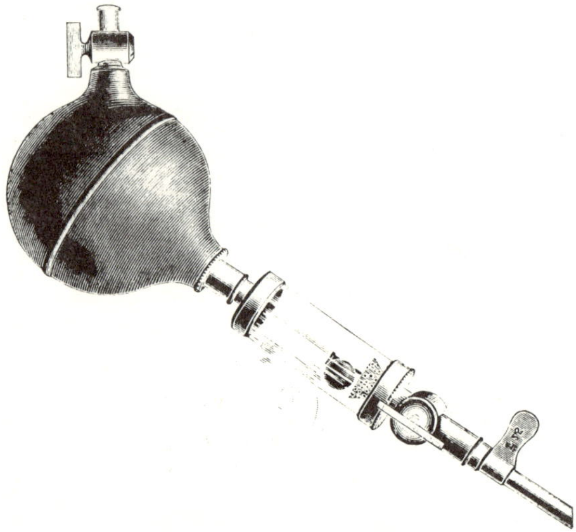

FIG. 4.[1]

I have made a convenient straight evacuator out of the evacuating sound by attaching to it a light receiver (like that of a breast pump) close to the catheter, adding also a flat

[1] A straight evacuator, made from the evacuating sound by adding below the valve a glass receiver to hold the fragments, and above the bulb a tap for the hose. Between the valve and the bulb, inside, is a flat strainer (not seen) to keep the fragments out of the bulb.

strainer[1] at the entrance of the bulb, to keep the fragments out of it, and a hose to manage the air and water (Fig. 4).

The same arrangement is here also shown (Fig. 5) in metal instead of glass.

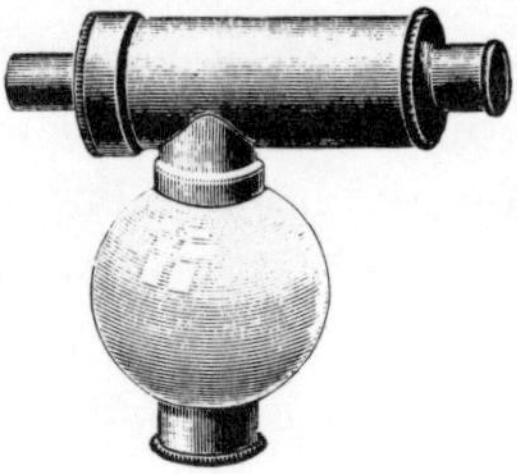

FIG. 5.[2]

In Fig. 6 the glass receiver has been transferred from the neighborhood of the catheter to the position it occupied in my first evacuator, below the bulb, to which the fragments are now of course admitted, by removing the flat strainer.

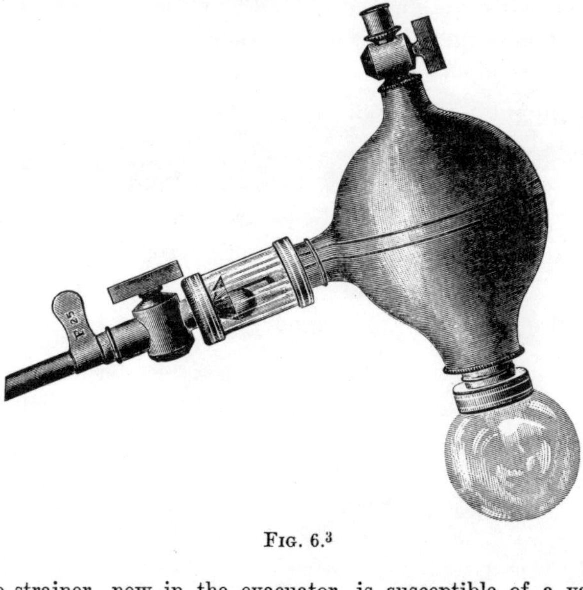

FIG. 6.[3]

[1] The strainer, new in the evacuator, is susceptible of a variety of applications and of forms. A long narrow slit in the tube answers as well as the perforations.

[2] The valve and trap of Fig. 4, made of metal.

[3] The same as Fig. 4, except that the receiver is here transferred to the bulb, and the flat strainer has been removed to admit the fragments to it.

All these are varieties of the straight apparatus. This is much the best, in the distribution of its parts, of the evacuators wholly supported by the hand. The centre of the bulb is in line with the catheter; and were it not so heavy when full of water, it would be a most convenient handle for the management of that instrument.[1]

In short, if the operator prefers to carry the bulb unsupported in his hand, straight instruments, such as have been described, are the best.

But I prefer a support or stand of some sort. If a flexible tube or joint is interposed between the bulb and the catheter, the former can be supported upon the patient, or on a stand at a height corresponding with the inclination which the prostate gland gives the catheter, while the latter has a free and independent motion. Such is the instrument I use for any considerable evacuation.[2]

It is no great matter where the catheter enters the wall of the bulb; but it should finally deliver inside at some point lower than the top, so that any air can rise out of the way. Mr. Berkeley Hill was quite right in saying that the catheter should not deliver into a narrow part of the apparatus

[1] By a straight Instrument is here meant one in which the catheter and bulb are fixed in line rigidly, so that one cannot move without the other. If the bulb, still retaining a metal connection, were bent down out of this line, it could be supported on the patient or the table. But when it is bent up and attached inflexibly, it seems to me more difficult to manage. It is then neither so convenient for the operator to support its weight, nor is it easy to keep the catheter from oscillating. The rigid short connection seems to have been adopted in the hope, by shortening their route, of preventing a return of fragments. It fails to do this, because most of the fragments come, not from the tube, but from the bulb.

[2] The mobility of the bulb in a stand can be provided for in a variety of ways, — by making a ball-and-socket joint of the spherical bulb and a ring (Fig. 7), or of its glass receptacle (Transactions of the Clinical Society, London, 1879, and Boston Medical and Surgical Journal, January 1, 1880. See pp. 277 and 285 of this volume.) The bulb can also be hung from a crane.

where fragments are crowded together, because then they go back to the bladder. It is the worst place, although if a valve or strainer is used the defect is less important.

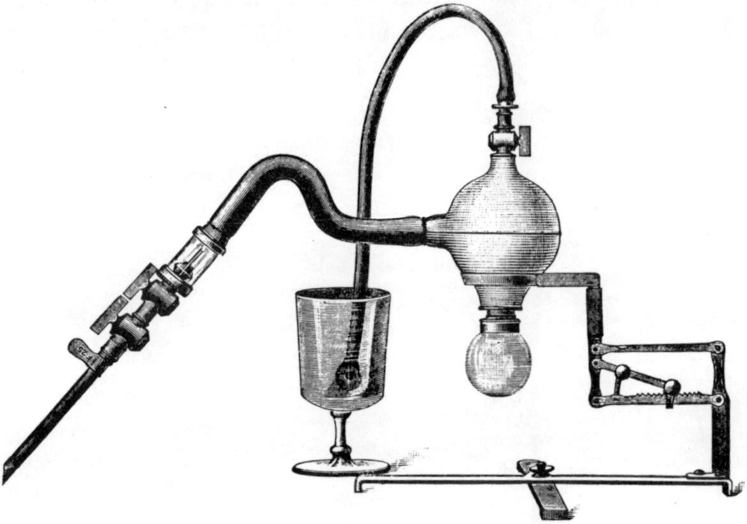

FIG. 7.[1]

But let me repeat it: a proper tube to deliver the fragments, with an effectual contrivance to prevent their return, are the essential parts of the new apparatus; what remains is a matter of convenience or perfection, and every operator can choose the arrangement which suits him best. *When the instrument is imperfect, the fragments will go backward and forward; but they always leave a certain number outside. The evacuation will be accomplished in the end by every evacuator that has the large catheter, which is the key to modern lithotrity.*

[1] A complete evacuator, used by the writer, — being the same as that represented in Fig. 5, with the addition of a stand and an elastic tube. Curves in the elastic tube make it less liable to flatten when bent. The hose is attached whenever it is needed.

What has here been said about the evacuator, an instrument which has been of late years so modified as to make it a chief factor in the operation of lithotrity, is intended rather to illustrate the principles which should guide the surgeon in its construction than to recommend any particular one. For although the instruments I showed at the Congress, and which I have described here, and use, accomplish the work of drawing out the fragments and preventing their return more perfectly than any previous apparatus for the purpose, this is not the only consideration which in practice determines the surgeon in the choice of such an instrument.

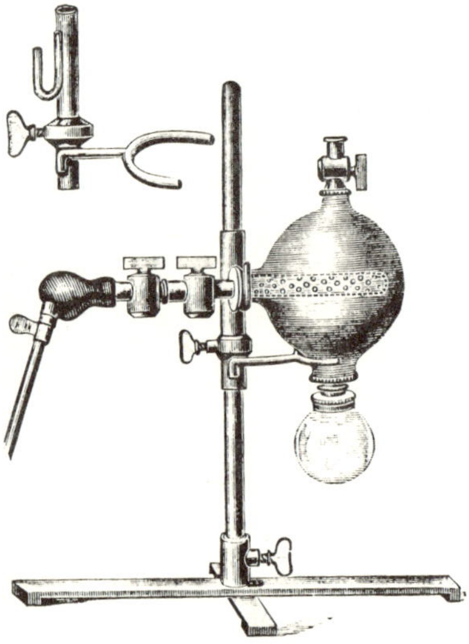

FIG. 8.[2]

I now recommend an evacuator on the ground of simplicity in construction and economy in price.[1] It works quite well enough, with or without a stand. It is, in fact, the instrument already described, with a strainer substituted for the valve. Several instruments shown by me were provided with strainers, but this one is arranged with reference to the fact

[1] The aspirators here described, and also the various lithotrites, are made by J. Weiss and Son, London.

[2] The "Simplified Evacuator" and Stand. The catheter is prolonged, by a long tubular strainer, into the bulb. This makes a catheter-valve, though still advantageous, less necessary. An elastic ball or universal joint, with a small tubular strainer, is also substituted at the head of the catheter for the elastic tube, and makes the instrument shorter. The stand is here a retort stand. The bulb hangs firmly in a fork (separately figured), and can be variously inclined.

that the return of fragments from the apparatus to the bladder is much greater from the bulb than from the tubes, to which it has been erroneously attributed. The strainer is here a perforated cylinder added to the catheter, passing inside the bulb and extending nearly across it. Through this the fragments are drawn into the bulb-cavity. They swirl there for a few seconds; but when the water goes back to the bladder, it strains them off, and they fall into a receiver. The lengthened tube adds little to the amount of the returned débris, and if obstructed is easily cleared by a rod (Fig. 11). The apparatus here described has the following advantages: —

1. As the bulb is spherical, whether a receiver is attached to it or not, the hand of the operator, grasping its centre, is in line with the catheter as if holding the handle of a long screw-driver, — which is better than if the hand were above it, out of line. This is an advantage common to all straight evacuators.

2. The instrument is a short one. A long inflexible apparatus is liable to irregular movements, which produce pain. Otherwise, the tubular strainer might be placed outside the bulb (in the glass trap, for example, described by Mr. Berkeley Hill, Figs. 9, 10). It is here fixed inside the bulb (Figs. 8, 11), which so shortens the apparatus that we have room for two connecting cocks, one for the bulb and one for the catheter. This makes the operation much drier than where there is no cock for the catheter.

3. There is a hose for air and water above the bulb, and a receiver for fragments below it.

Without a stand, this instrument belongs to the straight evacuators, with a rigid connection between the catheter and bulb. The operator then, of course, supports the weight of the bulb, which I find troublesome if the operation is more serious than that of washing out the bladder or securing a last fragment. We can easily have a stand here, steady enough to sustain the weight of the arm of the operator, and prevent the oscillation of the catheter. Three inches of elastic tube, or an elastic ball about an inch in diameter, can be interposed between the bulb and catheter to act as a universal joint.[1] It is then easy to rest the bulb in one hand on the patient's thigh, while the catheter is manipulated with the other, or upon the glass receiver flattened into a foot. The stand here figured is of simple construction, and can be adjusted at any convenient height with reference to the catheter (see Fig. 8).[3]

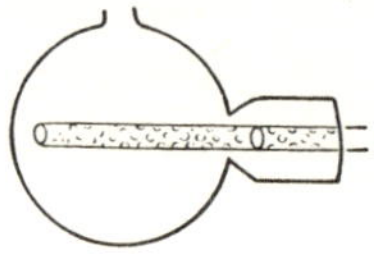

FIG. 9.[2]

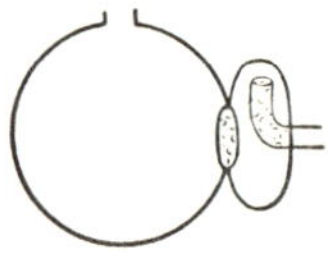

FIG. 10.

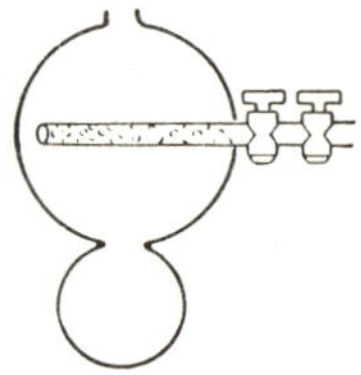

FIG. 11.

I have condensed the arrangement here described from the materials referred to in the preceding part of this paper, having been lately persuaded that a compact and inexpensive apparatus, performing as perfectly as this one, is a desideratum. To designate it appropriately, I have called it "The Simplified Evacuator." A stand and elastic joint can be had with it.

Within three years renewed attention has been given to the lithotrite, which was supposed to be beyond improvement. A

[1] A small metal drum with elastic ends makes a good joint. The metal sides cannot fall against the catheter and obstruct it.

[2] Figs. 9, 10, and 11, — diagrams intended to show how much a straight instrument (Fig. 9) is shortened by flattening the glass receiver (Fig. 10) or by removing it from the catheter (Figs. 4, 5, 9, 10) to the bulb (Figs. 6, 7, 8, 11). The space may be occupied by stop–cocks (Fig. 11). The body of the bulb is spherical, and lies in the axis of the catheter, with a hose and a receiver attached to it.

[3] If the patient lies on a soft bed, the bulb must be held in the hand, unless the stand be steadied, like a fracture box, by something under it. But I usually do this surgical operation, like others, on a table of some sort.

calculus may indeed be crushed by any lithotrite, if strong enough; but since decisive crushing has become more desirable, and the limit to the size of the stone has been extended, different lithotrites are more and more used for different stones. The old lithotrite, the combined work of Retoré, Costello, Charrière, and Weiss, underwent little change in half a century. A most convenient addition to it is the long handle described by Thompson.[1] It gives a better hold for the left hand. But the inconvenient button in the lock of Weiss, which it incloses, has never been changed. The thumb and the eye of the operator must search for it when the instrument is turned. By changing the lock a little I have been able to replace this button by a more convenient ring, which the fingers cannot miss (Fig. 12). To reach this ring-lock with the fingers, after the stone is seized, requires neither practice nor attention, while one or both are needed with the Weiss button.

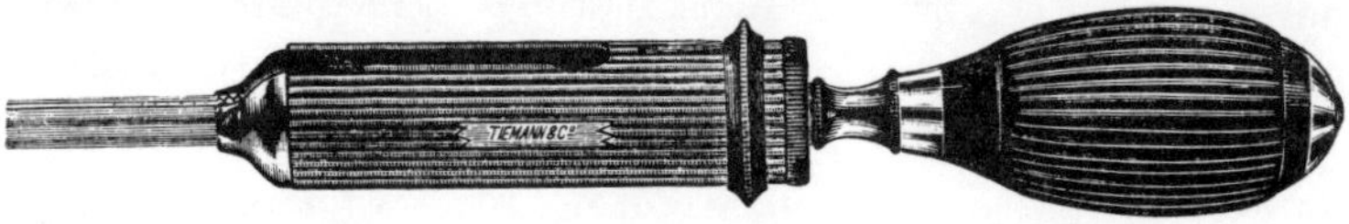

FIG. 12.[2]

The easiest movement of the right forearm or hand is rotation from left to right, — supination. I have adapted the locking of my lithotrite to this motion.[3] An instrument which can be thus locked and unlocked has this superiority, that not even the fingers of either hand relax their grasp until the stone has been screwed down between the blades. No other

1 Practical Lithotomy and Lithotrity, p. 157. London, 1863.

2 A lithotrite in which a ring is substituted for Weiss's button to operate the lock.

3 This was accomplished by making the usual guides, which prevent the screw from rattling against the sides of the lock, also turn and close it, by the action of the right hand upon the male blade. I have called it the *male-blade lock*.

lithotrite gives the surgeon this advantage. This lock is attached to the usual American instrument, and I have lately further improved it (Figs. 13 and 14).

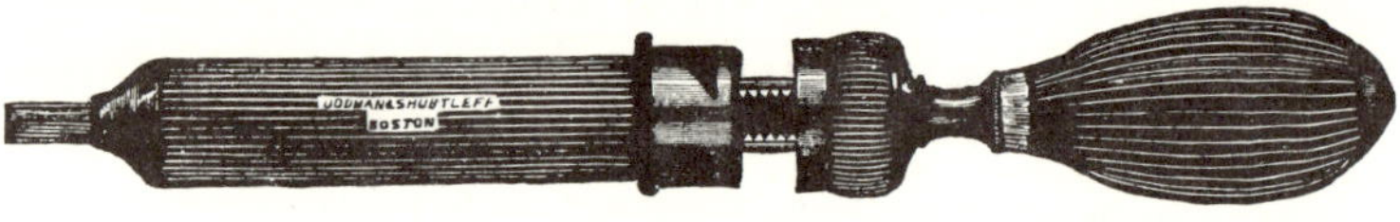

FIG. 13.[1]

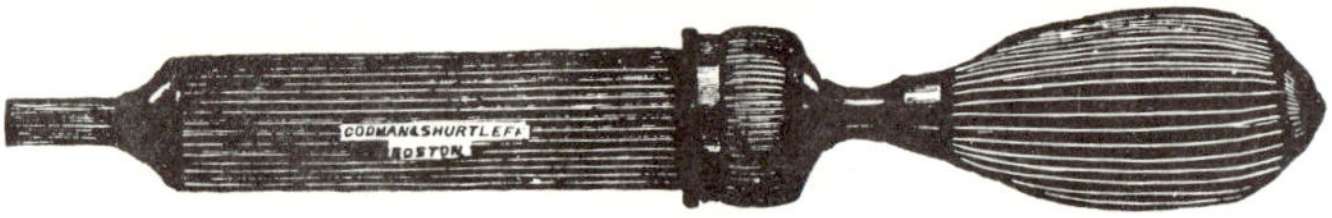

FIG. 14.

We may educate the movements of the hand to the piano, the violin, or some especial lithotrite, but the process is laborious. That instrument, therefore, is the most convenient, which, in accomplishing its object, is best adjusted to the readiest movements of the hand. Workmen may become, indeed, proficient in the use of any form of instrument; but the skill of the Japanese wood or metal worker, which is unrivalled, is not evidence of the convenience of his tools, which are rude.

In the "Lancet" of Nov. 2, 1878, p. 616, I pointed out the advantages of certain lesser modifications of the usually accepted lithotrite, partly new and partly not. Among these were, besides the increased calibre of the jaws, a large opening at the heel of the female blade into which the flanges of the male blade projected so as to drive out the débris and prevent impaction where it is likely to be greatest; jaws as much at right angles with the stem as can be safely introduced, whereby their efficacy is increased; a thicker toe to the female

[1] Figs. 13 and 14, — author's lithotrite, having a male-blade or right-hand lock, which is closed by a quarter revolution of the lock cover held between the thumb and fore-finger of the operator's right hand. It also has an elongated vulcanite handle shaped to fit the hand.

blade, elongated to prevent the bladder from being seized by the closing blades, and well rounded off to facilitate its introduction; a ball, or larger wheel or handle instead of the classical narrow wheel of Civiale, which had been retained for half a century although it excoriates the hands (see Figs. 13, 14, 15, 16). The adoption of all these changes in the most common American lithotrite, and their recent valuable indorsement, in his later instrument, by so skilful a lithotritist as Sir Henry Thompson, show their value.

Before choosing the instruments for an operation, I measure both the urethra and the stone. But the limit to the size of instruments is not merely mechanical; it is also related to the fact that the membranous urethra is peculiarly intolerant of injury.

The healthy urethra, according to Otis, has a calibre about 32 French, the meatus being about 24. I generally use a catheter about 29 French (18 English), but also smaller sizes, which are often more comfortable to the unetherized patient, and in a diseased subject safer. With 25 or 26 you can produce the click of a last fragment or of a small calculus, and easily deliver it when crushed. In fact, much of the débris of a stone is in the form of dust, and what is not can be further comminuted.

But when the stone is not a small one, and the urethra is of normal capacity, I use the size 29 or 30, or even 31,—as large as the urethra will comfortably admit, but no larger. The advantage in doing so is that the smaller fragments need not be crushed again.

Strong lithotrites are now in general use for large and hard stones. I like a large lithotrite on account of its powerful, rapid, and efficient action; but it by no means follows that it is essential to use a large instrument to break a small stone. Any small lithotrite answers for small stones. The average stone of these days is small. I always crush a last fragment with a small instrument. A large stone once broken can obviously be treated by an instrument of less size; but once in the bladder, I think the surgeon will generally continue to use the instrument with which he has successfully begun the crushing.

A calculus out of the bladder would be crushed best by a colossal instrument at a single grasp. It is the necessity of safely introducing and withdrawing the instrument that determines the size of its blades. The length has most to do with their introduction; the calibre at the heel, with their withdrawal through the prostatic and membranous urethra.

While long blades slide easily from the meatus as far as the triangular ligament, the delicacy and skill of a practised operator are needed at this part of the passage. On the other hand, once safely in a bladder of fair size, a long blade has a positive advantage in seizing and crushing the stone. The instrument can be readily turned down either way upon the oval floor, especially if the handle be inclined a little to the side toward which the blades are turned. Behind the perpendicular wall of a high prostate, short and blunted blades which can be inverted readily are the most convenient.

The calibre of the blades is a question by itself. Blades may safely be large at the heel, which is the largest part, if they do not become clogged with débris, and by their increased size endanger the neck of the bladder while being withdrawn. If they cannot be cleared of débris they should be small. Fergusson's method of removing débris with the lithotrite is not now generally in use. No lithotrite that can be cleared is drawn out loaded. It is almost universally agreed that fragments can be removed better through a catheter than in a lithotrite. This fact has led to renewed search for a lithotrite that can be completely emptied and closed before withdrawal, without danger of impaction. It can then be made stronger and larger,—at least as large as a smaller lithotrite when it is full of débris, or as the evacuating catheter (26 to 29 French) that is used at the same time,—and since it does not need to be repeatedly withdrawn to be emptied, crushing can be continued as long as it is desirable.

The dust of certain stones mixed with mucus clogs the lithotrite, especially at the heel, with a very hard composition. To prevent this, I have recommended a high floor at this part, or, what is the same thing, low sides in the female blade; and in the male blade, lateral notches steep enough to push off the débris laterally (Figs. 15 and 16). This plan has been adopted

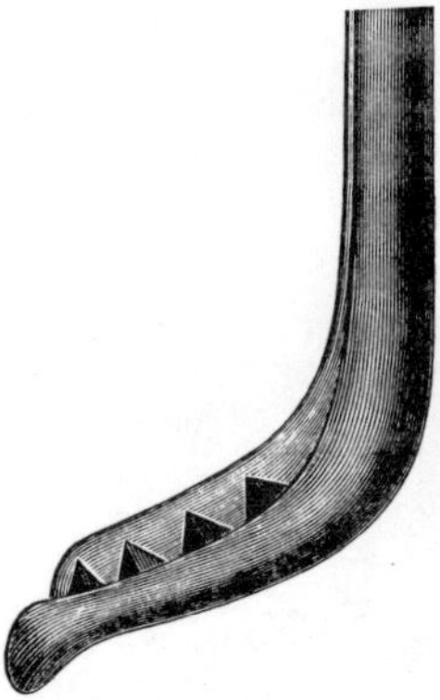

FIG. 15.[1]

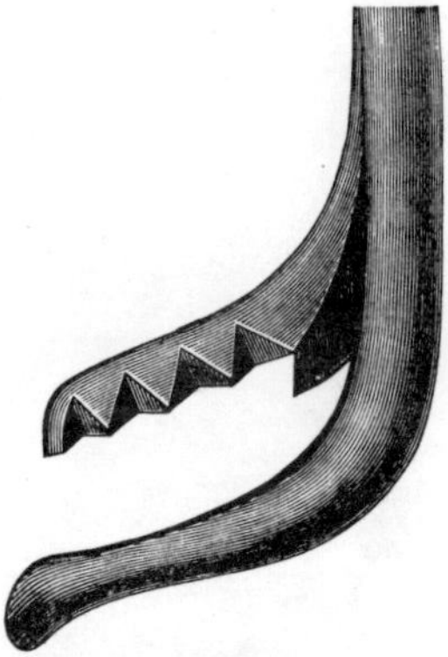

FIG. 16.

in the more common American instrument. I also think well of the fenestrated lithotrite in practised hands. An instrument of this kind will comminute the stone, especially a hard one, sufficiently to pass the catheters. When lithotritists, three years ago, were warning one another against the

[1] Figs. 15 and 16,—blades of the author's lithotrite. The notches, as here represented, are intended to be deep and steep enough to insure the blades against the usual impaction in front. At the heel, where clogging is always worst, the débris, divided by the spur of the male blade, falls off on each side from the high floor of the female blade. The female blade has a long blunted toe, curved forward. The size of the heel is 26 French.

danger of fatal cystitis, — which had been attested, as they supposed, by the experience of half a century, — my first precaution while making experiments was to protect the floor of the bladder by a solid female blade. A projecting splinter of stone, firmly set in the fenestra of an open female blade, while being crowded through it, is obviously a dangerous weapon. The blades should always be lifted off the floor as soon as the fragment is secured, before crushing it. But it is a great relief to the hand of the operator if the blades shut, at the last moment, quietly together. The old fenestrated instrument can be made to crush as well as cut the stone by widening the female blade and sharpening its rim inside so as to retain it (Fig. 17). This also protects the bladder

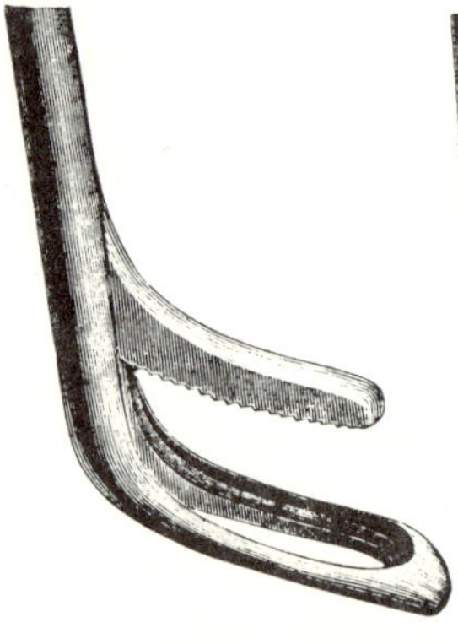

FIG. 17.[1]

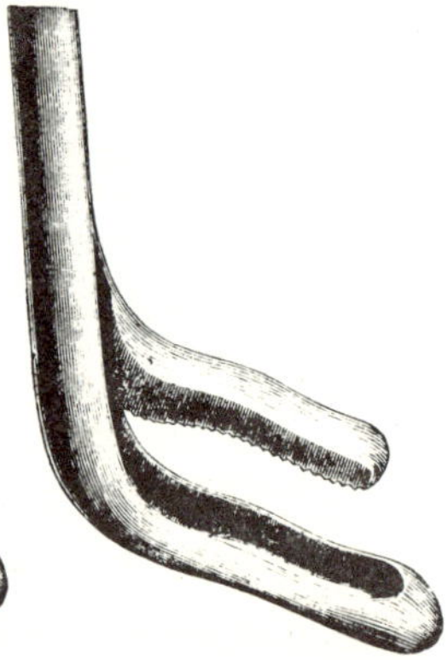

FIG. 18.[2]

from any scissors-like action of the edges. The sole of the male blade is grooved lengthwise, and serrated. In order to widen the hold upon the stone in another way and occupy less room in the urethra, I have used a zigzag fenestrated

[1] Fenestrated instrument, with a wide floor and high rim to hold the stone while being crushed. The toe is long and curved.

[2] Fenestrated instrument, with blades curved laterally to widen the grasp upon the calculus. The toe is also curved.

blade, which has proved quite efficient (Fig. 18). I have employed a fenestrated instrument with great success upon a hard stone, which it crushes and does not slice as it does a soft stone. Dr. Keyes first advocated the use of the fenestrated instrument to avoid impaction in the long sitting.

The toe of the female blade should be not only long and rounded, so that it shall not injure the upper wall of the prostatic urethra as it moves along, but I have also curved it

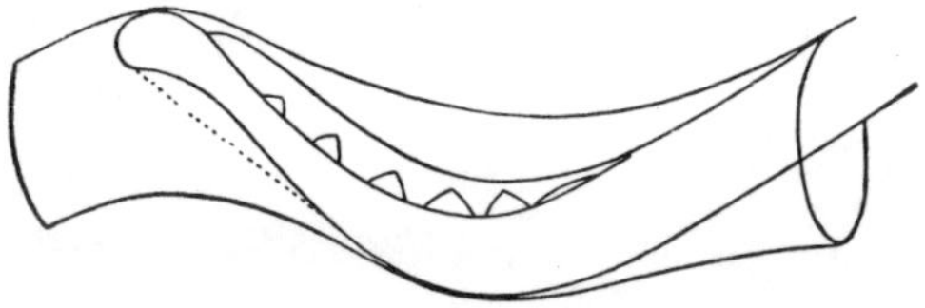

FIG. 19.[1]

forward. Its added length, besides protecting the bladder, then makes the passage easier (Figs. 15, 16, 17, 18, and 19).

Let me add a few general remarks. Lithotrites are of several sizes, and of two sorts,—the solid and the fenestrated. The latter of course cannot clog, and has been sufficiently described. Of the former it may be further said that it does not clog, the notches in the male blade being steep enough to deliver the detritus at the side. It is absolutely essential that the notches be deep and well slanted. This implies a thick male blade, to which I have no objection. The crushing is chiefly done at the front of the blades, where, so far as I know, every other lithotrite with solid blades clogs. The

[1] Diagram intended to show how the curved and blunted toe protects the roof of the membranous urethra, and also that the blades in passing occupy no more room with it than without it. The position of the instrument here represented is the proper one at this part of the urethra. The dotted line shows that the curve is the result of removing superfluous metal from the sole of a blunted blade.

heel, which never crushes advantageously, has here a long narrow fenestra, cleared by a projecting metal plate which passes through it. This divides the débris, one half of which falls off at each side from the high floor, and effectually hinders clogging where it is always worst. These lithotrites have the male-blade lock and long vulcanite handle figured in the previous pages. The blades represented in Figs. 15 and 16 are of the middle size. They measure at the largest part of the heel 26 French. The stem of the instrument is small, and moves freely in the urethra, but it communicates great power to the blades, which are strong, and adapted to general use.

A straight catheter, which I think evacuates best, generally passes with great ease. Sometimes a curved catheter passes better, and now and then the urethra is capricious about receiving any instrument. In passing an instrument, after dividing the meatus if necessary, or divulsing a stricture, we reach at once the triangular ligament, where the chief difficulty of the passage lies. Here the instrument should be insinuated with a light hand, not by depressing the handle in a quarter circle as if it were a catheter, still less by force; but the aperture should be carefully sought for. Beginners are very apt to strike above it. To avoid this mistake, after the instrument has been passed vertically down *quite as far as it will go*, it should be withdrawn a little before being pushed forward, and this manœuvre repeated till the point slides through the ligament. A surgeon may quickly acquire great skill in passing an instrument in the living urethra, by practice upon the dead subject, if he will twist a common tin sound into irregular angles and curves, and pass first one end and then the other through this opening. The ligamentous orifice is really the turning point in the successful passage of an instrument. Once safely beyond it, a catheter, if straight, can be rotated horizontally through the prostatic urethra.

But a curved catheter, or a lithotrite, should be lowered only to an angle of about 45° with the horizon, if the patient is on his back, and then urged carefully forward like a boat in the water upon an even keel. The floor of the canal is depressed by the heel of the instrument as it slides along, and this relieves its roof from the pressure of the toe (Fig. 19).

I usually search for a stone with a common tin sound bent extemporaneously to suit the case, and measure it with a lithotrite, which also makes an excellent sound. The search for a last fragment or a minute calculus is best done with a small evacuating catheter by which the fragment can escape, or, if too large to pass, is arrested with an audible click. A trap and bulb are attached to it (see Fig 3). In these days fragments are made to seek the sound rather than the sound the fragments, as has been the case heretofore. I think that the old method of sounding for a small calculus is generally abandoned, unless the calculous material is adherent or otherwise immovable.

Evacuation is a simple thing, and is usually successful, even with an imperfect evacuator. To secure the water I tie an elastic band round the penis after the catheter is in place, and judge of the distension of the bladder by ascertaining, from time to time, the tension of the urethra behind it. The pumping is an easy, continuous movement. There is no need of pausing after the stroke, which may be as rhythmical as the swing of a pendulum. If any pause is made, it is after compressing the bulb, to let the débris settle, when there are few left. Every fragment sooner or later finds the catheter, most of them at once and with surprising readiness. The most advantageous spot, higher at first, lower when fragments become fewer, is soon discovered by trial. A quarter of an inch higher or lower sometimes makes an unexpected difference. When the fragments cease to fall into the receiver, the catheter may be immediately withdrawn; but I often add to the evacuation a thorough sounding in pursuit of a possible last fragment, which perhaps does not exist, and thereby make the operation much longer. This search can be deferred if the condition of the patient makes it desirable, although I do not think it more important to abbreviate this surgical operation than any other. Without this prolonged attempt at complete evacuation, verified by a final careful sounding, evacuation is usually a short matter; and the number of grains evacuated in a unit of time, say in a minute, is large.

Let me illustrate with a single case how the catheter may be obstructed. A patient was relieved three years ago, by lithotomy, of about a gill and a half of stones of the uniform size of small marbles. A month ago I operated upon him by crushing. The operation occupied two and a half hours, and was tedious in the extreme. Neither the lithotrite nor the evacuator performed as usual. Afterward it was clear that the crushing was slow because I could never seize a piece larger than a marble; and evacuation was next to impossible, because the catheter was constantly obstructed by a similar marble. The patient did well. He was seventy-two years old. The quantity removed was nearly nine hundred grains.

Among diseases that obviously reduce the chances of a patient, surgical kidney, upon which Sir Henry Thompson has laid much stress, is perhaps the most common and most fatal complication of any operation for stone. Its symptoms have been of late so accurately defined by Professor Guyon and his disciple, Dr. Bazy, that perhaps the most important single question to be solved, if possible before operating, is whether the patient has surgical kidney or not.

I adopt no special preparatory treatment. If necessary, immediately before the operation, I enlarge the meatus or divulse a stricture. Rest after a journey, the relief of some obviously aggravated and temporary symptom, the antiseptic or other washing of the bladder when desirable, — all this belongs to the common principles and common practice of surgery.

After the operation, opiates and warm fomentations are often comforting and sometimes essential. The bladder should be left empty, and as far as possible kept so. Where complete retention is probable, and it is always possible, the patient should be within reach of the surgeon. The bladder may be washed out with water or mild antiseptic fluid, if the character of the urine suggests it. One of the most troublesome complications is a mass of mucus that creates tenesmus, and will not pass through the catheter.

I have been cognizant of four fatal cases in which the deep urethra, which is less tolerant of injury than the bladder, was lacerated. Such cases do not count against lithotrity, but show the need of habit as well as care in passing and withdrawing the instruments, especially the larger sizes. These, in the hands of the general surgeon, are less safe than the smaller ones. Within the bladder the entire wall can hardly be caught with impunity in the forceps-like extremities of the old lithotrite, though strips of mucous membrane have been torn from it without serious consequences.

I think I am justified in assuming it to have been demonstrated that where lithotrity has hitherto been the accepted rule of practice, as in the case of a healthy patient or of a small stone, the new method is better than the old one, and that the domain of lithotrity has been notably extended. I think we need no further statistics relating to small stones.

The question still remaining concerns lithotomy and its indications. It is whether modern lithotrity is not better than lithotomy in that class of cases hitherto claimed by lithotomy, comprising larger stones and surgical kidneys, conditions which are distinctly unfavorable to any operation at all. It will take time to decide this point. The practised surgeon may even find it so difficult to rid himself of a merely traditionary preference for lithotomy that the verdict may be unnecessarily delayed. But even when lithotomy is successful, I ask myself if the patient would not have encountered a less risk with the new lithotrity? I do not know any new indications that enable us to decide peremptorily when lithotomy is better than lithotrity. The latter does not, it is true, so completely drain and rest the bladder. In the case of a large stone it is perhaps likely to be done less skilfully than the operation of lithotomy by the general surgeon. But there is no danger of secondary hæmorrhage, nor is there a grave wound in a diseased prostate, communicating perhaps with a putrid catarrh of the urinary tract. As yet no disproportionately unfavorable results have set a limit to the new lithotrity for large calculi and diseased patients. On the contrary, its use is becoming more common. Extraordinary stones have been successfully removed by crushing.

I myself add to twenty-one cases I have already published of promiscuous stones, large and small, twenty-four other cases with one death. Of these I mention here only ten cases,—comprising six calculi weighing over two hundred grains and under five hundred, one over five hundred and under seven hundred, and three over seven hundred and under one thousand grains. The single death was by septic infection, in a patient sixty-six years of age, having a phosphatic stone of two hundred and seventy grains. There was no apparent injury of the canal or bladder sufficing to explain it. The only peculiarity of the case was an unusual vascularity of the urethra during the operation.

The manœuvres in a long sitting do not greatly differ from those in a short one; but they need more persistent care and patience, because the attention is rather apt to flag during the continued repetition of the same movements. The possession of a reflex skill, acquired by practice and acting without thought, as in swimming, bicycling, writing, or playing a musical instrument, is then of the greatest value. It insures to the patient, as no mere good intention can, the advantage of what Cadge has called "all the little knacks and tricks which go to make up successful lithotrity." I think, with the improvements here shown, the operation becomes safer for the general surgeon. I often hear of successful operations upon large stones by the new method in the hands of surgeons who have scarcely done lithotrity before; but I am satisfied that patients are yet safer in the hands of a surgeon who makes lithotrity in some measure a special study.

LITHOLAPAXY.

REMARKS MADE AT A MEETING OF THE BOSTON SOCIETY FOR MEDICAL IMPROVEMENT.[1]

Dr. Bigelow, in opening the discussion, said he had been much interested in the cases reported. Dr. Cheever's case was that of a hard stone, while Dr. Gay's was that of a large one. The results which they had obtained might be expected as a rule.

In reply to the inquiry how often it was necessary to slit the meatus, Dr. Bigelow said that the necessity was only exceptional. If the meatus is small, and the operation is to be a long one, it is a convenient and harmless expedient; it is well to take a little care afterward not to engage the mucous edge of the urethra upon the catheter and strip it up.

Air in the bladder does no harm. The amount contained in the catheter is legitimately there; beyond this amount no air can enter the apparatus unless from leaky joints. A little air is often as comfortably trapped for a time in the top of a large bladder as in the evacuator. The only harm the air does is to take up room which is better occupied by water if the bladder is not a capacious one. It is easy to remove it from the evacuator through a stop-cock and small hose at the top of the bulb, through which also the amount of water can be regulated.

Asked how long cystitis lasted after the operation, Dr. Bigelow replied that it depended on the relation it bore to the stone; that is, if the stone were the disease, and the cystitis were dependent on its presence, it would be cured. If, on the other hand, there were a previous cystitis with enlarged pros-

[1] The Boston Medical and Surgical Journal. March 23, 1882.

tate, and the stone were the result of these conditions, the relief, though often considerable, would be partial. Cystitis with a large secretion of mucus is a troublesome complication. The mucus plugs the urethral orifice, causing painful tenesmus until the tenacious mucus comes away in a mass, and the bladder is relieved.

In answer to further inquiries, Dr. Bigelow said that perhaps the most difficult part of the crushing operation is picking up pieces behind the vertical wall of certain forms of enlarged prostate. As a rule the stone is easiest secured by pressing down the floor of the bladder with the heel of the lithotrite, which then occupies a pocket into which the stone gravitates; or by carrying the instrument well back, opening it, turning it to one or the other side, and closing it. A stone or fragment behind the prostate can be usually caught by depressing the floor beyond it; although if the perpendicular wall of the prostate is high it may be difficult to reach it even by inverting a short blade. One difficulty with the old lithotrite was the obliquity of the heel, so that when the crushing force is applied the stone is urged forward in the blades. The clearing out of an obstruction in the straight tube can easily be accomplished by passing through it an ordinary tin sound. A curved tube sometimes gives more trouble, but can be freed by an elastic catheter. Any resistance, however slight, in withdrawing the tube should lead the operator to suspect that a dangerously large fragment is engaged in its extremity.

In reply to a question as to whether he had ever known injury to result from nipping the walls of the bladder, Dr. Bigelow said that he knew of one case in which he believed a fatal issue was due to that accident. In the ordinary instrument, with blades fitted at their extremities as accurately as forceps are, and with a female blade having no projection to keep away the wall of the bladder, the latter must often be seized. If only the mucous membrane were torn, no serious effect might ensue; but if, in a thin bladder, the whole thickness of the walls were pinched, he thought there must be danger. For this reason he himself felt easier in using his own instrument, which guards against this accident. The long female blade is especially useful to those not operating habitually.

In regard to the choice of a straight or curved tube, Dr. Bigelow thought neither was safer; the danger depends on the relation in size between the catheter and urethra. The tube, if large, must be introduced with great care and with a perfect understanding of the anatomy of the parts, directing it downward until it reaches the layer of fat lying between the urethra and the rectum, then coaxing it through the aperture in the triangular ligament, and finally reaching the bladder by a corkscrew motion of the straight tube in the axis of the body. In only two or three cases had Dr. Bigelow found any trouble in introducing a straight tube. Sometimes the curved tube can be easiest introduced by hugging the pubes, and thus passing the upper instead of the lower part of the opening in the triangular ligament. The introduction of the straight tube is usually easier to the surgeon, but perhaps not quite so comfortable to the unetherized patient. After the curved tube has entered the bladder the shaft occupies the urethra, and is of course straight.

Aided by the blackboard, Dr. Bigelow described at some length the difficulties of attaining a perfect and convenient evacuator, and explained the faults of all those now in use. The question is one of physics, and involves the separation of air, water, and fragments in the most effectual way by the simplest means. He believed that he had at last devised a satisfactory instrument. To suppose that experiments to this end, out of the bladder, have no value, is like supposing that the edge of a surgical knife can be tested only on the living tissues.

LITHOTRITY, WITH EVACUATION.

REMARKS MADE AT A MEETING OF THE NEW YORK ACADEMY OF MEDICINE.[1]

Dr. Bigelow said that when asked some time ago by the president to present this subject before the Academy, he felt that it was one which had already become old, and so familiar to most surgeons that he could offer but little of interest in connection with it; and it was only when the request was again urged, at a subsequent time, that he had reluctantly consented to do so. He believed, however, that his own accumulated experience, and especially that of the New York surgeons, had now thrown added light upon the operation. He could not forget also that it was in New York that the procedure which he had labored to perfect had received its first distinct approbation, and that at a time when it needed friends. The profession here had then tested the matter by practical experiments; and he could not refrain from mentioning his special obligation to the distinguished Professor Van Buren, among others, for his interest and assistance.

The subject, he continued, was one relating distinctly to operative surgery, a mechanical one; and it was to the mechanical part of it — a mere matter of physics — that whatever advances had been made in lithotrity of late were really due. He should confine himself therefore, during the limited time at his disposal, to the mechanical procedure, because he believed it was what the Academy would perhaps prefer now to discuss. There were a number of points in regard to which he would like to have an expression of opinion from some of

[1] The Boston Medical and Surgical Journal, May 25, 1882.

the gentlemen present. Any common lithotrite, he went on to say, would break a stone, and most evacuators will remove it; but it was an important question which special instrument would do it best. Although it was stated by Sir James Paget and other authorities, during the noted discussions which took place in London in 1878, that the subject of lithotrity had apparently gone as far as it could go, and that the operation would probably not be further improved, yet since that time all the lithotritists had been steadily at work, and distinct advances had been made. It was desirable at the present day to use instruments materially different from those formerly in use, although the whole question was still one of breaking up a stone and getting the fragments out through the urethra,—an operation that had been in vogue for many years.

When Civiale began to operate he required from twenty to thirty minutes; but as he improved his instruments he gradually reduced the time to three or four minutes,—a limit to the sitting generally accepted and taught since Civiale's day.

The means for removing the fragments completely, however, did not formerly exist. The sharp fragments remained in the bladder and did the damage, not the operation. When it came to be possible to remove them, it was found, to the surprise of everybody, that the bladder was a very tolerant organ. That this tolerance of the bladder had never been suspected up to that time, and the fact that such an error had existed for half a century, seemed to show the advantage of doubting everything in medicine of which we had had no personal experience. The single agent to which actual progress was due was the large catheter which held the urethra open while the fragments were drawn out through it: and it was a fact that the small catheter of Clover's instrument had retarded progress for a very long time. In 1846, Sir Philip Crampton had drawn out a large quantity of débris in the form of powder by means of a vacuum made in a glass globe. If fragments were completely pulverized, of course a small catheter would answer for the removal of the whole calculus; but the bladder could not afford to wait until pulverization was gradually accomplished.

A large catheter by itself was not a new device, since it had been in use in former times to some extent. Collin's instrument had a catheter of number 25 or 26; but it was found to be inefficient, and was soon pronounced impracticable. The distinctly new and important point in the apparatus now employed was the use of a large catheter — 25 to 31 — in combination with an efficient suction. This constituted the novelty of the thing. Having, then, the large catheter, the first question was, Should it be straight or curved? This was a matter concerning merely the introduction of the instrument; and Dr. Bigelow said that he preferred a straight one. As most of the passage was practically straight, it could be introduced with greater facility than a curved one. The choice was simply one of convenience, and was related to the habit of the operator, or sometimes to the individual case.

Dr. Bigelow next described the character of the extremity of the catheter which he preferred, and drew a diagram of it upon the blackboard. It was oblique and blunted, and had a projecting lip of considerable length below, while the orifice was above. The orifice, he said, should be about the size of the calibre of the tube, for if it were larger than this a fragment was liable to become engaged there; and in this connection he mentioned a death which occurred in consequence of the orifice of the catheter employed being disproportionately large. A fragment had thus become fixed; and as a result of the laceration of the urethra occasioned in its withdrawal the patient died of septicæmia. Dr. Bigelow also recommended that the tube-wall above the orifice should be thickened, so that no injury might be inflicted by its edge.

The next point involved the important matter of retaining the fragments when they had been once withdrawn from the bladder. It was a curious fact that until now all evacuators, so far as he knew, returned to the bladder something like one third to one half of all fragments evacuated. This had been attributed to the length of the elastic tube sometimes employed; but the length of the tube was not the main difficulty. As a fact, it was found on investigation that the fragments were really returned from the bulb, and that a little additional prolongation of the tube made very slight difference. Nevertheless he had tried to devise a trap at the extremity of the tube. It consisted of a little glass cylinder containing a valve in the shape of a loose rubber ball, which worked backward and forward, and thus closed and opened the orifice alternately, while the water returned through a strainer. This he had found to work very well; but as the objection had been made that it was too complicated an arrangement, he had afterward employed a simpler one, which also acted perfectly, and which he had not as yet published. This was nothing more or less than half an inch of cotton tube fastened at the end of the metal tube, in such a way that it acted as a valve in closing and opening the orifice. Still, as even this might be thought complicated by some surgeons, he had tried quite a number of other valves. An objection to a metal valve was that it was liable to become obstructed by fragments. Consequently he had been obliged to resort to a variety of expedients, which he would refer to in a moment.

He would first go a step further, and speak of the evacuator as a whole. We are to dispose by means of it of air, water, and fragments. The receptacle for the fragments might be placed either between the catheter and the bulb or below the bulb itself. For his own part, Dr. Bigelow considered it better to place the receptacle immediately below the bulb, especially for the reason that it materially shortened the instrument; and this of itself was a very important advantage. It was also an important matter to place the axis of the bulb in a line with the axis of the catheter; otherwise there would be a leverage causing the instrument to work at a great disadvantage. The moment the bulb and the receptacle were combined in one piece the question arose whether or not the catheter should be detached by an elastic tube to allow its freer motion. The ordinary straight elastic tube was liable to double on itself, and thus obstruct the flow of water; but a curved tube of proper construction was not open to this objection. In regard to the use of a stand, Dr. Bigelow said that his preferences had been in favor of it. Perhaps his present opinion might be best expressed in this way: if the stone were a small one, and the operation short, it was better to dispense with the stand; but if it were large, the stand was a considerable help, since the two or three pounds' weight of the instrument made quite a difference to the operator if it had to be supported by the hand. Still, the general belief in such matters was often the correct one, and the prevailing practice, which was opposed to the use of the stand, he was willing to adopt.

Dr. Bigelow then exhibited the first instrument which he employed, and remarked that it made no sort of difference at what point the catheter entered the bulb, provided it did not finally deliver directly at the top where the air collects. If the tube penetrated even for a short distance into the bulb from above, an air chamber was at once formed. The only air that belonged legitimately in the bulb was that which came from the catheter, and the amount of air varied with the calibre of the catheter. The best rule was to have the catheter deliver as near the centre of the bulb as possible; and when this was the case, the greatest possible facility was afforded for the uninterrupted passage of the fragments into the receptacle below. If the tube entered the lower narrow part of the bulb where the fragments accumulated, it was important that it should be prolonged above this point, or else they would be returned in great quantity to the bladder. This brought him to the point of showing how regurgitation of the fragments from the bulb took place in almost all instruments. He then exhibited an evacuator which he said had been abandoned by its author, and beneath the bulb of which he had attached a short glass tube so that the course of the currents might be observed. It was clearly demonstrated that a considerable portion of the fragments went directly back into the bladder. How then, it might be asked, was evacuation ever accomplished by such an instrument? Simply by washing the fragments backward and forward between the bladder and the instrument until all of them had been finally dropped into the receptacle. This has been, till now, a serious defect of many evacuators. There was in this instrument also a current, which actually lifted the fragments out of the glass receptacle and sent them back to the bladder. In other words, the general fact held good, that wherever the water goes in an evacuator the fragments go also, unless they are prevented by means of a strainer.

Dr. Bigelow exhibited the latest instrument devised by Weiss, of London, which he had received during the past winter, and remarked that the first difficulty about it was that, as in Clover's evacuator, the bulb was not stiff enough. In his own instruments, a special point was made of having the bulb sufficiently stiff. A second difficulty was that some of the fragments, following as usual the course of the current, were collected in the bulb and thence carried back into the bladder. Dr. Bigelow also exhibited one of his own instruments with a valve, which worked perfectly well, although he said that it was not as simple in construction as was desirable. It was provided with a stand. He had often felt it a relief to stop once in a while in a long operation to see how things were going on, which the self-supporting character of the instrument enabled him to do with ease. With regard to the rubber hose which was attached to the top of the bulb and provided with a stop-cock, he regarded the device as a great advantage, and had continued to employ it in all his evacuators up to the present time. Its purpose was not only to dispose of the air, but especially to add or remove water. As had been stated, the only air legitimately held in the bulb was that contained in the catheter. If it were desirable to get rid of even this amount of air, it could be promptly accomplished by compressing the bulb and filling its place with water by means of the hose. Another point in this connection was, that all bladders were not of the same size or the same elasticity. In a small bladder it was difficult to evacuate completely because the walls were liable to fall against the catheter. This was owing to the fact that there was not enough water in the bladder. It could easily be added by means of the hose, and the quantity graduated exactly according to the desire of the operator. Sometimes during the operation the patient strained or vomited, so that everything became very tense; and in that case we had only to open both stop-cocks and deliver the water temporarily. He believed, therefore, that the hose was a valuable addition, both for the purpose of getting rid of air and of regulating the amount of water according to the circumstances arising from time to time during the operation.

Finally, Dr. Bigelow exhibited the new and simple instrument which he said he had now settled down upon, and which could be used with either a single stop-cock or with two, as might be preferred. In the first place, it had a spherical bulb acting as a handle in the axis of the catheter. In the second place, it was quite short from end to end. In the third place, the obliquity of the tube carried the receptacle high in the air, one advantage of which was that it brought it nearer the level of the eye of the surgeon. In the fourth place, the whole thing fitted well into the cavity of the hand which held it. In regard to the use of stop-cocks, he preferred to have two instead of a single one. He then gave a demonstration of its manner of working, — it being shown, after a moment or two, that there was not a fragment left remaining in the glass vessel used to represent the bladder. The simple method by which this desirable result was accomplished, he said, could readily be understood. There was a cylindrical strainer that prolonged the catheter inside the bulb; and inasmuch as any strainer may get clogged with fibrin, resulting from an inflamed state of the bladder, this was so arranged that it could be readily removed and cleaned by brushing. The strainer could be replaced in an instant. The fragments enter the bulb from the bladder through the main orifice, by reason of the momentum which the current has acquired in coming from the bladder. But the combined area of the small apertures along the tube being much larger than that of the principal orifice at its extremity, most of the water returns by these apertures, and is strained.

Dr. Bigelow then spoke briefly in regard to the lithotrite. He stated that the most convenient instrument of any sort was that which was best adapted to the movements of the hand. In devising his own instrument, therefore, he had first considered which was the easiest motion of the latter, and had arrived at the conclusion that this was its rotation. He had, therefore, not only made the handle of a size adapted to the hand, but so that it could be worked by rotation. He had also provided the lithotrite with a lock, by means of which any position of the blades could be maintained as long as desired, without the necessity of changing the position of the hand. The blades were made at as near a right angle as would admit of their introduction into the bladder with convenience and safety, and are thus found to work at a much greater advantage than the more oblique blades formerly sometimes employed. As the greatest impaction always took place at the heel of the instrument, he had abandoned the idea of crushing much at this point, and passed a flange through it, in order to bisect the detritus and discharge it laterally. The crushing was mainly done in front of the heel. When the patient was in good health, he believed that the safety of the procedure depended simply upon the surgeon's skill; and that with the facilities now at our command, if proper care were observed, there would very rarely be any bad consequences. In cases where the kidneys were affected, however, favorable results were not, of course, always to be anticipated.

A SIMPLIFIED EVACUATOR FOR LITHOLAPAXY.[1]

The operation for the immediate removal of a calculus through a catheter, like many other surgical operations, can be accomplished more or less satisfactorily by any one of several instruments which much resemble one another. But it can be done better by employing a more perfect apparatus than those now generally in use. It has been said that "no new form of instrument is required by this operation," which is true so far as it implies that neither a lithotrite nor an evacuator is a new instrument. But it would be a mistake to infer that the operation could have been done with the instruments of the old lithotrity, and that they needed no change to adapt them to what is now required of them, or that they cannot be still further modified to advantage. The new operation cannot be performed with the old instruments. It requires a larger evacuating catheter than that of Clover, through which the usual product of the lithotrite could not pass, except as powder and sand, and then only in limited quantities, because the other detritus obstructed the entrance of the tube.[2] Though at first received with a good deal of

[1] The Lancet, January 6 and 13, 1883.

[2] Sir Henry Thompson says (Diseases of the Urinary Organs, Philadelphia and London, 1882): "The evacuating catheter to be attached to the aspirator should be as large as the urethra will admit; usually No. 15 or 16 of the English scale [26 to 28½ French] may be used without any danger. Sometimes No. 17 or 18 [30 and 31 French] are admissible; but such sizes are quite unnecessary for small stones, and may produce mischief; hence they are only to be used where the presence of a large stone demands corresponding instruments." Or, it might be added, to expedite the operation, when the urethra is large and healthy. The size of the normal urethra, according to Otis, is, if we except the meatus, 32 of the French scale. Clover's evacuating catheter was 21. Those now in use

distrust, the large catheter has been finally adopted by all the surgeons who have performed the operation, and in fact cannot be dispensed with. It should be combined with a thoroughly efficient aspirator. But no particular form of aspirator has so far met with general approval. Though improvement has been made, surgeons have no aspirator which entirely satisfies all requirements of the operation, and is at the same time compact and convenient to handle and simple in construction. This part of the evacuator still needs improvement.

The usual parts of an evacuator, not including the catheter, are these: —

1. The exhaust, the best form of which is an elastic bulb.

2. A space or trap for air, at the upper part of the instrument.

3. A glass receiver at the lower part, to collect and show the débris.

In drawing out fragments from the bladder through the large catheter, one bulb or aspirator, if strong enough, is about as efficient as another. An aspirator of almost any shape and having almost any combination of its parts will do this. So will a mere elastic bulb attached directly to the catheter, without joints or receiver, if it is placed lower

range from 26 to 31. Care, however, and often special skill may be required to introduce safely the largest sizes; 31 is very rarely needed, and the French sizes 28 and 29 are generally the most convenient. For a final washing or sounding without anæsthesia, when it is desirable to give the patient the least discomfort, even so small a calibre as 26 is sometimes useful. Through a catheter of this calibre Mr. Teevan has removed calculi weighing six or eight hundred grains; but such cases should be regarded as showing what is possible, rather than as establishing a rule of practice. Here I may add that although no lithotrite compares in size with the larger tubes, it is yet true that long-bladed lithotrites, especially if they have the sharp extremity of the old instruments, are more difficult than tubes to introduce with safety. Although since 1878 my lithotrites have been made in three sizes, I have rarely had occasion to employ any other than the middle size.

than the catheter, and bent down like the body of a retort, so that the fragments can fall to the bottom of it; and the instrument will still work well if it has joints made, for economy, of cork or rubber instead of metal. But, however otherwise arranged, a satisfactory aspirator should have —

4. Some device, near the catheter, to act as a trap for débris and secure every fragment that has passed it.

The chief difference among evacuators now is in the degree of certainty with which they retain the fragments they have aspirated. Any instrument will draw out the fragments, but few hold them securely; for the débris do not always fall into the glass receiver, nor do they always remain in it. On the contrary, they are easily carried back to the bladder. This defect in the action of the evacuator has received little attention from surgeons, although it is the only point connected with the evacuator which offers any difficulty whatever. Until recently it has been remedied only by sacrificing simplicity in the apparatus.

In endeavoring to make a satisfactory evacuator for litholapaxy, many experiments have to be tried. It is quite possible that a perfectly satisfactory instrument might have been contrived some time ago if it had been generally understood that an evacuator that works best with pieces of broken coal in a vessel of water will succeed best with the fragments in the bladder.[1] So also will the surgeon if he is otherwise well qualified. It is true that the living tissues are easily injured, but in other respects the experiment can be made sufficiently like the operation to give it great value. Aspirating débris from the bladder is not a question of pathology, but of operative surgery, — of physics; and in view of the fact that we fail, in some bladders, to discover a last fragment even by repeated washing, an evacuator should be so constructed that

[1] The specific gravity of hard coal is 1.575. That of a urate calculus is 1.510, and of a mulberry calculus, 1.262.

it will absolutely prevent a fragment that has once passed the catheter from returning to the bladder to become the nucleus of another calculus.

It is not altogether easy to meet this requirement, because the solid particles are usually borne back and forth with the current of water. In a common evacuator, they are carried wherever the current goes, — first from the bladder to the bulb, and then, when it is reversed, back to the bladder, a part only falling into the receiver at each aspiration. As we may fairly assume that a surgeon would not deliberately inject foreign bodies into a patient's bladder, there must be something wrong in a system which obliges him to do this, and makes it necessary to aspirate the same débris twenty times over in order to remove it. In short, the apparatus as commonly arranged is still a defective one, and needs some special contrivance to assist the action of gravity in securing the débris.

Surgeons have long felt this. The use of an elastic tube connected with the catheter has been more than once criticised, and with some reason, on the ground that it might contain fragments which would be returned to the bladder; and again, in order to shorten by an inch the route from the bladder, a less convenient stop-cock has been substituted for the usual one. But lithotritists should be fully aware of the fact that whether there is an elastic tube or not, a tenfold greater quantity of fragments is generally driven back out of the bulb itself, and that the difficulty lies almost wholly in that part of the instrument. At each expansion débris are drawn from the bladder into the bulb, where they are delayed until, when it is compressed, they are injected back into the bladder. Only a part of them, sometimes only the larger half (the quantity varying in different instruments), settle into the glass receiver. This important fact, so little recognized, should not be accepted without demonstration.

An instrument which Sir Henry Thompson has lately abandoned (Fig. 1) can be made to demonstrate exactly how the currents act upon the fragments, in an evacuator which is unprovided with a catheter-trap to prevent them from re-entering the bladder. It is here selected because the peculiar form of this instrument makes it easy to fit a glass tube to it so that we can see what takes place in the interior. Let a piece of glass tube an inch in diameter be inserted at the joint *JJ*, between the bulb *B* and the catheter, to show what passes with the current from one to the other in either direction. If the end of the catheter be now placed in a suitable vessel of water containing fragments of coal of different sizes, while the bulb is alternately compressed and allowed to dilate, a continued stream of fragments will be seen rising from the vessel into the bulb, and then returning to the vessel, as they inevitably would do to the bladder. The back-flow of débris can be still better watched if a glass tube be also substituted for the catheter, as in the figure.

But there is another important fact illustrated by this instrument. Fragments do not always stay in a receiver after they have been deposited there. When the glass receiver *R* of this evacuator is half filled with fragments, a part of these are easily carried back into the vessel or into the bladder. They are first lifted up from the receiver into the bulb, and then driven out through the catheter; for though the orifice of this glass receiver is small and protected by a special trap, the current and débris pass out of it as well as into it. It could not have been foreseen that fragments would escape from a receptacle apparently so well arranged; but it will be found that in any instrument, if the bulb or catheter directs the current into the glass receiver, whether directly or obliquely, fragments are easily carried out again.

The general result is little better, if, to avoid stirring the fragments which lie in the receiver, the current is directed

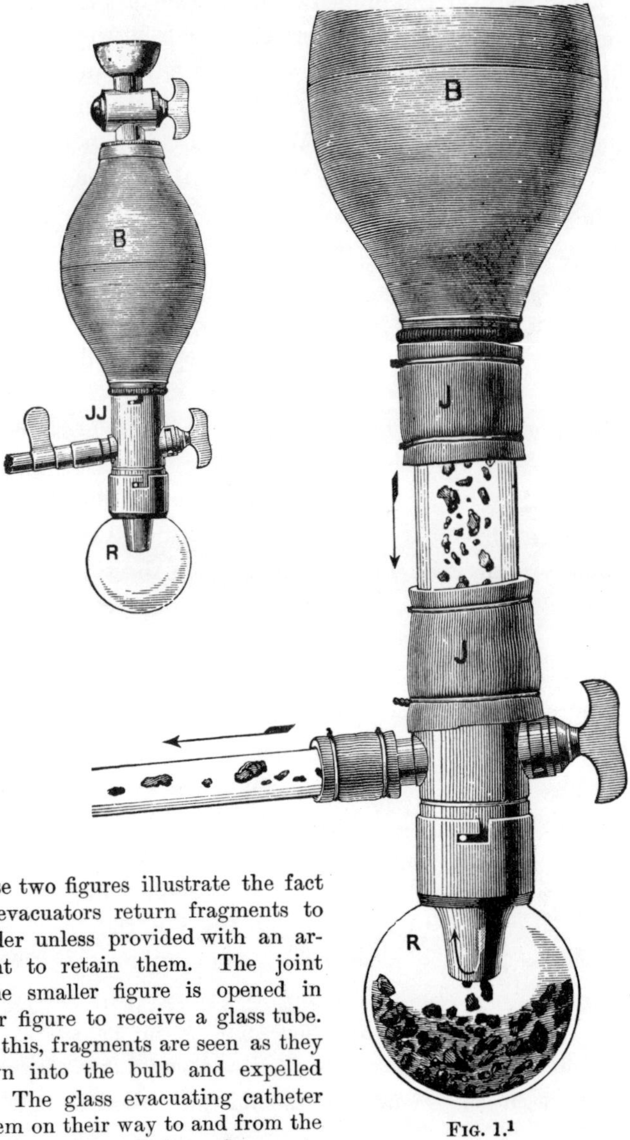

FIG. 1.[1]

These two figures illustrate the fact that all evacuators return fragments to the bladder unless provided with an arrangement to retain them. The joint *JJ* of the smaller figure is opened in the larger figure to receive a glass tube. Through this, fragments are seen as they are drawn into the bulb and expelled from it. The glass evacuating catheter shows them on their way to and from the bladder. The receiver *R* shows fragments in the act of being lifted by the current and returned to the bladder.

horizontally over the mouth of it instead of into it. Some of them then pass directly back and forth between the bladder and the bulb, over the receiver, without falling into it. This defect can be shown in an instrument recently employed by Sir Henry at the suggestion of Weiss and Co.,[1] where the stream from the catheter passes horizontally through an empty chamber on its way to the bulb. As the stream enters it, its velocity is so diminished that fragments fall to the bottom into the receiver, and in greater number when the bulb is weak. Many fragments are of course secured. But, to be wholly effectual, the chamber intended to retard and break up the current by its size would have to be inconveniently large, in order to give time to the floating débris entering on one side to settle into the receiver without passing farther. The principle here involved is quite different from that of the evacuator represented in the above figure. This instrument is not unlike one formerly figured in the "Lancet;"[2] but the valve and strainer which there act as a trap have been omitted, and, in consequence, not a few fragments escape back to the bladder.

In Weiss's evacuator again, some of the fragments which enter the bulb gather in the bottom of it, which is lower than its outlet, and where there is no receiver to collect them. The chief difficulty, however, is not that these fragments stray into the bulb, but that for want of a trap they are afterward liable to escape out of it and back to the bladder.

This difficulty is not wholly obviated by placing a strainer across the mouth of the bulb to prevent the fragments from entering it, as has been done in some other evacuators. Let me mention in this connection the results of a former experiment. It might be supposed that if the passing fragments were arrested by a flat strainer placed across the current, whether at the orifice of the bulb or elsewhere, they would

[1] Lancet, January 7, 1882.

[2] Lancet, September 21, 1881, Fig. 5. (See pp. 300, 301, of this volume.)

fall into a glass receiver placed directly below them; but this is not the case. Though a large part will fall into it, others collect upon the strainer; and unless the operator pauses after each aspiration till they have settled quietly into the receiver, they are liable to be carried back by the current, unless it is a very feeble one. This has happened, in my own experience, whether the strainer was horizontal, vertical, or oblique. The fragments do not glance from it down into the receiver, but some of them cling to it until the current is reversed, and then go back. To make a strainer act as a trap, the fragments should pass freely beyond it and be intercepted only on their return. They will then be strained away from the bladder and not toward it. It is very desirable that the current should be obstructed while the bulb is expanding, whether by a strainer or by curves and angles in the tubes. A simple flat strainer, placed anywhere across the whole current, retards it, especially if the urine is flocculent.

I find that the simplest expedient for collecting the fragments so that they will settle undisturbed into the glass receiver, is to admit them into the bulb and prevent their escape from it. After many experiments, I have found nothing more effectual for this purpose than a straight cylinder with perforated walls, which is practically a prolongation of the catheter into the bulb. The water after bringing the fragments from the bladder is strained as it returns. To the open end of this perforated cylinder a valve might be attached,— either a ball-valve moving loosely,[1] which is less liable to obstruction than a valve with a hinge; or still better, half an inch of cotton tube at the same point, which opens, allowing the fragments to pass up through it, and collapses with the reversed current, cutting off their retreat, the water, as it returns, passing back through the perforated walls. In operating with this arrangement I have found it to work perfectly;

[1] Lancet, September 24, 1881. (See p. 298 of this volume.)

but a valve is not necessary, and the apparatus is more simple without it.[1]

The evacuator described below is less complex in construction and aspirates more perfectly than any I have used. It is shown in Fig. 2, and is a compact modification of one formerly published in the "Lancet"[2] as "a simplified evacuator," but without the stand of that instrument, which is not essential, and has been omitted because operators seem to prefer to do without it.

The catheter is made to enter a spherical bulb obliquely upward, and is prolonged to the centre of the cavity by the tube just referred to, open at its end and perforated on its sides with numerous holes, which act as a strainer. The catheter, tube, and elastic bulb are in a straight line. This arrangement has the great advantage of *not deflecting the current* and thereby diminishing its force. During aspiration the current bearing the débris is drawn straight from the bladder through the tube, into the widest part of the bulb, and the fragments, spreading there, fall toward the receiver. But when the bulb is compressed, the water returns mostly through the perforations in the side of the tube, because their area is collectively larger than the opening at the end of it,

[1] A hinged or other valve strainer at the mouth of the catheter, if it opens to allow the water and the débris to pass through, works well enough as a substitute for the tube-strainer. The catheter then opens directly into the bulb, and the route is the shortest possible one. But the tube-strainer is much more simple, and the two inches which it adds to the length of the catheter are quite unimportant. In fact the usual length of the catheter itself might be reduced two inches to shorten the route if desired. For strainers and strainer traps, see "Lancet," September 21, 1881. (See pp. 298, 301, of this volume.) As there described, they are used in pairs, — one protecting the entrance of the bulb, while the other, furnished with a valve and placed at the head of the catheter, acts as a trap. The former, for reasons already given, is not always advantageous; but an effectual catheter-trap to arrest returning fragments is necessary.

[2] Lancet, September 21, 1881, Figs. 8 and 11. (See pp. 304, 306, of this volume.)

and because they are nearer the point at which the water passes out of the bulb. By means of this simple contrivance the water is strained, and *the return of fragments is practically prevented.* The tube-strainer can be removed, cleaned, and replaced in a moment; and this is an advantage when there is much mucus, coagulum, or shreddy material in the urine by which the holes of any strainer may be partly obstructed. Even then this tube continues to work well; but it is better to pass a brush over it if mucus adheres to it. It can be examined as often as the receiver is emptied. After the water has once been changed, less mucus will be found.

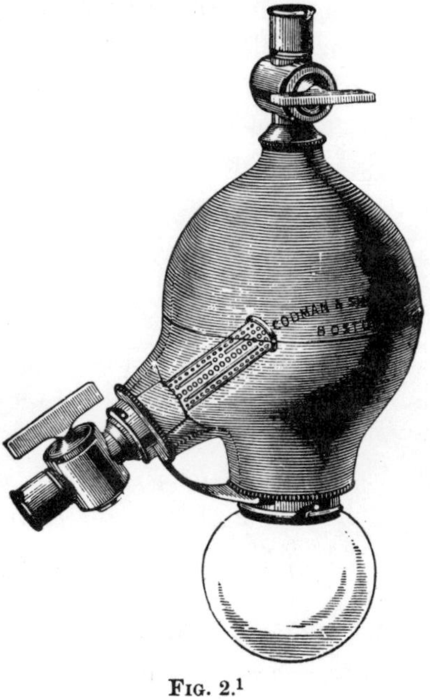

Fig. 2.[1]

The action of the perforated tube meets all requirements. In fact, if the catheter is prolonged into the bulb by a tube which has no perforations in its sides, the instrument will perform very fairly. Such a tube might be fastened permanently in the bulb; but the apparatus can be kept cleaner if there is a joint through which it can be removed. The cavity of the bulb cannot be made too accessible.

[1] The writer's Evacuator. It has an elastic bulb, glass receiver, and stop-cocks. Below, there is a metal brace between the collar of the glass receiver and that of the catheter to steady the latter. Within the bulb, and open at the end, is a tube strainer to prevent the return of débris. The bulb forms a concentric handle to the catheter.

The above arrangement has several other advantages.

1. With the trap placed inside the bulb, the instrument is more compact, shorter, and more easily held; and as the spherical bulb is here placed in a straight line with the catheter, it forms a concentric handle, which enables the surgeon to direct the catheter better than when this handle is placed above it, at an angle with it.

2. The glass receiver is here attached immediately below the bulb, and is easily seen. A glass cylinder shows fragments better than a globe, but is less capacious.

3. It is well known that the bulb in action, especially when placed above the catheter, at an angle with it, communicates an oscillation to the latter, of which some patients complain. By a special device, the catheter is here made so steady while the instrument is in use that a separate stand is not needed. This consists of a brace uniting the metal collar of the catheter with that of the glass receiver, and so steadying it that *the catheter no longer feels the movement of the bulb.* The conical projection of the bulb at the point where the catheter is attached contributes to the same result.

4. An elastic hose (Fig. 3) which can be quickly connected with the top of the bulb facilitates the operation. We can then, with a single compression of the bulb, get rid of any air or discolored water, and replace it with clean water without delay and without uncoupling the catheter. Besides, no matter how the bulb may have been filled at first,[1] it is better to be able to vary the quantity of water at any moment afterward; and although without a hose we can add water through a tunnel, we cannot as easily withdraw it in the same way. We should be able to regulate the amount of water carefully, not only at the outset, according to the capacity of the par-

[1] We can quickly fill the evacuator from a pitcher, if we invert the bulb and detach the receiver. The little remaining air can afterward be made to escape through the hose or tunnel.

ticular bladder, but also during the operation. For example, it is sometimes desirable to draw it quickly away to allow for the muscular strain of retching, or to relieve the expulsive efforts of the bladder, which sometimes becomes very tense, and ejects water at the side of the catheter, even of

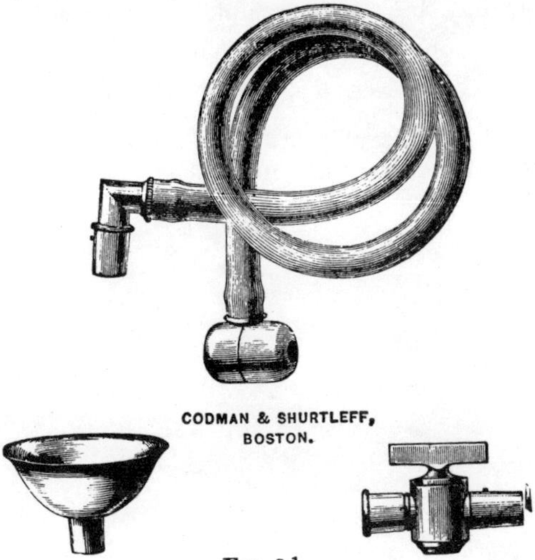

FIG. 3.[1]

the large ones. More water is required at first, while fragments are numerous, to separate them and prevent their being wedged in entering the catheter. Later in the operation, less water makes it easier to find the last fragment, the minimum being reached when the wall of the bladder vibrates against the orifice of the catheter as the bulb expands, painfully so if the patient is conscious. It is then important to add water again, just enough to prevent this obstruction and no more. In short, there is no doubt that we can evacuate better by trying a little more or a little less water from time to time during the operation, and that this can be done more

[1] Apparatus belonging to the evacuator but not essential to it; namely, a tunnel and a hose, both of which fit on to the top of the bulb, and an extra stop-cock for the evacuating catheter.

accurately and more readily by means of a hose than in any other way. With one end attached to the bulb, the other can conveniently remain in a vessel placed between the patient's knees, or in any convenient position, or remain unattached till wanted.

The hose may be used or not. For those who prefer a tunnel (Fig. 3), one is furnished with the instrument; as also a second stop-cock (Fig. 3), which I find useful if attached to the head of the catheter, in keeping the bed-clothes dry when the bulb is to be removed.

INDEX.

INDEX.

PART I.—DISLOCATIONS OF THE HIP.

A.

Abduction, 34.
Abstract, 4.
Acetabulum, unchanged in old luxation, 101.
  fracture of rim of, 109.
  head of femur driven through, 111.
  asserted fracture of, 112.
Amblard, case of perineal luxation, 73.
Anæsthesia in reduction, 30.
  by wine, 30.
Angular extension, 114.
  apparatus for, 114, 116.
  useful in old luxations, 102.
Annandale, reduction of pubic dislocation, 87.
Arthritis, dry chronic, after dislocation, 52.
Aubry, autopsy of pubic dislocation, 81.
  reduction of pubic dislocation, 85.

B.

Beraud, case of fractured acetabulum, 111.
Bertin, ligament of, 16.
Bidard, two autopsies of dislocation below the tendon, 58.
Bouisson, case of dislocation on the tuberosity with slight flexion, 72.
Boyer, on resistance of capsular ligament, 14.
Broca, M., 102.
Brodhurst, B. E., resistance to reduction not capsular, 101.
Brodie, fracture of socket inferred, 112.
Buck, reduction of thyroid dislocation, 76.
Busch, W., resistance to reduction ligamentous and capsular, 14.

C.

Cabot, case of reduction by rotation, 52.
Cadge, N., autopsy of supra-spinous dislocation, 91.
Callender, G. W., capsule no obstacle to reduction, 49.
Capsular orifice to be enlarged, 32.
  case of enlargement of, 53.
Capsule of the hip, 20.
  its condition in autopsies of dislocations, 10, 16.
Chapplain, on superficial and deep iliac luxations, 43.
Chassaignac, resistance to reduction purely muscular, 13.
Circumduction, varieties of, 35, 50, 52, 119, 132.
Cock, his rule for reduction, 47.
Collin, reduction of dorsal dislocation, 46.
Colombot, his method of reduction, 46.
Cooper, Sir Astley, cases of reduction by pulleys, 11, 12.
  resistance to reduction muscular, 12.
  his erroneous method of reduction, 27.
  case of dislocation below tendon, 61.
  case of dislocation near tuberosity, 71.

Cooper, Sir Astley (*continued*).
case of thyroid dislocation reduced by extension in sitting posture, 78.
cases of fractured acetabulum, 110, 111.
Bransby, autopsy of pubic dislocation, 81.
Cummins, case of supra-spinous dislocation, 90.

D.

Després, his method of reduction, 64.
Devilliers, reduction of pubic dislocation, 85.
Dislocation, regular, 4, 26, 35.
in dead subject, 9.
cause of difficulty in reducing, 13.
confinement of limb in final position of reduction of, 31, 53, 105, 109.
partial, 24.
varieties of, 24.
dorsal, varieties of, between the rotator muscles, 35, 42.
unimportant in reduction by flexion, 37.
mutually convertible, 37.
signs of, 37.
inversion in, 38.
autopsy of, 38.
congenital, 38.
shortening in, 40.
apparent, 39.
limited by Y ligament, 39.
mobility in, 41.
differential diagnosis in, 41.
apparent reduction of, 41.
reduction of, by traction, 45.
by rotation, 48.
lateral swing of femur how hindered in, 48.
above the obturator, how to reduce, 49.
depression of pelvis in reduction of, 50.
reproduced after reduction, 53.
how to prevent reproduction of, 53.
muscles subcutaneously divided in, 54.
Dislocation (*continued*).
dorsal, case of, at 3½ years, 55.
below tendon, 56.
why so called, 57.
Cooper's case, 57.
Malgaigne's case, 58.
autopsies of, 58.
identified in living subjects, 65.
signs of, 59.
mechanism of, 61.
reduction of, 64.
reproduced by sitting up, 58, 59.
on "ischiatic notch," not worthy of the name, 56.
erroneously supposed irreducible, 56.
alleged difficulty of reducing, 57.
Cooper's case, 57, 130.
thyroid and downward, 66.
thyroid, reduction of, 75.
downward, reduction of, 79.
readily converted into others, 66.
vertical downward, 66, 69.
on tuberosity, 66.
perineal, 66, 71.
autopsy of, 71.
on the pubes, 80.
autopsy of, 81, 91.
reduction of, 85.
sub-spinous, 82, 86.
supra-spinous, 90.
anterior oblique, 87.
posterior oblique, 93.
everted dorsal, 94.
reduction of, 96.
irregular, 4, 26, 97.
Y ligament wholly broken in, 4, 26, 97.
positions of femur in, 97, 98.
upward, 99.
downward, 100.
reduction of, 101.
old, reduction of, 101.
from hip disease, 104.
with fracture of femur, 105.
spontaneous, 105.

E.

Extension, straight, by pulleys, obsolete, 117, 123.

F.

Flexion, 34.
Flexion method of reduction, 28.
Fountain, E. J., two cases of pubic dislocation reduced by manipulation, 85.
Fournier, case of acetabulum unchanged in old dislocation, 102.
Fracture of neck of femur, 6, 22, 34.
from manipulation, 34.
better than unreduced dislocation, 102.
of shaft of femur, with dislocation, 105.
of pelvis, 108.
simulating dislocation, 113.

G.

Gay, case of fractured acetabulum, 141.
Gellé on capsular slit, 32.
Gely, case of sub-spinous dislocation, 83.
Gordon, case of everted dorsal dislocation, 95.
Graves, case of fracture of femoral neck during reduction, 102.
Guersant, on superficial and deep iliac luxations, 43.
Gunn, capsular ligament capable of producing the signs of luxation, 14.
route of bone in reduction, 32.
Gurney, cases of dislocation downward, 69.

H.

Hamilton, F. H., on fractures and dislocations, 41.
cases of spontaneous dislocation, 106.
Harlow, E. A. W., case of dorsal dislocation, 50.
Hayward, G., case of deformity from arthritis, 52.
Head of femur, excision of, 104.
driven through acetabulum, 111.
Hip disease, with dislocation, 104.
after reduction of dislocation, 105.
Hippocrates, on flexion method, 27.
on shaking the limb in reduction, 27.
on dislocation downward, 70.

I.

Iliac luxation, on change of, to ischiatic, 63.
Immobility of thigh, its indications, 49.
Irregular dislocations, 4, 26, 97.
Irvine, J. M., case of pubic dislocation reduced, 87.
Ischiatic notch, prejudice against, 43, 56.
femur never slips into, 56.
dislocations into, erroneously supposed irreducible, 56.
easier than dorsal to reduce, 102.
changed to iliac, 63.

J.

Jerk, upward, in reduction, 48.
Jones, semi-flexed thigh in reduction, 49.

K.

Keate, case of dislocation on tuberosity, 74.
case of fracture of socket inferred in, 100, 112.

L.

Langmaid, case of spontaneous dislocation, 106.
Larrey, his method of reduction, 78.
case of pubic dislocation at a right angle, 81.
case of pubic dislocation reduced by, 87.
Lendrick, case of head of femur driven through acetabulum, 112.
Lente, case illustrating mechanism of supra-spinous luxation, 94.
Ligamentum teres, 20.
Limb, confinement of, as reduced, 31, 53, 103, 109.
how to be held in reduction, 32.
Lisfranc, case of reduction of dislocation below tendon, 64.

Luke, case of thyroid dislocation, 72.
Lyman, G. H., case of spontaneous dislocation, 107.

M.

Maisonneuve, fracture of acetabulum, 110.
union of broken acetabulum, 111.
Malespine, account of Lisfranc's case of reduction by Després's method, 64.
Malgaigne, route of bone in reduction, 32.
on ischiatic and iliac luxation, 63.
Mann, B., case of dorsal dislocation reduced by depressing pelvis, 51.
Markoe, semi-flexed thigh in reduction of dorsal dislocation, 31.
cases of thyroid luxation reduced by rotation, 76.
Mobility, degree of, an important sign in dorsal dislocation, 41.
Moore, E. M., case of spontaneous dislocation, 107.
case of head of femur driven through acetabulum, 111.
Morel-Lavallée, case of head of femur driven through acetabulum, 112.
Morgan, case of everted dorsal dislocation, 96.
Muscles, their action in dislocation, 15, 23.
subcutaneous division of, 54, 55.

N.

Nunneley, incomplete anæsthesia to be preferred in reduction, 30.
reduction of ischiatic luxation by manipulation, difficult, 64.

O.

Oblique extension, 117.
Obturator internus muscle, 21.
source of its strength, 21.
its importance in fracture of the femoral neck, 22.
its normal position, 61.
its position in dislocation below the tendon, 61.
Old dislocations, 101.
Cooper's case, 101.
Oldknow, case of anterior oblique luxation, 89.
Ollivier, case of dislocation below the tendon, 59.
Oscillation in reduction, 29.

P.

Papers, author's, on dislocation, 10.
Parea, Annibal, his method of reduction, 48.
Parker, W., case of perineal luxation, 73.
Parmentier, case of luxation between pyriformis and obturator internus, 43.
Pelvis, fracture of, 113.
often inferred without adequate proof, 112.
Perineal luxation, case of, with autopsy, 71.
Pope, case of perineal luxation, 73.
Position of patient and surgeon, 30.
Pouteau, on disadvantage of straight extension, 114.

Q.

Queen, case of sciatic nerve engaged on femoral neck, 58.

R.

Reduction, general remarks on, 26.
cases of, where limb requires to be confined, 31, 109.
Regular dislocations, 4, 26, 35.
Reid, W. W., muscles the chief source of resistance in reduction, 14.
his method of reduction, 29.
anæsthesia a detriment to reduction, 30.
incision in capsule, 33.
Richet, case of fractured acetabulum, 111.
Ridge, intertrochanteric, 7.
Rim of acetabulum, fracture of, 109.
Rotation, 28.
explained, 34.
Rotator muscles, their breaking weights, 21.
Roux, case of thyroid luxation, 68.

S.

Sciatic nerve engaged on femoral neck, 44, 58.
Servier, case of dislocation above the pyriformis, 43.
Shrady, case of everted dorsal dislocation, 96.
Smith, N. R., muscles the chief agents in dislocation and reduction, 13.
his method of reduction, 29.
Sophocles, Prof., signification of a term in Hippocrates, 27.
Spontaneous dislocation, 106.
Square, W. J., case of dorsal dislocation reduced by flexion, 47.
Stanski, case of dislocation near tuberosity, 72, 73.
specimen of anterior capsule ossified, 74.
Struthers, on the ligamentum teres, 20.
Sub-spinous dislocation, 80, 82.
Supra-spinous dislocation, 90.
reduction of, 96.
Surgeon to have definite plan of reduction, 29.
Sutton, G., method of reduction, 47.
Swing, lateral, of femur, hindered by capsular attachments, 48.
Syme, James, on dislocation on dorsum and ischiatic notch, 43.
Symes, G. R., case of everted dorsal dislocation, 95.

T.

Theory, author's, 15.
Thomas, case of dorsal dislocation, 52.
Thyroid dislocation, signs of, 67.
case of, in child six months old, 67.
Tillaux, on capsular resistance in dorsal dislocation, 63.
Traction, 28.
Travers, case of fracture in reduction of ischiatic luxation by pulleys, 64.
case of supra-spinous dislocation, 91.
Tyer, M., cases of fractured acetabulum, 110.

V.

Van Buren, W. H., case of everted dorsal dislocation, 96.
Verneuil, case of fracture in reducing pubic dislocation, 34.
case of dislocation reproduced by sitting up, 58.
Vertu, case of thyroid dislocation reduced by flexion, 77.

W.

Weber, G. and E., on the Y ligament, 19.
Weitbrecht, J., on the Y ligament, 19.
Winslow, J. B., on the Y ligament, 18.
Wormald, case of irreducible dislocation on ischiatic notch, 43.
case of dislocation towards the tuberosity, 59.
case of sub-spinous dislocation, 84.

Y.

Y ligament, description of the, 16.
its fasciculi, 17.
its breaking weight, 18.
its great strength, 18, 19.
to be tightened in certain cases of reduction, 31.
its external band produces inversion in dorsal dislocation, 37.
ruptured in supra-spinous dislocation, 90.
ruptured in everted dorsal dislocation, 94.

FRACTURES OF THE HIP.

A.

Anatomical structure of the neck of the femur, 141, 158, 161, 178.
Merkel on the, 159.
Meyer, 159.
pathological results due to the, 142.
rotation, 142.
shortening, 142, 179.
Wyman, on the, 159.

B.

Bony union of "intra-capsular" fracture, 140, 145, 150, 183.
impacted fracture near the head, 140, 145, 150, 183.

C.

Comminuted fracture of the trochanters, with eversion, 154.
with inversion, 154, 184.
without impaction, 154, 172, 184.
less common than impacted, 154.
Crack in the neck of the femur, 156.
Crepitus, 181.
Cushing, case of impacted fracture near the head, 152, 183.

D.

Diagnosis, differential, 147.

E.

Eversion, 146, 154, 179, 180.
Examination, protracted, is unjustifiable, 146, 185.
Extension, object of, 141, 187.

F.

Femur, anatomical structure of its neck, 141, 158, 161, 178.
false joint in neck of, 155.
true neck of, 143, 158, 162.
Fractures of the neck of the femur, 6, 22, 34, 118.
anatomy of, 144, 160, 178, 179.
characteristics of, 139.
classification of, 145, 154, 175.
comminuted, of the trochanters, 172.
with eversion, 154.
with inversion, 155.
without impaction, 154, 184.
crepitus in, 181.
danger in manipulating, 154, 168, 174, 185.
frequency of, 139, 175, 177.
"within" and "without" the capsular ligament, 145, 150, 172, 176.
distinction difficult, 145.
unimportant, 145.

G.

Gay, case of impacted fracture near head of femur, 150, 151, 182.

H.

Hamilton, impacted fracture with inversion, 146, 147.

I.

Impacted fractures, anatomy of, 144.
common, 139, 175, 177.
eversion in, 142.
identification of, essential, 140, 177, 181.

Impacted fractures (*continued*).
importance of, 140.
injury from over examination of, 154, 168, 174, 182.
near the head of the femur, 146, 150, 170, 182.
of the base of the neck, with eversion, 139, 167, 177.
with inversion, 146, 147, 172.
of the small part of the cervix, 146, 172, 176.
common in elderly persons, 172, 175.
prognosis unfavorable, 176.
resulting in false joint, 155.
of neck into head, 146.
shortening in, 142, 155, 179.
signs of, 140.
Impaction explained, 179.
Intertrochanteric ridge, 143, 144.
Inversion explained, 142, 147, 155, 180.

J.

Joint, false, 155.

M.

Manipulation, protracted, unjustifiable, 146, 154, 168, 174, 182, 185.
Merkel, on the structure of the neck of the femur, 159.
Meyer, 159.
Mutual impaction of head and neck, 152.

N.

Neck of femur, true, 143, 158, 162.

O.

Object of extension in treatment, 141, 147, 187.

P.

Pathology of neck of femur, 167.
Prognosis of fractures of the hip, 174, 176.
generally favorable, 140.

R.

Robert, on posterior impaction, 142.
Rotation in impacted fractures, 142.

S.

Shortening, mechanism of, 142, 179.
Signs of fracture of the hip, 140, 146, 168.
Smith, R. W., impacted fracture with inversion, 147, 149.
comminuted fracture with inversion, 155.

T.

Treatment of fractures of the hip, 147, 173, 185, 186.
Trochanter, comminuted fracture of, 154.
True neck of the femur, 143, 158, 162.
pathology of, 167.

U.

Unimpacted fractures, 172.
signs of, 146.

W.

Wyman, on structure of the neck of the femur, 159.
Wolff, 159.

PART II. — RAPID LITHOTRITY.

A.

Adherent stone, 219.
Anæsthesia in lithotrity, 199, 296.
Artificial bladder, 206.
Aspirator. *See* Evacuator.

B.

Bladder, artificial, 206.
capacity of, 200, 237.
casts of, 216.
cystitis of, 320.
damage to, by angular fragments, 193, 265.
injury to, by lithotrite, 194, 214, 321.
interior view of, 215.
over-distension of, 200, 235, 238.
how to avoid, 200, 237.
position of bulb affects the, 235.
removal of air from, 273, 320.
shape of, 216, 218.
modifications in, 218.
tolerance of, 193, 221, 265, 296, 324.
Bulb. *See* Evacuator.

C.

Clover's apparatus, 196, 202, 243, 281.
Connection, elastic, between evacuator and evacuating tube, 276, 284.
Crampton's apparatus, 196.
Cystitis, 320.

D.

Divulsor for stricture, 294.
Duration of sittings in old operation, 194, 214, 246, 296.
in new, 194, 214, 246, 261

E.

Elastic bulb. *See* Evacuator.
connection between evacuator and evacuating tube, 276, 284.
Evacuating instruments, antiquity of, 196.
old, valueless, 195, 243.
varieties of, 196.
sound, 299, 315.
tubes, advantages of, 232, 236, 325.
calibre of, 202, 232, 283.
curved, 270, 275, 322, 325.
how to pass, 196, 236, 270, 280.
large, absolutely essential, 201, 232, 269, 275, 297.
obstruction in, 238, 272, 321, 325.
recognition of, 208, 209.
removal of, 208, 238, 321.
straight, 236, 270, 322, 325.
easiest to introduce, 197, 236, 270.
Evacuation, position of operator during, 199, 206.
process of, 204, 205, 248, 272, 276, 279, 323.
prevention of the return of fragments, 301, 304, 326, 335.
quantity of water to be used in, 204, 271.
Evacuator, air in, removal of, 278, 320.
air space in, 278.
details of construction, 268, 275, 297, 322, 333.
hose attachment of, 278, 283, 299, 329, 342.
improved, 274.
manipulation of, 204, 205, 237, 248, 315.
receiver of, for fragments, 301, 326.

Evacuator (*continued*).
simplified, 306, 332, 342.
Sir H. Thompson's, 280, 336.
stand for, 269, 283, 302, 327.
strainer in, 298, 301, 304, 328, 330, 340.
trap in, 301, 326, 339.
used as a sound, 299, 315.
valve in, 29, 301.

F.

Fatal cases of litholapaxy, 222, 233, 317.
Fergusson's operation, 310.

H.

Handerson's catheter scale, 256.
Harmlessness of long sittings, 232, 318.
Hose, 205, 278, 283, 299, 329, 342.
How to pass the triangular ligament, 197.
pass an enlarged prostate, 198.
remove obstruction in the tube, 208, 238, 321.

L.

Large calculi, 241, 282.
instruments, introduction of, 197.
Litholapaxie, prix d'Argenteuil, 285.
Litholapaxy, adapted to large calculi, 215, 221, 241, 282.
cases of, 219, 228, 249, 261, 316.
dangers of, 192, 213, 317, 321.
derivation of term, 228.
experience valuable in, 194, 274, 318.
fatal cases of, 222, 233, 317.
harmlessness of long sittings, 232, 318.
instead of lithotomy, 221, 233.
in the female, 225.
mortality attending, 222, 225, 233, 261, 274, 317.
object of, 226, 245.
theory of, 232, 235.
time required in operation of, 194, 226, 238, 249, 262, 280.
Lithotrite, blades of, 212, 267, 310.
non-impacting, 229, 311.
triangular notches of, 213, 231, 311, 314.
description of, 210, 229, 239.
fracture of, 258, 260.
handle of, 211, 268, 307.
large, 231, 254, 260, 267, 309.
advantages of, 239, 252, 309.
lock of, 211, 232, 267, 307, 330.
manipulation of, 214, 239.
passage of, 199, 280, 314.
province of, 210.
shoe of, 212.
modified tip of, 311, 313.
protects the bladder, 213.
the new, 210, 239, 252, 254, 258, 306, 313, 330.
to comminute, not to pulverize, 210, 215.
importance of, 210, 225.
with fenestrated blades, 210, 229, 266, 311.
Lithotrity, anæsthesia in, 199, 296.
Civiale's, 191, 296.
compared with lithotomy, 224, 233, 242, 317.
limitations of, 192, 224, 233, 246.
modern, 194, 296, 324, 332.
modification in, 226.
Sir H. Thompson's, 222, 242, 255.
time required in operation of, 194, 214, 246, 264, 296.
traditions of, 191.

M.

Male blade lock of lithotrite, 267, 307.
Meatus, incision of, 275, 320.

O.

Obstruction in the evacuating tube, 208, 238, 271, 316, 321.
at the external meatus, 320.
inner meatus, 198, 261.
triangular ligament, 197.
prostate, 198.
Otis's discovery, 201, 246, 265, 281, 309, 332.

P.

Position of the operator, 199.
Preparatory treatment, 316.
Prostate, obstacle of, 198.

R.

Rapid lithotrity. *See* Litholapaxy.
Right hand lock of lithotrite, 253.

S.

Sir H. Thompson's views, 242, 254.
Sir P. Crampton's aspirator, 196.
Stone, adherent, 219.
Stricture of the urethra, 222, 233, 293.
Surgical kidney, 316.

T.

Trap to intercept returning fragments, 298, 303, 305, 326, 328, 334.
Treatment, preparatory, 316.
 after operation, 273, 317.
Triangular ligament, obstruction at, 197.

U.

Urethra, injury to, 309, 317.
 measurement of, 197, 309.
 size of, 246.
 stricture of, 222, 233, 293.
  divulsion of, 233, 237, 293.

V.

Valve in evacuator, 29, 301.

W.

Water in bladder, changed or regulated by a hose, 205, 278, 283, 342.
 to be injected before crushing, 200, 209.
 tube for injecting, 212.
 quantity needed, 204.
 retained by an elastic band, 201, 238.